BEYOND CLINICAL PATHS

ADVANCED TOOLS

FOR

OUTCOMES

MANAGEMENT

EDITOR

Patrice L. Spath

Beyond Clinical Paths

ADVANCED TOOLS

FOR

OUTCOMES

MANAGEMENT

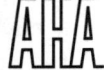 American Hospital Publishing, Inc.
An American Hospital Association company
Chicago

This publication is designed to provide accurate and authoritative information in regard to the subject matter covered. It is sold with the understanding that neither the author nor the publisher is engaged in rendering legal, accounting, or other professional service. If legal advice or other expert assistance is required, the services of a competent professional should be sought.

The views expressed in this publication are strictly those of the authors and do not necessarily represent official positions of the American Hospital Association.

AHA is a service mark of the American Hospital Association used under license by American Hospital Publishing, Inc.

© 1997 by American Hospital Publishing, Inc., an American Hospital Association company. All rights reserved. No part of this publication may be reproduced, stored in a retrieval system, or transmitted, in any form or by any means, electronic, mechanical, photocopying, recording or otherwise, without the prior written permission of the publisher. Printed in the United States of America.

Library of Congress Cataloging-in-Publication Data

Beyond clinical paths : advanced tools for outcomes management /
    Patrice L. Spath, editor.
        p.   cm.
    Includes bibliographical references and index.
    ISBN 1-55648-201-9
    1. Medical care—Quality control.   2. Medical protocols.
3. Outcome assessment (Medical care)   I. Spath, Patrice.
    [DNLM: 1. Quality Assurance, Health Care—organization &
administration.   2. Critical Pathways.   3. Outcome Assessment
(Health Care)   4. Information Systems.   W 84.1 B573 1997]
RA399.A1B49   1997
362.1'068'4—dc21
DNLM/DLC
for Library of Congress   97-16430
                                                                                    CIP

ISBN: 1-55648-201-9   Item Number: 027105

Discounts on bulk quantities of books published by American Hospital Publishing, Inc. (AHPI), are available to professional associations, special marketers, educators, trainers, and others. For details and discount information, contact American Hospital Publishing, Inc., Books Division, 737 North Michigan Avenue, Suite 700, Chicago, Illinois 60611-2615 (Fax: 312-951-8491).

This book is dedicated to my friend, Jill Fainter, assistant vice president of quality management, Columbia/HCA Healthcare Corporation. She has a special talent for helping people become what they are capable of being.

CONTENTS

	List of Figures and Tables	ix
	About the Editor	xiii
	Contributors	xv
	Preface	xix
CHAPTER 1	**Taking Clinical Quality Improvement Beyond Paths** Patrice L. Spath	1
PART I	**Clinical Process Improvement Initiatives**	
CHAPTER 2	**Using Performance Measurement as a Quality Improvement Tool** Meg Kistin Anzalone and Michael D. McGee	9
CHAPTER 3	**Improving Outpatient Care with Clinical Practice Guidelines** Gail O'Mahaney VanZyl and Gary Goby	35
CHAPTER 4	**Reducing Practice Variation in Open Heart Surgeries** Mary Lu Gerke	53
CHAPTER 5	**Creating a Multidisciplinary Disease Management Initiative** Lisa M. Zavorski and Barbara Taptich	71
CHAPTER 6	**Integrating Geriatric Evaluation and Management with a Multidisciplinary Care Planning Process** Jacquelyn Paynter, Katherine Ambrose, and Katherine Dolan	103
CHAPTER 7	**Mapping Home Care Services** Sheila Hawley and Bonnie Davis	129
CHAPTER 8	**Incorporating Case Management into Home Care** DeAnne Mosher	145
CHAPTER 9	**Reducing Length of Stay and Improving Outcomes** Kevin Turley and Kerry M. Turley	163
PART II	**Information Technology Solutions**	
CHAPTER 10	**Selecting an Automated Case Management and Clinical Path Information System** Sherry Lee	181

CHAPTER 11	**Building a Cost-Efficient Path Variance Database** *Darice M. Grzybowski*	199
CHAPTER 12	**Automating Clinical Pathway Variance Analysis** *Beth Weber, Linda Ratzlaff, Tom Hearn, and Joan McCanless*	213
CHAPTER 13	**Designing Information Systems for Disease Management** *Dianne J. Anderson, Christine W. Freire, and Patricia Hale*	225
CHAPTER 14	**Linking Expert Systems to Outcomes Analysis** *H. Edmund Pigott, Greg Alter, and Deborah L. Heggie*	253
	Index	263

LIST OF FIGURES AND TABLES

Figure 2-1.	Audit Worksheet Used to Gather Information from Client Records	16
Figure 2-2.	BASIS-32 Form	18
Figure 2-3.	Sample BASIS-32 Report	20
Figure 2-4.	Patient Satisfaction Survey	21
Figure 2-5.	Chart Audit Tool	23
Figure 2-6.	Provider Log	26
Figure 2-7.	Patient Information Sheet	27
Figure 2-8.	Provider Performance Measurement Process	28
Figure 2-9.	Sample Aggregate Performance Report for One Provider Facility	29
Figure 2-10.	Noncompliance Report	31
Table 2-1.	Performance Management Process	11
Table 2-2.	Pilot Project Measurements for the Four Performance Dimensions	13
Table 2-3.	Performance Management Profile Ranking Categories and Criteria	30
Figure 3-1.	Clinical Practice Guideline Development Process Applied to the Shewhart Cycle	37
Figure 3-2.	FirstCare Health Organizational Structure, 1993	38
Figure 3-3.	FirstCare Health Organizational Structure, 1995	41
Figure 3-4.	Acute Pharyngitis-Tonsillitis Clinical Practice Guideline	42
Figure 3-5.	Acute Pharyngitis-Tonsillitis Clinical Outcome Measurement	44
Figure 3-6.	FirstCare Health Organizational Performance Improvement Report Elements, 1997	45
Figure 3-7.	Clinical Practice Guideline Development Process	46
Figure 3-8.	Serous Otitis in Pediatrics Clinical Practice Guidelines	48
Figure 4-1.	Manual Data Collection Worksheet	56
Figure 4-2.	Sedation Management Practices for Coronary Artery Bypass Graft Patients: Process Flow	58
Figure 4-3.	Cause-and-Effect Diagram Used to Determine the Cause of Decreased Mental and Mobility Statuses in Coronary Artery Bypass Graft Patients	59
Figure 4-4.	Mayo Mini-Mental Status Worksheet	60
Figure 4-5.	Ramsey Sedation Scale	61
Figure 4-6.	Lutheran Hospital Falls Risk Scoring System	61

Figure 4-7.	Sedation Protocol for Open Heart Surgery Patients	62
Figure 4-8.	Falls Risk Standard/Treatment Flowsheet	63
Figure 4-9.	Data Elements	64
Figure 4-10.	Coronary Artery Bypass Graft Clinical Path	66
Table 4-1.	Preproject Baseline Performance Data	57
Table 4-2.	First Postimplementation Study Results Compared with Baseline Data	64
Table 4-3.	Second Postimplementation Study Results Compared with Baseline Data and First Study Results	68
Figure 5-1.	Congestive Heart Failure Pathway	74
Figure 5-2.	Generic Medical Pathway	76
Figure 5-3.	Development Model	80
Figure 5-4.	Multidisciplinary Team Members	81
Figure 5-5.	Cause-and-Effect Diagram for the Management of Congestive Heart Failure	82
Figure 5-6.	Defined Process of Care	85
Figure 5-7.	Admission, Exclusion, and Discharge Criteria	87
Figure 5-8.	Congestive Heart Failure Short-Stay Pathway	88
Figure 5-9.	Clinical Algorithm for Evaluation and Care of Patients with Heart Failure	89
Figure 5-10.	Excerpt from Congestive Heart Failure Patient Pathway	94
Figure 5-11.	Patient Instruction Sheet	95
Figure 5-12.	Program Statistics, Initial Year of Operation	98
Table 5-1.	Improvement Strategies Chosen and Rationale for Choices	84
Figure 6-1.	Integration of Multidisciplinary Care Management Program into Organizational Structure	105
Figure 6-2.	Nutritional Screening and Assessment	109
Figure 6-3.	Discharge-Planning Assessment	110
Figure 6-4.	Physical Therapy Screen	111
Figure 6-5.	Patient Education Assessment	112
Figure 6-6.	Variance Action Response Record	113
Figure 6-7.	Pressure Ulcer Potential Scoring System	116
Figure 6-8.	Falls Risk Scoring System	119
Figure 6-9.	Geriatric Multidisciplinary Care Plan Interventions and Outcomes	122
Figure 6-10.	Sample Geriatric Evaluation and Management Program Functional Outcome Indicator Report	124
Table 6-1.	Assessing Functional Status in Clinical Settings	115
Table 6-2.	Geriatric Evaluation and Management Program Benchmarks	118
Figure 7-1.	Standardized Home Visit Form	132
Figure 7-2.	Care Plan for Congestive Heart Failure Patients	134
Figure 7-3.	Assessment Visit Checklist	135
Figure 7-4.	Nursing Visit Note Form for Congestive Heart Failure Patients	136
Figure 7-5.	Copath for Insulin-Dependent Diabetes Mellitus Patients	138
Figure 7-6.	Variance Report Form	139

Figure 7-7.	Occupational Therapy Visit Note Form	142
Figure 7-8.	Occupational, Physical, and Speech Therapy Care Path for Patients with Nervous Disorders	143
Table 7-1.	Comparison of Prepath and Postpath Outcome Measures	140
Figure 8-1.	Nurse Case Manager Job Description and Performance Evaluation	149
Figure 8-2.	Visit Nurse Schedule Board	152
Figure 8-3.	Patient Update Form	153
Figure 8-4.	Case Manager Schedule Board	154
Figure 8-5.	Patient Calendar Showing Wound Care Path	158
Figure 8-6.	Face Sheet	159
Figure 8-7.	Use of PRN Nurses	161
Table 8-1.	Number of Possible Nurse Home Health Visits per Month	156
Table 8-2.	Case Management vs. Paths vs. Prepath Performance for Congestive Heart Failure Patients	160
Figure 9-1.	Standard Radical Outcome Grid	167
Figure 9-2.	Simple Pathway (Radical Outcome Method 1)	168
Figure 9-3.	Patient Progress Chart	170
Figure 9-4.	Job Description for Clinical Nurse Coordinator–Case Manager	172
Table 9-1.	Actual vs. Estimated Length of Stay: Cumulative Results for Total Bypass Patients	175
Figure 10-1.	Two Organizations' Goals for Automated Information Systems	189
Figure 10-2.	Software Package Feature Priority-Setting Form	191
Figure 10-3.	Sample Request for Information	192
Table 10-1.	Standard Variance Reports	186
Figure 11-1.	Care Guide Development Process	201
Figure 11-2.	Standard Care Guide Format for Cardiac Catheterization or Percutaneous Transluminal Coronary Angioplasty	202
Figure 11-3.	Standardized Care Guide Variance Reporting Form for Cardiac Catheterization or Percutaneous Transluminal Coronary Angioplasty	204
Figure 11-4.	Screen Display of Active Care Plan	205
Figure 11-5.	Screen Display of Admission, Discharge, or Transfer Care Plan	206
Figure 11-6.	Preprinted Physician Orders for Cardiac Catheterization or Percutaneous Transluminal Coronary Angioplasty Patients	207
Figure 11-7.	Care Guide Data Inventory	209
Figure 11-8.	Average Length of Stay Comparison for Percutaneous Transluminal Coronary Angioplasty Patients, 1995	210
Figure 11-9.	Average Charge Comparison for Percutaneous Transluminal Coronary Angioplasty Patients, 1995–96	211
Figure 11-10.	Care Guide Data Report for Percutaneous Transluminal Coronary Angioplasty, June 1996	212
Figure 12-1.	Stakeholders in the Clinical Path Process	215
Figure 12-2.	Clinical Path Variance Report	216

xii LIST OF FIGURES AND TABLES

Figure 12-3.	Variance Tracking Screen Display	218
Figure 12-4.	Variance from Expected Outcome (VEO) Pop-Up Table	219
Figure 12-5.	Sample Variance Report	219
Figure 12-6.	Sample Outcomes Analysis Report	221
Figure 12-7.	Chest Pain Pathway	223
Figure 13-1.	Components of the Regional Disease Management Model	227
Figure 13-2.	Case Manager Education Topics	229
Figure 13-3.	Case Manager Job Description	230
Figure 13-4.	Case Management Screening Criteria	231
Figure 13-5.	Clinical Path Work Plan	234
Figure 13-6.	Preliminary Statistical Analysis of Patients with Community-Acquired Pneumonia, June 1, 1994, to May 31, 1995	236
Figure 13-7.	Emergency Care and Inpatient Community-Acquired Pneumonia Clinical Pathway	237
Figure 13-8.	Plans for Information System Links	240
Figure 13-9.	Input Screen in PatRec for Hospital History and Physical	242
Figure 13-10.	Information Flow Using Computerized Patient Records	244
Figure 13-11.	Community-Acquired Pneumonia Data Summary Screen	245
Figure 13-12.	Hospitalization Threshold Screen	245
Figure 13-13.	Outpatient Treatment Selection Screen	246
Figure 13-14.	Inpatient Physician Order Sheet for Patients with Community-Acquired Pneumonia	247
Figure 13-15.	Outcomes Data Collection Screen	248
Figure 13-16.	Algorithm for Management of Community-Acquired Pneumonia	249
Table 13-1.	Length-of-Stay Comparative Data	228
Figure 14-1.	Clinical Quality Improvement Model That Links Expert Systems to Outcomes Analysis	256
Figure 14-2.	Crisis Triage Rating Scale	257

ABOUT THE EDITOR

Patrice L. Spath, BA, ART, a health care consultant based in Forest Grove, OR, has extensive experience in quality and resource management initiatives. She was previously a regional councilor for the Health Care Division of the American Society for Quality Control and chairman of the Quality Management Section of the American Health Information Management Association. A sought-after speaker, Ms. Spath has presented more than 250 educational programs on performance improvement, utilization review, case management and clinical paths, and outcomes management. She is the author of several books, video programs, and journal articles on these subjects. For American Hospital Publishing, Inc., she was the editor of *Clinical Paths: Tools for Outcomes Management,* published in 1994, and *Medical Effectiveness and Outcomes Management: Issues, Methods, and Case Studies,* published in 1996.

Ms. Spath is a regular columnist for *Hospital Case Management* and *Hospital Peer Review* and is editor for *The Quality Resource,* the newsletter of the Quality Management Section of the American Health Information Management Association. She served on a work group of the Agency for Health Care Policy and Research to develop a model for translating clinical practice guidelines into medical review criteria. She was a member of the Clinical Practice Guidelines Panel of the Veterans Health Administration and a member of the Clinical Path Work Group of the Association for Operating Room Nurses.

CONTRIBUTORS

Greg Alter, PhD, is principal at Pacific Applied Psychology Associates in Berkeley, CA.

Katherine Ambrose, RN, MS, is Medicare QA/UM project director at Next Stage Healthcare, Inc., in Melville, NY. She was previously professional resources administrator at Catholic Medical Center of Brooklyn & Queens, Inc., in Flushing, NY.

Dianne J. Anderson, MS, RN, is vice president of patient services and chief nursing officer at Glens Falls Hospital in Glens Falls, NY.

Meg Kistin Anzalone, PhD, is vice president of quality management at Massachusetts Behavioral Health Partnership. She was previously clinical director and area quality director at Merit Behavioral Care in Burlington, MA.

Bonnie Davis, BSN, RNC, is manager at Clinton Memorial Hospital Home Health Agency in Wilmington, OH. She has 8 years of experience in the home health field. She is coauthor of the Clinton HomeCare-Paths and has spoken nationally on this topic. She is a member of the Intravenous Nurse's Society.

Katherine Dolan, BA, MBA, is director of planning for Daughters of Charity National Health System–East Central Region. She is also an outcomes management consultant and is a Health Care Forum, Healthier Communities Fellow. She was previously executive director of St. Joseph's Hospital in Flushing, NY. She has more than 20 years of experience in hospital management.

Christine W. Freire, MSW, CSW, is director of case management at Glens Falls Hospital in Glens Falls, NY.

Mary Lu Gerke, BSN, MSN, is director of the intensive care unit at Gundersen Lutheran hospital in La Crosse, WI. She has pioneered with Hewlett Packard the implementation of the CAREVUE 9000 system and has spoken internationally on clinical information systems and on clinical quality improvement efforts related to such systems.

Gary A. Goby, MD, a diplomate in family practice, has an ongoing 23-year practice at the Albany Family Medical Clinic, a division of FirstCare Physicians in Albany, OR. He also serves as coordinator of clinical services on the Managing Council of FirstCare Health. For the past 20 years, he has been associate clinical professor at the Family Practice Clinic of Oregon Health Sciences University.

Darice Grzybowski, RRA, is the director of health information management at Hinsdale Hospital in Hinsdale, IL, where she has been employed for the past 12 years. She is also adjunct associate professor of health informatics at University of Illinois at Chicago.

Patricia Hale, PhD, MD, is a primary care internal medicine physician in private group practice in Glens Falls, NY. She has extensive experience in the application of informatics and computers in medical practice.

Sheila Hawley, MSN, RN, CS, is clinical supervisor at Clinton Memorial Hospital Home Health Agency in Wilmington, OH. She conceived of and developed the Clinton HomeCare-Paths and copaths and has spoken nationally on this topic.

Tom Hearn, MBA, MPH, is cofounder and principal of Decision Support Systems in Charlotte, NC. He previously held two titles at Carolinas Medical Center, serving 7 years as vice president of administration and as administrator of the Carolinas Heart Institute.

Deborah L. Heggie, PhD, is director of managed care for Capitol Region Mental Health Center, Connecticut State Department of Mental Health in Hartford, CT. She was previously founding partner and director of outpatient services at PATH, P.C., and was director of the psychology internship at Mount Sinai Hospital in Hartford, CT.

Sherry Lee, BSN, RN, MEd, is an information systems and clinical pathway consultant based in Matthews, NC.

Joan McCanless, RN, is cofounder and principal of Decision Support Systems in Charlotte, NC. She has over 20 years of experience in hospital management, quality improvement, utilization management, and nursing management.

Michael D. McGee, MD, is medical director of Merit Behavioral Care in Burlington, MA.

DeAnne Mosher, RN, MA, CCM, CNAA, is director of Clinton Memorial Hospital Home Health Agency and Corporate Health Services in Wilmington, OH. She has 12 years of experience in home care. She has contributed to the books *Home Care and Clinical Paths: Effective Care Planning Across the Continuum, Documentation and Information Management in Home Care and Hospice Programs,* and *Orientation to Home Care Nursing.*

Gail O'Mahaney VanZyl, RN, BSN, CNA, CHRM, is director of the MASH (Measurement, Analysis, and Support for Healthcare Improvement) Division at FirstCare Health in Albany, OR. Her past nursing experience includes critical care, emergency room, PACU, operating room, home infusion, trauma, and nursing education. She has spoken nationally on health care applications of continuous improvement concepts.

Jacquelyn R. Paynter, BS, MPH, is director of customer and government relations at Fidelis Care New York, a statewide managed care plan located in Flushing, NY. She was previously professional services administrator at St. Joseph's Hospital Division, Catholic Medical Center of Brooklyn & Queens, Inc., in Flushing, NY. She has 18 years of experience in health care, including progressive administrative responsibility for operations, strategic planning, quality improvement, case management, and health information management services.

H. Edmund Pigott, PhD, is founder and president of PATHware, Inc., in Columbia, MD. He was previously founding partner and president of PATH, P.C. He is a licensed psychologist and has published extensively in the area of expert systems and treatment outcome research.

Linda Ratzlaff, RN, BSN, MS, has been director of case management at Bristol Regional Medical Center in Bristol, TN, since 1994. She was previously catastrophic case manager for Intracorp in Little Rock, AR. She also held several administrative positions with St. Mary's Hospital in Russellville, AR, including vice president of nursing and director of home health, and has served on the faculty of Arkansas Tech University in Russellville.

Barbara Taptich, MA, RN, is director of education at McFaul and Lyons, Inc., in Trenton, NJ. She was previously senior director of critical care and cardiopulmonary services at St. Francis Medical Center in Trenton.

Kerry M. Turley, MSN, MPA, RN, is clinical nurse coordinator and case manager in pediatric cardiovascular surgery at California Pacific Medical Center in San Francisco and consultant at Kaiser Permanente Foundation of Northern California.

Kevin Turley, MD, is chief of pediatric and congenital cardiovascular surgery at California Pacific Medical Center in San Francisco and is the former professor of surgery and pediatrics and chief of pediatric cardiac surgery at the University of California, San Francisco. He is a consultant in pediatric cardiac surgery for Kaiser Permanente Foundation of Northern California.

Beth Weber, RN, MHA, is vice president of clinical systems at Decision Support Systems in Charlotte, NC. She was previously manager for process improvement initiatives at the Charlotte-Mecklenburg Hospital Authority in Charlotte, NC. She has over 10 years of experience in clinical and administrative health care.

Lisa M. Zavorski, RN, is director of utilization management at St. Francis Medical Center in Trenton, NJ.

PREFACE

This book is about improving clinical quality—not the kind of improvement that comes from a single patient management tool, but the kind that comes from new attitudes and knowledge. There is probably no better way to introduce the material in this book than to ask you to read the following passage:

Excellence can be attained if you . . .
- Care more than others think is wise.
- Risk more than others think is safe.
- Dream more than others think is practical.
- Expect more than others think is possible.

The organizations represented in this book exemplify excellence—not just because they designed innovative patient care tools, but because their people cared, risked, dreamed, and expected more of themselves. In this era of change, it is all too common to see the "program of the month" overpower the importance of relationships, mind-set, and environment.

If you are looking for a "quick fix" for your cost or quality problems, you may be disappointed with this book. None of the authors claim to have rapidly achieved significant measurable gains. In some instances, repairing breached relationships between disciplines and providers took the better part of a year. Only then could the health care team begin to tackle the challenges of clinical quality improvement.

If you are looking for a silver bullet, you also may be disappointed. No *one* outcomes management tool is ideal for every organization. You will find that, like all tools, they are a means to an end. Knowing what you are trying to accomplish is the first, most important question to be answered. From there, caregivers pick the tool or tools they need to achieve their goals.

Much has been written recently about how caregivers have successfully implemented clinical paths. For the period from January 1988 through December 1996, more than 800 pathway-related citations can be found in the medical and allied health literature. These reports have prompted many managed care organizations to mandate certain clinical paths or seek affiliations only with health care organizations that are willing to develop them. Unfortunately, considerably less has been written about failed clinical path initiatives.

In 1994, when *Clinical Paths: Tools for Outcomes Management* was published by American Hospital Publishing, Inc., caregivers were just beginning to embark on clinical quality improvement initiatives. *Clinical Paths* described many first attempts. As the demand for cost-efficient, high-quality patient care intensified, so did clinical quality improvement activities within the health care industry. Many organizations that had developed traditional, nurse-driven clinical pathways realized the need to move to a multidisciplinary model. Organizations that had not yet introduced clinical paths in 1994 saw the need to initiate some kind of clinical quality improvement, and some chose pathways as the tool for achieving their goals. As would be expected, when the numbers and types of professionals involved in designing improvement strategies increased, so did the amount of innovation. Thus, in 1997 (only three years after *Clinical Paths* was published) health care organizations can select from a wide variety of outcomes management tools and techniques. The intent of this book is to broaden everyone's understanding of the array of clinical quality improvement tools, besides and in addition to paths, that clinicians and managed care organizations can use to achieve their cost containment and quality improvement goals. This book builds on what was written in 1994, and rather than superseding, it complements the fundamentals outlined there.

Chapter 1 introduces the book, giving an overview of the components of a successful clinical quality improvement initiative. Interestingly, a total quality managed environment appears to be the most important predictor of success. Quality planning, quality control, and quality improvement are inseparable elements of clinical quality improvement. The remaining 13 chapters are grouped into two parts: Part I, Clinical Process Improvement Initiatives, and Part II, Information Technology Solutions. In Part I, readers are provided a look at the elements of clinical quality improvement and the variety of initiatives being undertaken by health care organizations.

In chapter 2 Meg Kistin Anzalone and Michael D. McGee describe the quality improvement initiative at Merit Behavioral Care (MBC), a managed care organization based in Burlington, MA. After reviewing outcomes management techniques used by other groups, MBC chose to design a comprehensive performance measurement process as its improvement step. This managed care organization worked closely with its providers to design a measurement system that would make valid and reliable data available to provider facilities for their use in managing their own quality systems for care delivery.

In chapter 3 Gail O'Mahaney VanZyl and Gary Goby recount the experience of FirstCare Health, a physician-driven integrated health network in Albany, OR, in developing and implementing clinical practice guidelines. Initial efforts were less than successful because of organizational and ideological barriers. The authors describe how these hurdles were overcome with eventual implementation of several outpatient care guidelines.

In chapter 4 Mary Lu Gerke describes why Lutheran Hospital in LaCrosse, WI, believed it was necessary to improve its coronary artery bypass postoperative sedation practices *before* implementing a clinical path. The caregivers realized that, by itself, the path tool would not effect change. Reducing significant practice variation required a continuous quality improvement approach.

The transition of a traditional, nurse-driven clinical path model into a multidisciplinary disease management initiative is described by Lisa M. Zavorski and Barbara Taptich in chapter 5. Although the original pathway initiative at St. Francis Medical Center in Trenton, NJ, had helped prepare caregivers for the disease management initiative, they soon realized that paths alone were not sufficient to guide patient management decisions. This initiative demonstrates the importance of interdisciplinary teamwork in improving patients' quality of life and reducing resource use.

In chapter 6 Jacquelyn Paynter, Katherine Ambrose, and Katherine Dolan outline the steps taken by St. Joseph's Hospital in Flushing, NY, in developing its multidisciplinary care planning process for patients with specific diagnoses or procedures. Building on this model, the caregivers at St. Joseph's next designed a collaborative approach for managing and improving care for high-risk frail elderly patients.

Clinical quality improvement has become an important component of service in home health care. In chapter 7 Sheila Hawley and Bonnie Davis describe how Clinton

Memorial Hospital Home Health Agency in Wilmington, OH, developed clinical paths to guide the delivery of home care services. Reflecting an outcome-driven approach, these tools helped ensure that patients achieved the most desirable outcomes within a reasonable time period. It soon became apparent, however, that paths alone were not enough. In chapter 8 DeAnne Mosher recounts the next evolutionary step for Clinton Home Health Agency. The addition of case management to the already existing pathway program proved to be a challenge, albeit worth the effort.

In chapter 9 Kevin Turley and Kerry M. Turley recount the clinical path transitions of cardiovascular caregivers at California Pacific Medical Center in San Francisco. Their pathway experience began with an interactive approach, which decreased variation while optimizing patient care. The pathway initiative then progressed to a proactive model, which reduced negative variance while encouraging positive variances. This innovative, collaborative patient management approach has markedly reduced hospital stays for even the most complex and heterogeneous groups of cardiac surgery patients.

Part II of the book, Information Technology Solutions, begins with an overview of the desirable components of a computerized case management and clinical path information system. In chapter 10 Sherry Lee outlines the issues to be considered in selecting an automated information system and provides a step-by-step procedure for evaluating vendors and their products.

Sometimes low-cost information system solutions can be found within the organization. In chapter 11 Darice M. Grzybowski describes how Hinsdale Hospital in Hinsdale, IL, used its preexisting automated charge system to capture path variance data and other outcome measures. Grzybowski emphasizes the importance of involving health information management professionals in designing efficient clinical path data management systems.

In chapter 12 Beth Weber, Linda Ratzlaff, Tom Hearn, and Joan McCanless describe how Bristol Regional Medical Center in Bristol, TN, teamed up with Decision Support Systems to provide an automated framework for gathering and analyzing path-generated process and outcomes data. The improvement opportunities identified through sophisticated computer analysis of path variances have helped caregivers achieve even higher levels of patient care effectiveness.

In chapter 13 Dianne J. Anderson, Christine W. Freire, and Patricia Hale report on the progress of a disease management initiative in Glens Falls, NY. To overcome the challenges of implementing disease management, the physicians and other caregivers in the Glens Falls Hospital community are designing a computerized patient record system to augment their deployment of clinical practice guidelines. This move away from paper-based medicine is requiring a significant effort on the part of physicians, hospital staff, and other entities involved in patient care.

Recent advancements in information technology are making it easier to build expert systems that improve the clinical decision-making process. Unlike traditional clinical paths, an expert system contains rules and decision algorithms that incorporate knowledge and judgment about the health problem at hand and alternative tests and treatments for it. In chapter 14 Edmund Pigott, Greg Alter, and Deborah L. Heggie describe a clinical quality improvement model that links an expert decision support system with outcomes analysis. By integrating the prospective focus of expert systems with the retrospective rigor of outcomes analysis, Pacific Applied Psychology Associates in northern California hopes to accelerate advances in all aspects of health care service delivery.

It is the nature of the health care system to change. The initiatives shared in this book will evolve, and further innovation, perhaps within your organization, will expand the limits of outcomes management tools as we know them today. Coupled with a continuing dedication to improvement, this evolution and innovation will bring higher aspirations and greater possibilities.

CHAPTER 1

Taking Clinical Quality Improvement Beyond Paths

Patrice L. Spath

In 1992, when the book *Total Quality Management: The Health Care Pioneers* was published by American Hospital Publishing, Inc. (AHPI), health care providers were just discovering what seemed to be a powerful patient care management tool: the clinical path. In this book Karen Zander of the Center for Case Management in Methuen, MA, describes a path as a tool for operationalizing total quality management (TQM) at the direct patient care level.[1] Unfortunately, it was the *tool*, not the *message*, that many clinicians embraced. For whatever the reason (perhaps our innate search for a quick fix), health care leaders latched onto paths as the solution to their cost and quality dilemmas. They overlooked the importance of the underlying TQM environment and its impact on outcomes management tools such as clinical paths.

Over the ensuing years, clinical paths became very popular patient management tools. A July 1993 survey conducted by AHPI and Medicus Systems Corporation revealed that 42 percent of the 328 hospitals surveyed had implemented clinical paths, with a mean of 7.5 paths per facility.[2] Most (82 percent) of the hospitals had begun pathway development after January 1992. In 1994, when *Clinical Paths: Tools for Outcomes Management* was published by AHPI, health care organizations nationwide were in various stages of clinical path design and implementation. As of 1995, the percentage of facilities using paths had increased. A survey conducted by Andersen Consulting for Decision Support Systems in Charlotte, NC, revealed that 81 percent of the 187 responding health care organizations said they use clinical paths.[3] Today paths are moving into nontraditional areas, such as home health care, perioperative services, and ambulatory care.[4-6]

Despite the growing interest in clinical paths, select organizations that started their initiatives prior to January 1992 are questioning the value of their pathways as outcomes management tools. Some, such as Rhode Island Hospital, a chapter contributor to *Clinical Paths: Tools for Outcomes Management*, have stopped using their original pathways. Cardiovascular caregivers at Carondelet St. Joseph's Hospital in Tucson (another contributor to the book) have reportedly found preprinted physician orders to be a better tool than pathways for reducing practice variations. Nonetheless, other organizations, such as Abbott Northwestern Hospital in Minneapolis, continue to find their pathways (known as *clinical progressions*) to be a valuable patient care management tool.[7]

Is this disparity of opinion the fault of the pathway tool itself, or is it merely caused by our rush to find the silver bullet rather than fix the problems at hand? To answer this question, consider the following scenario, which illustrates the steps in a typical clinical pathway initiative:

> The leaders of the health care organization establish clinical path implementation as a strategic care management goal. It is not uncommon for the leaders to define the minimum number of paths to be completed for high-volume patient groups. A pathway project coordinator is named and given the responsibility for the initiative. Clinical path development teams are formed. Their charge is to design a path for a particular patient population.
>
> The coordinator may provide the team with a "draft" pathway based on how this group of patients is usually managed by the caregivers. After discussion the team agrees on the pathway content, and clinicians begin using it for patient management. A new tool is introduced into the health care delivery process, and the organization's strategic goals are met—caregivers now have clinical pathways!

Whether these pathways will actually improve the clinical decision-making process is unclear. They may enhance the efficiency of patient care documentation. They may help the organization comply with the Joint Commission on Accreditation of Healthcare Organizations' multidisciplinary care-planning standards. They may provide a framework for data collection. However, reduced practice variations and improved patient outcomes may not be realized. The clinical paths at this organization are likely to be less successful at improving clinical quality than the paths used by other organizations. Why? Because the organization's leaders in the scenario overlooked two basic quality improvement principles:[8]

1. *The administrative and medical staff leaders should define the improvement goals together. Let the process improvement team select the actions necessary for achieving the goals.* In other words, pathways are tools, not end goals, of care management. Instead of telling the project team to suggest needed changes, the leaders tell the team to develop a clinical path. Entitling the group a "clinical path design team" gives the impression that a path is the only desired solution. A pathway may be the right tool for improving the process of care. If so, let the team arrive at this conclusion after they have studied current care management practices and identified improvement opportunities. The team members should be free to recommend whatever actions they believe are most likely to achieve desirable results.

2. *All involved caregivers must agree that it is important to study and improve the care management process.* Normal vaginal delivery is a high-volume reason for hospital admission. For this reason vaginal delivery pathways are found in many hospitals.[9] However, it is not uncommon to learn that the pathway did not cause significant improvements in care. Why? Because the process did not need improving in the first place! Clinical quality improvement projects should focus on known or suspected problem areas that caregivers are interested in resolving. Improving a care management process is hard work. Unless the physicians and other team members are rooting for project success, their interest in the initiative will be short lived.

Through trial and error, health care organizations are realizing that Zander's 1992 remark about TQM was much more important than the CareMap™ model she introduced. TQM is a structured system for creating organization-wide participation in continuous quality improvement. Joseph Juran originally coined the term *total quality management*. According to Juran, TQM involves three important management functions: quality planning, quality control, and quality improvement.[10] A *clinical path* is a quality control tool that can be used to clarify and illuminate process variation, foster awareness of the impact of different clinical decisions, and encourage reduction in undesirable practice variation.[11] Paths, guidelines, algorithms, and other quality control techniques complement the TQM environment, but they do not stand alone. Planning and improvement are equally important. Without these factors in place, any quality control tool will be less than effective. According to Juran, the three TQM components are "an inseparable package."[12]

This book is about organizations that have "gone beyond" traditional clinical paths to improve clinical quality. Some began their journey with a very narrow, prototypical pathway initiative and through experience learned the importance of the TQM triad. Other organizations had the luxury of time and did not launch a full-blown clinical quality improvement program until recently. To say that all of the initiatives detailed in this book are "advanced" would be a fabrication. Many of the clinical quality improvement techniques described by these organizations have been tried before. What is "advanced" about all of these initiatives is that they were undertaken in a environment committed to continuous improvement, and they incorporate all three elements of the TQM triad. Most important, the clinical quality improvement tools were selected only after administrative and clinical leaders clearly understood what they were trying to accomplish. Rather than ending up with "solutions in search of a problem," these organizations have made measurable quality strides.

COMMON CHARACTERISTICS OF A SUCCESSFUL CLINICAL QUALITY IMPROVEMENT INITIATIVE

Although the tools are different and the techniques varied, all health care organizations that successfully achieve their clinical quality improvement goals have certain characteristics in common.

Administrative and Clinical Leaders Are Involved

The leaders have a nondelegable role in ensuring the success of improvement activities. They collaboratively establish organization-wide quality goals, including clinical quality improvement goals, and communicate them to their constituents. Leaders regularly review results against these goals and personally intervene when individual or organizational biases hinder innovation at the caregiver level.

Goals Are Environmentally Aligned

The leaders carefully consider their organization's current financial and collaborative environment when defining organization-wide quality goals and strategies. In health care markets in which the providers' financial incentives are not aligned or few cost containment pressures exist, radical changes are less likely to be supported by the caregivers.

Fundamental Solutions, Not Short-Term Fixes, Are Sought Out

Leaders maintain their focus on the fundamental changes in attitudes and systems that are most likely to produce positive long-term gains. They do this by establishing quality goals and incrementally investing in the strategies necessary to achieve these goals.

Interdisciplinary Collaboration Is Rewarded

Clinical quality problems and challenges are confronted by a *team* of the most appropriate people and disciplines, regardless of their levels or jobs within the department. This team meets face-to-face to learn the value each discipline brings to the health care delivery process and to sculpt user-friendly patient management tools. The organization realizes that more can be accomplished by working together to *improve* the system than by having individual contributors work *around* the system.

Caregivers Make Fact-Based Decisions

The health care team members manage by facts and know how to analyze problems by using simple tools to understand variability and data. Whenever possible the patient care recommendations are based on evidence from current medical literature rather than "the way we've always done it."

Measurement Is an Important Improvement Tool

Each initiative involves timely feedback of process and outcome measures to the clinicians. The validity and reliability of the data are confirmed *before* the data are reported. The information is not used for purposes of judgment but for purposes of learning.

STAGES OF CLINICAL QUALITY IMPROVEMENT

Clinical quality improvement should be a major component of a health care organization's performance improvement strategy. However, it would be foolhardy to suggest that clinical quality initiatives are easily integrated into the culture of an organization. The change process moves through five stages: apathy, realization, confirmation, action, and consolidation.[13]

Apathy

At this stage there is little concern or involvement by the caregivers in formal quality initiatives. The leaders of the organization do not recognize the benefits of fundamental solutions, focusing instead on "quick fixes." It's business as usual.

Realization

There is a general recognition of the need to change attitudes and formalize a commitment to long-term quality goals. Quality improvement priorities are established jointly by the medical staff and administrative leaders. The organization becomes focused on those clinical processes that, if improved, are likely to result in improved patient outcomes.

Confirmation

During this phase it is time to get the caregivers' attention with data. Multidisciplinary clinical quality improvement teams are formed. They are provided with information about current practices to substantiate practice variation and its impact on patient outcomes (both cost and quality).

Action

Once the opportunities for improvement are evident and the caregivers recognize the need for change, the clinical quality improvement teams search for solutions. This is the time to evaluate the care processes of other organizations and review feedback from patients regarding what is important to them. The teams may acquaint themselves with the quality control tools that have been used by other groups, for example, clinical paths, algorithms, flow charts, protocols, standing physician orders, interdisciplinary care plans, preprinted encounter forms, and so on. Ultimately, the teams reach consensus on the best change strategies for their caregivers.

A component of the action stage is the selection of measures. How will the team know when the desired goals have been achieved? The teams select process, outcome, cost, and satisfaction measures to show clinicians that change resulted in improvements. Collection of measurement data is incorporated into the implementation plan.

Consolidation

At this point clinical quality improvement has been fully integrated into the ongoing activities of the organization and supports the organizational mission, vision, and values. Data on the effectiveness of clinical quality improvement are an important component of the organization's continuous performance improvement effort.

CONCLUSION

Clinical quality improvement should not be a separate organizational agenda. It should be part of an explicit, evidence-based process for evaluating and improving clinical practice. Any quality improvement effort requires change, and it is important to listen to the change process and act accordingly. Do not jump to the action stage without first convincing caregivers of the value of change. Lasting success is more likely if the clinical quality improvement projects are based on a thorough understanding of the causes of variation and the potential effect of proposed remedies.

References

1. Zander, K. Critical pathways. In: M. M. Melum and M. K. Sinioris, editors. *Total Quality Management: The Health Care Pioneers.* Chicago: American Hospital Publishing, 1992.
2. Lumsdon, K., and Haglund, M. Mapping care. *Hospitals and Health Networks* 67(20):34–40, Oct. 20, 1993.
3. Andersen Consulting. *Clinical Path Survey: A Study of Clinical Path Trends in Healthcare.* Charlotte, NC: Decision Support Systems, 1995.
4. Gooldy, J., and Duncan, B. Home care's role in clinical pathways. *Journal of Home Health Care Practice* 6(2):63–69, Feb. 1994.
5. Spath, P. L. Critical paths: maximizing patient care coordination. *Today's OR Nurse* 17(2):13–20, Mar.–Apr. 1995.
6. Czaplijski, T. J. Critical pathways: broad implementation in an ambulatory service division. *Outreach* 15(2):4–5, Mar.–Apr. 1994.
7. Dixon, M. D., Burton, C. V., Graham, K. J., and others. Outcome and effectiveness models in cardiovascular and spine services. In: P. L. Spath, editor. *Medical Effectiveness and Outcomes Management: Issues, Methods, and Case Studies.* Chicago: American Hospital Publishing, 1996, pp. 161–89.
8. Scholtes, P. R. *The Team Handbook.* Madison, WI: Joiner Associates, 1988.
9. Andersen Consulting.

10. Juran, J. M. *Juran on Leadership for Quality.* New York City: Free Press, 1989.
11. Goonan, K. J. *The Juran Prescription: Clinical Quality Management.* San Francisco: Jossey-Bass, 1995, p. 122.
12. Juran, J. M. Made in USA—A renaissance in quality. *Harvard Business Review* 71(4):42–50, July–Aug. 1993.
13. Spath, P. L. Keep guideline implementation orderly. *Hospital Peer Review* 20(11):158–60, Nov. 1995.

PART I

Clinical Process Improvement Initiatives

CHAPTER 2

Using Performance Measurement as a Quality Improvement Tool

Meg Kistin Anzalone and Michael D. McGee

When health care providers do the *right thing,* at the *right time, every time,* optimal clinical and financial outcomes should be achieved. Clinical paths that define what is to be done, by whom, and when have become popular outcomes management tools in addition to their use in quality control. Indeed, paths would be the ideal solution to the quality puzzle if every patient care situation could be predicted objectively and if the health care team and patients could be counted on to perform reliably. However, a health care event is an extraordinarily complex process that is impossible to forecast accurately using a clinical path or any other patient management tool. Several factors produce legitimate variations in the health care process:[1]

- Diversity in the training, experience, and personal judgment of clinicians
- Differences in patients' biological states, illness severities, socioeconomic conditions, cultures, and personal health care preferences
- Variability in delivery system models, available community resources, and other provider- and community-related factors

These variations contribute to differences in practice decisions that may or may not affect the end results. To reduce variant practices that harm patient outcomes, many tools, including clinical paths, must be brought to bear.

FROM MICROMANAGEMENT TO SYSTEMS MANAGEMENT

In 1995 Merit Behavioral Care (MBC), a national managed care organization with headquarters in Park Ridge, NJ, faced the task of managing the performance of a statewide behavioral health provider network for an HMO in Massachusetts. To meet this challenge MBC sought to design a performance management system that was practical, user friendly, interactive between MBC and its providers, and valuable for patients, providers, and payers. After reviewing performance management systems used by other organizations, including clinical practice guidelines and clinical paths, MBC chose to focus on performance measurement as its *first* step toward managing patient outcomes. Performance measurement was seen as the most sensible focus for several reasons. MBC of Massachusetts had already established service standards across all levels of care, which, together with MBC's clinical necessity criteria, are intended to specify MBC's provider expectations regarding quality service delivery. Further, MBC wanted to move as rapidly as possible away from the micromanagement of individual cases toward managing systems. In this model data would be made available to provider facilities for use in managing their quality systems for care delivery. The provider community in Massachusetts is for the most part quite sophisticated and interested in collaborating with managed care organizations in delivering cost-effective, quality behavioral health services, with micromanagement of cases held to a minimum. In this environment performance measurement can be an effective quality improvement tool.

The purpose of the project was to design an effective performance measurement system that eventually could be used by all MBC providers throughout Massachusetts and that would allow for objective, reliable comparisons among providers. The intent was to develop a process that would enable providers to obtain real-time outcome data on individual patient progress, allow them to compare their performance with a network aggregate, and influence performance improvement activities at the facility level. Performance measurement results were not intended to be used by MBC to credential providers, channel referrals, or exclude certain caregivers or facilities from the managed care network.

The project described in this chapter focused on agencies and facilities across all levels of care for mental health and substance abuse. MBC conducted a similar corporate project that focused on individual outpatient providers. Using the Behavior and Symptom Identification Scale-32 (BASIS-32)[2] clinical outcomes measure and internally designed chart audit and patient satisfaction surveys, as well as utilization data, MBC Massachusetts developed a measurement system to evaluate provider performance across four dimensions: clinical outcomes, utilization, technical performance, and patient satisfaction.

The initial project was begun as a pilot with facilities providing inpatient and outpatient mental health and substance abuse services. These providers were selected based on geographical and level-of-service representation. After analyzing the results of the pilot project, MBC plans to expand the pilot to its inpatient and group provider network in Massachusetts. There are no plans to extend this project to other states.

Before quality improvement could occur, several elements had to be in place. MBC first selected its overall performance improvement strategy. Borrowing from the industrial quality improvement literature, MBC leadership chose the Plan-Do-Check-Act model of process improvement.[3] This model was used to illustrate MBC's performance management process. (See table 2-1.)

The project was divided into six phases:

1. Define objectives
2. Identify performance measurements
3. Select measurement tools
4. Define measurement processes
5. Transform data into information for analysis
6. Use the information to improve performance

TABLE 2-1 Performance Management Process

Process Improvement Model	MBC Performance Management Steps
Plan	1. Define objectives
	2. Identify performance measures
	3. Select measurement tools
Do	4. Define measurement methods and collect data
Check	5. Transform data into information (data analysis)
Act	6. Use information to improve performace

At the time of this writing, the pilot project was complete through and into phase 5. These first steps are described in this chapter. It is our hope that other health care delivery systems and managed care organizations will find MBC's experiences useful in designing similar networkwide performance management systems.

DEFINE OBJECTIVES

As Laurence Peter notes, "If you don't know where you're going, you will probably end up somewhere else."[4] The goal of the MBC project was to develop a performance management system that:

- Gathers valid performance data from multiple providers to allow them to evaluate the quality of patient care
- Encourages providers to initiate meaningful quality improvement initiatives at the caregiver level

When determining the objectives for their performance management system, MBC leaders had to confront the question, What is quality? Theoretically, *quality* is most closely associated with the concept of *value*. The value equation consists of some optimal balancing of utilization and clinical outcomes. Too little or too much utilization may diminish the value of care. The use of inappropriate treatment modalities or unnecessarily costly patient care at delivery sites can also decrease the value of the health care experience. Correlations between appropriate versus inappropriate utilization and other quality dimensions have yet to be fully explored in the behavioral health literature. There is some suggestion, however, that patient satisfaction may correlate with clinical outcomes, raising the question of whether one must always measure both satisfaction and clinical outcomes.[5] Another important and as yet unanswered question is how different aspects of technical performance, including compliance with clinical paths, correlate with patient satisfaction and clinical outcomes.

In the end, behavioral health caregivers may find that the most important dimension of performance will be that of patient and family satisfaction: if patients are treated effectively, efficiently, and with warmth and respect, they will have an optimal outcome and will be satisfied with that outcome. However, as of today, the question of which health care dimension is the best indicator of quality in terms of optimal clinical and fiscal outcomes remains unanswered. MBC therefore chose to assess performance in all four major health care dimensions: clinical outcomes, utilization, technical performance, and patient satisfaction.

In addition to establishing the performance dimensions to be evaluated, MBC leaders also agreed that the aggregate results of this "report card" effort should be made available to the network for use in improving patient care delivery systems. While the performance measurements were not intended to focus on an individual's performance or to be used by the managed care organization to evaluate the care provided to a particular patient, the BASIS-32 results were nonetheless intended to be made available to treating providers in real time. This was to be accomplished by having providers purchase scanning devices or by having MBC scan in the information and then fax patient-specific results to providers.

Working over an 8-month period in 1995, the overall objectives for this pilot provider performance management project were developed and set by the MBC Massachusetts medical director and area quality director in collaboration with the MBC corporate quality department and chief clinical officer. A task force of providers invited to participate in the project was convened in late 1995 to help refine the data collection processes and feedback loops.

IDENTIFY PERFORMANCE MEASUREMENTS

After defining the performance management goals and the scope of the project, measurements addressing the four dimensions of performance were selected. In reviewing the variety of measurements being used by other health care providers and managed care organizations, MBC found there were many possible performance rates that could be used to evaluate each important health care dimension. Commonly used behavioral health performance indicators for the four health care dimensions chosen by MBC are summarized below:

- *Clinical outcome measurements:* Clinical outcome measurements fall into two general categories: patient-reported outcomes and clinician-reported outcomes.[6]
  - *—Patient-reported outcomes* generally address attitudinal, somatic, and behavioral components such as physical function, role function, bodily pain, general health, vitality, social function, emotional function, and mental health. Patient-reported outcomes are considered to be subjective clinical measures.
  - *—Clinician-reported outcomes* generally address patients' biological and physiological functioning, diagnoses, achievement of therapeutic goals, presence or absence of complications, relapse and retreatment rates, incidence of adverse events such as patient death or crises, unexplained discharges from treatment, or unsuccessful completion of treatment.
- *Utilization measurements:* Indicators of utilization can include units of service, average cost per unit, days of treatment, total cost of a treatment episode, and annual cost per patient. These utilization data might be stratified by patient type, impairment severity, site, and setting.
- *Technical performance measurements:* Measurements of technical performance focus on the health care delivery process. One measurement would be the extent to which the actions of a health care practitioner conform to a clinical practice guideline or clinical path.[7] In managed care settings, measurements of providers' compliance with utilization review policies and procedures would be considered a technical performance measurement. In general, technical performance measurements are useful for evaluating compliance with defined standards of care and practice, clinical and administrative performance standards, policies, procedures, and other regulatory requirements.
- *Patient satisfaction measurements:* With the patient being the principal customer of health care services, most satisfaction measurements focus on the patient.[8] Patients may be asked to respond to questions such as: Do the caregivers treat you well? Do the caregivers respond quickly when you need to see them? Do you have confidence in your caregiver's abilities? How satisfied were you with the length of time

TABLE 2-2 Pilot Project Measurements for the Four Performance Dimensions

Dimension	Measurement
Clinical outcomes	Changes in clients' functional status
Utilization	Number of service units per treatment episode
Technical performance	Completeness of client record documentation
Patient satisfaction	Patient-reported satisfaction

spent waiting at the office before you were seen by the caregiver? The managed care organization can also measure patient satisfaction by evaluating complaints or grievances received and by monitoring patient transfers from one provider to another. Further, satisfaction data can be solicited from providers, case managers, employers, or family members.

MBC leaders agreed it was important to select performance measures that would provide objective, statistically valid results. Also deemed important was starting with data elements that were routinely collected or, if new collection processes were necessary, would not burden facilities with extraordinary requirements. Another important objective was to provide real-time feedback of treatment progress to the treating provider. Considering these objectives, the measurements shown in table 2-2 were selected by MBC for each of the four performance dimensions.

SELECT MEASUREMENT TOOLS

To ensure reliability of performance measurement results, it was important to select validated tools. Therefore, MBC turned to the literature to identify suitable behavioral health measurement instruments. Another important criterion in selecting measurement tools was to minimize the data-gathering burdens for MBC providers.

Utilization Measurement Instruments

For the utilization measures, no additional data collection was necessary. Utilization rates could be captured from claims data. However, measuring performance in the other dimensions required the introduction of new tools. Several options, including the commonly used measurement instruments listed below, were considered.

Clinical Outcome Measurement Instruments

Tools to measure patients' initial and posttreatment status include both patient-reported and clinician-reported evaluation instruments.

Patient-Reported Instruments For patients, researchers have designed many different self-rating scales to measure the severity of the patient's symptoms and functional impairment. These measurement instruments can be administered pretreatment and posttreatment or at other planned intervals. Changes in impairment can be evaluated according to provider, patient population, setting, or treatment modality and compared with a larger treatment population. Commonly used tools are listed below:

- *The Beck Depression Inventory* is a 21-item self-rating questionnaire (or 13 items in short form) that is used to assess attitudinal, somatic, and behavioral components.[9]

- *The Center for Epidemiologic Studies Depression* self-rating scale measures severity of stroke patients' depressive symptomatology. This 20-item questionnaire investigates the patient's perceived mood and level of functioning within the past week.[10]
- *The SF-36,* developed by the Medical Outcomes Trust, Boston, measures nine patient-reported health concepts: physical function; role function, physical; bodily pain; general health; vitality; social function; role function, emotional; mental health; and reported health transition.[11]
- *The OQ-45.1,* a psychological research tool developed by Intermountain Health Care, Salt Lake City, evaluates three categories of patient function: psychological symptoms; ability to perform in world, school, or household roles; and functioning in interpersonal relationships. It also flags any tendencies toward substance abuse, suicide, or other dangerous behavior.[12]
- *The Brief Symptom Inventory* (BSI) is a 53-item, self-report symptom inventory.[13] It is designed to measure the following dimensions: somatization, obsessive-compulsive, interpersonal sensitivity, depression, anxiety, hostility, phobic anxiety, paranoid ideation, and psychoticism. The BSI was developed from its longer parent instrument, the Symptom Check List-90-R.
- *The BASIS-32* is a 32-question survey tool used to gather patient-reported outcome data in mental health services.[14] This self-rating scale provides subjective measures of patient symptoms, distress, and functional impairment.

Clinician-Reported Instruments   Clinician-reported measures of patient outcomes include the following:

- *The Global Assessment of Functioning* (GAF) scale is an instrument used by the clinician to rate the patient's illness severity on a scale of 0 to 100; it has also been found to be useful in evaluating family members' social functioning. Since the development of the modified GAF by Richard Hall, the fourth edition of the *Diagnostic and Statistical Manual of Mental Disorders* (*DSM-IV*) has redefined the GAF from a 0–90 scale to a 0–100 scale. Consequently, Hall and Parks recalibrated the GAF to a 0–100 scale.[15] The scale can also be found in the *DSM-IV,* published in 1994 by the American Psychiatric Association.
- *The Psych Sentinel,* developed by Hal Mark, is a public-domain outcomes assessment tool based on symptom reduction.[16] It is a nonproprietary user-supported system. Data collected are sent to the University of Connecticut, where the forms are scored. In addition, patients are classified relative to diagnosis and adjusted by illness severity, length of stay, and expected level of improvement.
- *The Psychiatric Symptom Assessment Scale* was developed by Bigelow and Berthot for the National Institutes of Mental Health at St. Elizabeth's Hospital, Washington, DC, with a population of persons with chronic schizophrenia.[17] It is a twice-daily scale administered by one primary nurse in consultation with all nursing staff on duty who had contact with the patient. It measures 22 items according to the quality of a given behavior as opposed to presence or absence of that behavior. It can be a sensitive instrument when used to assess treatment-induced change in clinical studies.

Instruments Completed by Clinician and Patient   Some outcome measurement tools combine clinician observation and patient self-reporting. Two commonly used tools of this variety are the following:

1. *The Addictions Severity Index* developed by MacLellan and others is a 60- to 75-minute interview appropriate for all substance-abusing and psychiatrically im-

paired adult populations with the exception of schizophrenia.[18] It is an interview format intended to be administered by a research technician or clinician and measures seven functional areas that may contribute to a person's substance abuse syndrome, including medical status, employment, drug use, alcohol use, legal status, family social status, and psychiatric status. Within each area there is an interviewer 10-point severity rating of lifetime problems as well as a composite score reflecting recent severity (within the past 30 days).

2. *The Depression Technology of Patient Experience* developed by the Health Outcomes Institute, Bloomington, MN, and the University of Arkansas for Medical Sciences includes baseline and follow-up survey instruments that are completed by the patient and the clinician.[19] The patient survey provides information about diagnosis, prognostic factors, patient functioning, health status, and personal characteristics. The clinician survey provides information about diagnosis and treatment recommendations, patient compliance with treatment recommendations, and medications.

Technical Performance Measurement Instruments

Check sheets and audit worksheets are the traditional tools for gathering technical performance measurement data.[20] An example of an audit worksheet for collecting data found in client records is shown in figure 2-1. Careful design of data collection forms and procedures is critical for ensuring both the reliability and the validity of a performance measure. To reduce variation in data collection procedures, the data-gathering tool should be accompanied by written instructions or decision rules for the abstractors.[21]

When patient care information is computerized and sufficiently detailed, the database can be a useful source of technical performance measurement data. For example, "Guidelines for Treating Dissociative Identity Disorder (DID) in Adults," published by the International Society for the Study of Dissociation, recommends that the minimum frequency of therapy sessions for the average DID patient be twice a week.[22] To measure compliance with this technical performance measure, the researcher need only query the patient care database to determine whether this minimum treatment standard was met.

Patient Satisfaction Measurement Instruments

Health care providers use a wide range of techniques for gathering patient satisfaction data. These methods include telephone and mail surveys, focus groups, structured interviews, open-ended interviews, and analysis of complaint or praise letters. A comprehensive analysis of patient satisfaction should include an interactive combination of these various methods.[23]

Because the more comprehensive focus group or interview techniques are costly, patient satisfaction data are typically gathered through custom-developed mail or telephone surveys. These surveys include Likert-type questions about satisfaction with treatments, clinicians, and treatment environment and about satisfaction with other aspects of the health care experience, including access, waiting times, and treatment by nonclinical personnel.[24] Several options are available for classifying satisfaction scores. Feedback is better if the patient is given more than two answer choices, that is, more than yes or no.[25] Ware and Hays, in studies of patient satisfaction with outpatient visits, found *excellent-to-poor* ratings superior to direct satisfaction ratings such as *very satisfied* to *not at all satisfied*.[26]

FIGURE 2-1 Audit Worksheet Used to Gather Information from Client Records

---
Objective Setting for Substance Abuse Clients

Chart No. _____ Date of Review: _____ Reviewer's Name: _____

Is there documentation in the client's record that confirms the following issues were taken into consideration during the discussion of treatment objectives?

	Yes	No
1. The client set the objectives with assistance of staff	___	___
2. Objectives included provision for the client's:		
a. Physical requirements	___	___
b. Maintenance of emotional stability	___	___
c. Reduction of the use of pathological defense mechanisms	___	___
d. Understanding and acceptance of substance abuse/dependency disorder	___	___
e. Identification with peers	___	___
f. Hope for recovery	___	___
3. Objectives addressed:		
a. Resocialization and increased interpersonal skills	___	___
b. Development of increased self-worth and self-esteem	___	___
c. Establishment of alternative coping skills	___	___
d. Improvement of motivation to continue treatment	___	___
e. Prevention of noncompliance	___	___
f. Involvement of family and significant others	___	___

Reviewer's Comments:

Source: Reprinted, with permission, from Kibbee, P., and Spath, P. L. *Quality Management in Psychiatric, Alcohol and Substance Abuse Treatment Facilities.* Forest Grove, OR: Brown-Spath and Associates, 1991.

The structured interview involves active listening to the patient. Open-ended questions are asked about the patient's experience, for example, "Describe what happened when you were admitted to the hospital." These surveys invite more candid discussions of the patient's satisfaction with the treatment experience. Structured interview tools can also be used in focus group interviews, where feedback is solicited from different categories of patients. Focus groups strengthen the communication channels between the provider and the patient.

Satisfaction measurement tools may also be designed to obtain information from the patient's family, for example, "What did you view as best or worst about the patient's treatment and what do you think could have been improved?"[27]

Measurement Instruments Chosen by MBC

In keeping with the objectives of the provider performance management project—to create valid performance measures and to minimize data-gathering burdens—the following measurement instruments were selected.

BASIS-32 The BASIS-32 was chosen for measuring *clinical outcomes* because it is brief, practical, psychometrically sound, and inexpensive, in addition to providing meaningful information about patient distress and impairment.[28] This 32-item scale, developed at McLean Hospital in Massachusetts, measures symptoms across five subscales: relation to self and others, daily living and role functioning, depression and anxiety, impulsive and addictive behavior, and psychosis. Primarily developed for inpatient populations, it has been found to be reliable for all but seriously schizophrenic adults. Although it has been utilized with outpatients, its usefulness with this population remains to be finally established.

Designed to assess psychiatric outcome from the patient's viewpoint, the BASIS-32 can be self-administered or used as an interview instrument that lends itself to an automated scanning or scoring technology. The BASIS-32 consists of a two-sided questionnaire (figure 2-2) with a perforated response column that tears off for easier handling. The completed questionnaire form can be scanned electronically and the results evaluated through the use of a computer software package developed by HCIA Response Technologies, East Greenwich, RI.

In its self-administered form the BASIS-32 takes about 5 to 10 minutes to complete. As such it is user friendly in that the administrative burden is low and caregivers can be provided real-time feedback on the success of an ongoing treatment episode. A sample report is shown in figure 2-3.

MBC Corporate Patient Satisfaction Survey The MBC Corporate Patient Satisfaction Survey (figure 2-4) was chosen for evaluating *patient satisfaction*. This survey has been in use since 1993 and has been widely accepted by MBC client organizations as a meaningful measurement of patient satisfaction. Past survey return rates have averaged 18 to 20 percent. MBC's corporate quality department distributes the survey by direct mail to a selected sample of patients who are enrolled in the managed care organization and have received services in the prior 6 months. To streamline the process and increase the rate of return during the pilot project, providers agreed to distribute the survey directly to clients. MBC will be evaluating the extent to which this change in distribution affects results.

Chart Audit Tool For assessing *technical performance* a chart audit tool (figure 2-5) was developed. This tool includes each of the MBC performance standards, which were developed in the Massachusetts office by the medical, clinical, and quality directors in collaboration with senior management and the clinical department. In developing these standards the MBC Massachusetts medical director utilized a consensus process involving input from network providers and medical directors. MBC Massachusetts providers are contractually obligated to adhere to these standards.

DEFINE MEASUREMENT PROCESSES

The project advisory group was actively involved in designing the measurement data collection processes. Careful consideration had to be given to data collection timing and data abstraction methods. Because performance measurement procedures would eventually affect all MBC providers in the state, issues such as patient confidentiality, provider routines, data system requirements, and provider resources needed to be considered.

It was important to develop data collection processes that would yield reliable and valid performance measurements. For example, if a facility does not administer the satisfaction survey in a manner that reassures patients that the responses will be kept confidential, the resulting data will not convert to meaningful information.

FIGURE 2-2 BASIS-32 Form

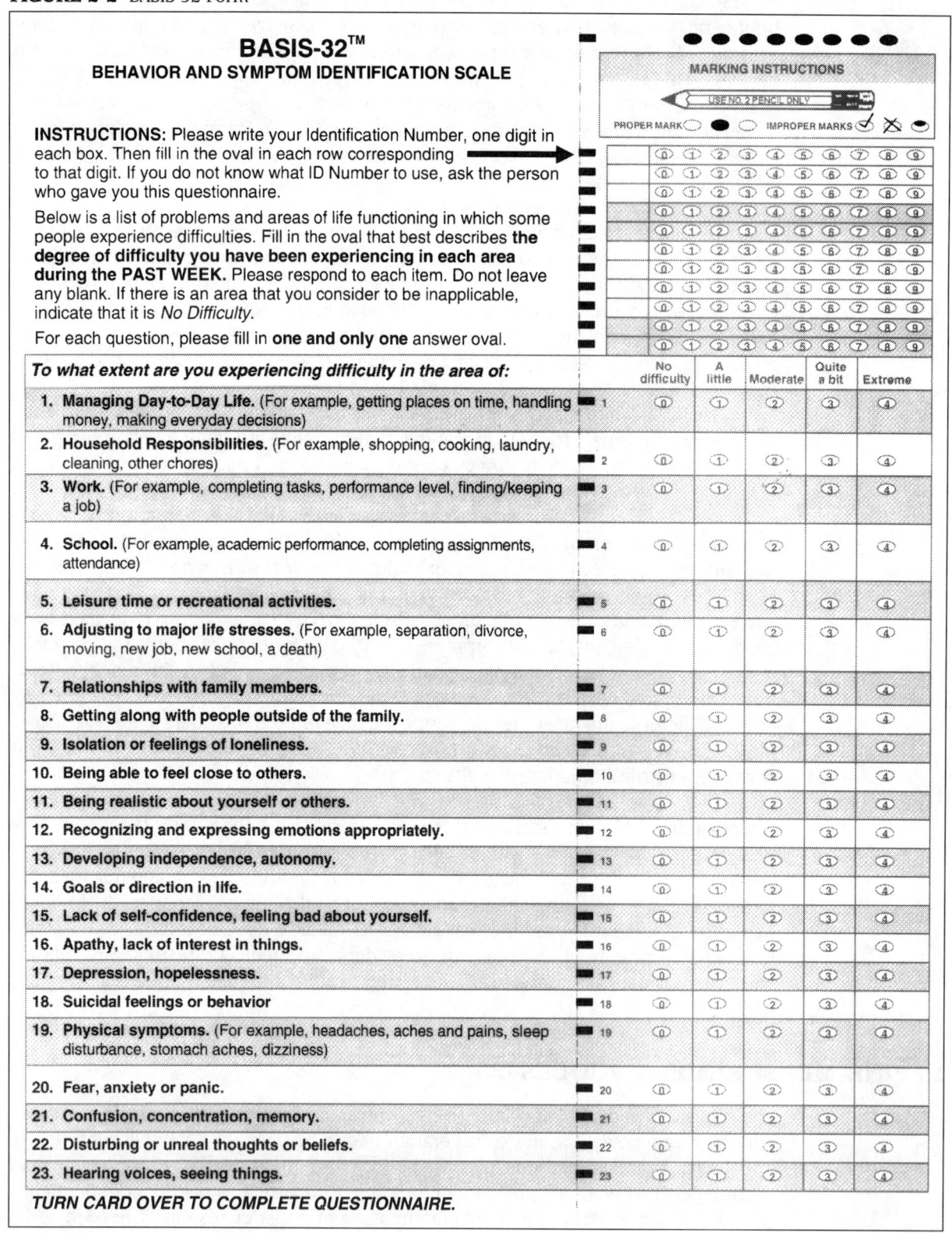

BASIS-32™
BEHAVIOR AND SYMPTOM IDENTIFICATION SCALE

INSTRUCTIONS: Please write your Identification Number, one digit in each box. Then fill in the oval in each row corresponding to that digit. If you do not know what ID Number to use, ask the person who gave you this questionnaire.

Below is a list of problems and areas of life functioning in which some people experience difficulties. Fill in the oval that best describes **the degree of difficulty you have been experiencing in each area during the PAST WEEK.** Please respond to each item. Do not leave any blank. If there is an area that you consider to be inapplicable, indicate that it is *No Difficulty*.

For each question, please fill in **one and only one** answer oval.

MARKING INSTRUCTIONS
USE NO. 2 PENCIL ONLY
PROPER MARK ●   IMPROPER MARKS ✓ ✗ ◐

To what extent are you experiencing difficulty in the area of:	No difficulty	A little	Moderate	Quite a bit	Extreme
1. **Managing Day-to-Day Life.** (For example, getting places on time, handling money, making everyday decisions)	0	1	2	3	4
2. **Household Responsibilities.** (For example, shopping, cooking, laundry, cleaning, other chores)	0	1	2	3	4
3. **Work.** (For example, completing tasks, performance level, finding/keeping a job)	0	1	2	3	4
4. **School.** (For example, academic performance, completing assignments, attendance)	0	1	2	3	4
5. **Leisure time or recreational activities.**	0	1	2	3	4
6. **Adjusting to major life stresses.** (For example, separation, divorce, moving, new job, new school, a death)	0	1	2	3	4
7. **Relationships with family members.**	0	1	2	3	4
8. **Getting along with people outside of the family.**	0	1	2	3	4
9. **Isolation or feelings of loneliness.**	0	1	2	3	4
10. **Being able to feel close to others.**	0	1	2	3	4
11. **Being realistic about yourself or others.**	0	1	2	3	4
12. **Recognizing and expressing emotions appropriately.**	0	1	2	3	4
13. **Developing independence, autonomy.**	0	1	2	3	4
14. **Goals or direction in life.**	0	1	2	3	4
15. **Lack of self-confidence, feeling bad about yourself.**	0	1	2	3	4
16. **Apathy, lack of interest in things.**	0	1	2	3	4
17. **Depression, hopelessness.**	0	1	2	3	4
18. **Suicidal feelings or behavior**	0	1	2	3	4
19. **Physical symptoms.** (For example, headaches, aches and pains, sleep disturbance, stomach aches, dizziness)	0	1	2	3	4
20. **Fear, anxiety or panic.**	0	1	2	3	4
21. **Confusion, concentration, memory.**	0	1	2	3	4
22. **Disturbing or unreal thoughts or beliefs.**	0	1	2	3	4
23. **Hearing voices, seeing things.**	0	1	2	3	4

TURN CARD OVER TO COMPLETE QUESTIONNAIRE.

FIGURE 2-2 *Continued*

Please respond to each item. Do not leave any blank. If there is an area that you consider to be inapplicable, indicate that it is *No Difficulty*.

To what extent are you experiencing difficulty in the area of:	No difficulty	A little	Moderate	Quite a bit	Extreme
24. Manic, bizarre behavior.	⓪	①	②	③	④
25. Mood swings, unstable moods.	⓪	①	②	③	④
26. Uncontrollable, compulsive behavior. (For example, eating disorder, hand-washing, hurting yourself)	⓪	①	②	③	④
27. Sexual activity or preoccupation.	⓪	①	②	③	④
28. Drinking alcoholic beverages.	⓪	①	②	③	④
29. Taking illegal drugs, misusing drugs.	⓪	①	②	③	④
30. Controlling temper, outbursts of anger, violence.	⓪	①	②	③	④
31. Impulsive, illegal or reckless behavior.	⓪	①	②	③	④
32. Feeling satisfaction with your life.	⓪	①	②	③	④

33. How old were you on your last birthday?
    - ○ 14 - 18   ○ 19 - 24   ○ 25 - 34
    - ○ 35 - 44   ○ 45 - 54   ○ 55 - 64
    - ○ 65 - 74   ○ 75 or more

34. What is your sex?   ○ Male   ○ Female

35. Marital status.
    - ○ Never married   ○ Married
    - ○ Separated / divorced / widowed

36. In the past 30 days, what were your usual living arrangements?
    - ○ Alone   ○ With family
    - ○ Halfway house/Treatment setting
    - ○ With non-relative   ○ Other

37. In the past 30 days, were you working at a paid job?   ○ Yes   ○ No

38. If YES, how many hours per week? (If NO, leave unanswered.)
    - ○ 1 - 10 hours   ○ 11 - 20 hours
    - ○ 21 - 30 hours   ○ More than 30 hrs.

39. In the past 30 days, were you a student attending a high school, vocational training program, college or graduate degree program?   ○ Yes   ○ No

END OF SURVEY. THANK YOU VERY MUCH.

THE FOLLOWING SECTION IS FOR OFFICE USE ONLY.

40. Visit Type
    - ○ Admission/Intake   ○ Mid-Treatment
    - ○ Discharge/Termination
    - ○ Post Treatment Follow-up

41. Level Of Care
    - ○ Inpatient   ○ Outpatient
    - ○ Partial Hospitalization/Day Treatment

42. Episode Of Care/Visit #

43. Date Form Was Completed
    - Day ⑩ ⑩ ⑳ ㉚
    - Year ⑲ ⑳

FOR OFFICE USE ONLY   Ⓐ Ⓑ Ⓒ Ⓓ Ⓔ Ⓕ

Source: Reprinted, with permission, from McLean Hospital, Department of Mental Health Service Research.

FIGURE 2-3 Sample BASIS-32 Report

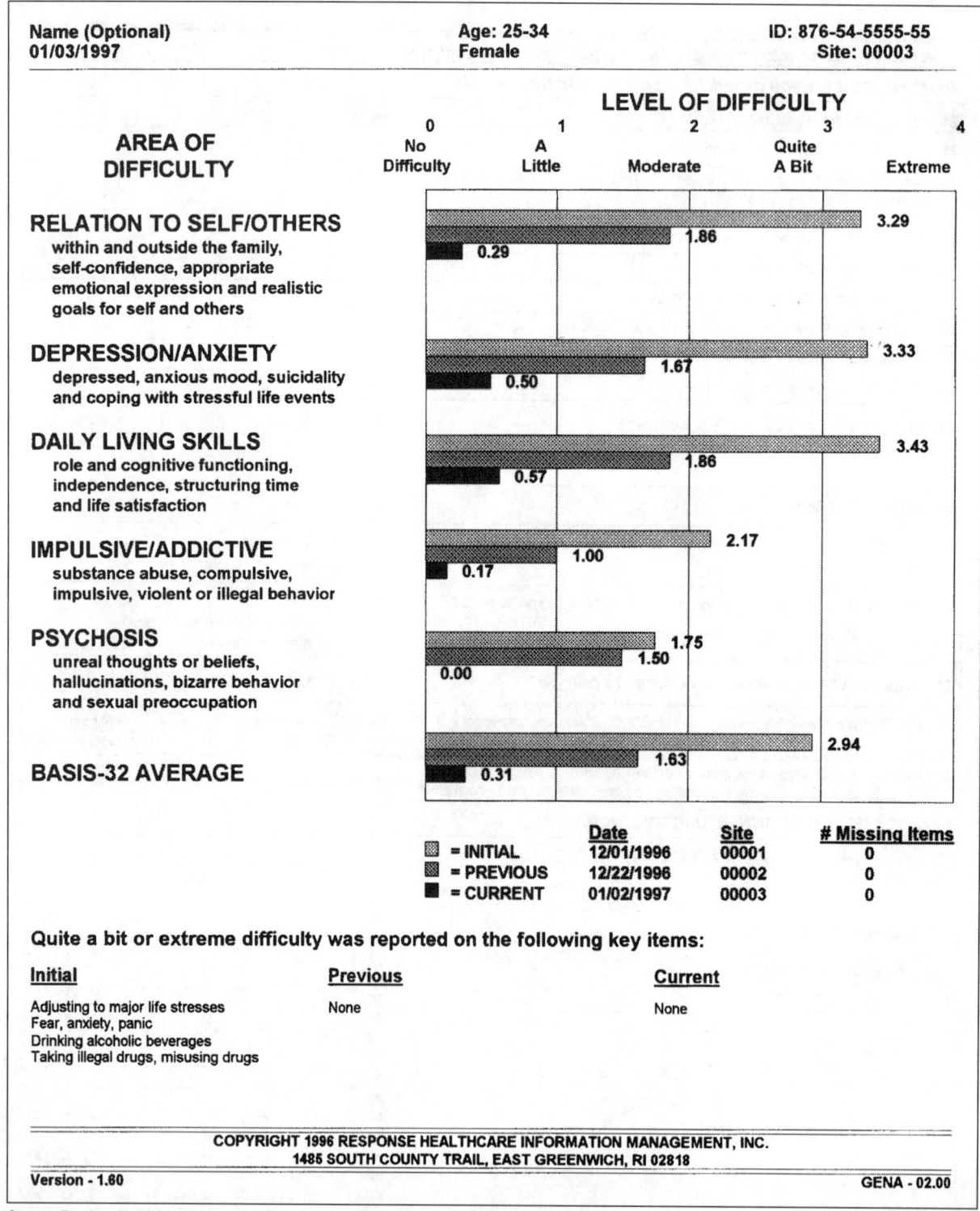

Name (Optional)	Age: 25-34	ID: 876-54-5555-55
01/03/1997	Female	Site: 00003

LEVEL OF DIFFICULTY

	0	1	2	3	4
AREA OF DIFFICULTY	No Difficulty	A Little	Moderate	Quite A Bit	Extreme

RELATION TO SELF/OTHERS
within and outside the family, self-confidence, appropriate emotional expression and realistic goals for self and others
- Initial: 3.29
- Previous: 1.86
- Current: 0.29

DEPRESSION/ANXIETY
depressed, anxious mood, suicidality and coping with stressful life events
- Initial: 3.33
- Previous: 1.67
- Current: 0.50

DAILY LIVING SKILLS
role and cognitive functioning, independence, structuring time and life satisfaction
- Initial: 3.43
- Previous: 1.86
- Current: 0.57

IMPULSIVE/ADDICTIVE
substance abuse, compulsive, impulsive, violent or illegal behavior
- Initial: 2.17
- Previous: 1.00
- Current: 0.17

PSYCHOSIS
unreal thoughts or beliefs, hallucinations, bizarre behavior and sexual preoccupation
- Initial: 1.75
- Previous: 1.50
- Current: 0.00

BASIS-32 AVERAGE
- Initial: 2.94
- Previous: 1.63
- Current: 0.31

	Date	Site	# Missing Items
= INITIAL	12/01/1996	00001	0
= PREVIOUS	12/22/1996	00002	0
= CURRENT	01/02/1997	00003	0

Quite a bit or extreme difficulty was reported on the following key items:

Initial	Previous	Current
Adjusting to major life stresses	None	None
Fear, anxiety, panic		
Drinking alcoholic beverages		
Taking illegal drugs, misusing drugs		

COPYRIGHT 1996 RESPONSE HEALTHCARE INFORMATION MANAGEMENT, INC.
1485 SOUTH COUNTY TRAIL, EAST GREENWICH, RI 02818

Version - 1.60　　　　　　　　　　　　　　　　　　　　　　　　　　　　GENA - 02.00

Source: Reprinted, with permission, from Response Healthcare Information Management, Inc.

DEFINE MEASUREMENT PROCESSES   21

FIGURE 2-4 Patient Satisfaction Survey

Please answer each question by filling in the oval for the response that best answers each question. Use a #2 pencil and make your marks dark and solid.

Correct mark / Incorrect marks

FORM #

IDENTIFICATION #

SEX: MALE / FEMALE

If your care involved treatment in a therapist's office, please complete this section. Please rate your experience with the following items:
(1) Excellent (2) Very good (3) Good (4) Fair (5) Poor

Your Therapist:

1. Listened closely to you
2. Described how you would work together (your treatment plan)
3. Was on time for your appointment(s)
4. Understood your problem and how you felt about it

How Satisfied Were You With:

5. The time you waited between calling for your first appointment and the appointment time you received
6. The time you waited between appointments after your first one
7. The convenience of appointment times for your schedule
8. The waiting time between your need to see a psychiatrist (if needed) and the appointment time you received
9. The ease in which you got through to the therapist's office on the telephone
10. The number of appointments you have received
11. The therapist's office staff's courtesy and responsiveness
12. The pleasantness of the physical environment
13. The amount of paperwork you were asked to complete
14. The match between the therapist's skills/specialty and your concerns
15. The coordination of services among the therapist, those making your appointments and others involved in your care
16. The willingness of the therapist to help you obtain other care (if needed)

© 1992 Response Technologies, Inc. East Greenwich, RI 02818   CP92-0258   © 1992 Response Technologies, Inc. East Greenwich, RI 02818

FIGURE 2-4 *Continued*

If your care involved an overnight stay, please complete this section. Please rate as follows: (1)Excellent (2)Very good (3)Good (4)Fair (5)Poor.

19.	The pleasantness of the physical environment
20.	The courtesy and responsiveness of the facility's staff
21.	The competence of the facility's staff
22.	**Considering your entire treatment experience, please complete this section.**
23.	Compared to previous experiences with other healthcare companies, this company and their staff understood and administered your benefits
24.	(1) Worse than others (2) About the same (3) Better than others ========>
25.	To what extent has our program met your needs (1) Almost all (2) Most of (3)Only a few (4)None of (my needs been meet)
26.	Have the services you received helped you to deal more effectively with your problems?
27.	(1)Yes, helped a great deal (2)Yes, helped somewhat (3)No, they really didn't (4)No, seemed to make things worse ===============>
28.	In an overall, general sense, how satisfied are you with the services you received?
29.	(1)Very satisfied (2)Mostly satisfied (3)Indifferent/mildly dissatisfied (4)Quite dissatisfied ===============>
30.	If you were to seek help again, would you come back to our program? (1)No, definitely not (2)No, I don't think so (3)Yes, I think so (4)Yes, definitely
31.	How many times have you seen a therapist in his/her office during this course of treatment? (1)1-6 (2)7-12 (3)13-18 (4)19+ (sessions)
32.	Did you receive care from more than one therapist during this treatment episode? (1) Yes (2) No
33.	Are you still being treated by a therapist? (1) Yes (2) No
34.	Did your most recent course of care include: **(mark all that apply)**
35.	(1)Individual Therapy (2)Group Therapy (3)Family Therapy (4)Treatment with medication ==================>

A. Therapist's Name _____

B. Is there anything you especially want us to know about the care you received in the therapist's office or facility?

C. _____

D. Thank you for completing this survey and your interest in helping make our services even better.

For Office Use Only

© 1992 Response Technologies, Inc. East Greenwich, RI 02818

Source: Reprinted, with permission, from HCIA Response, copyright 1992.

FIGURE 2-5 Chart Audit Tool

MBC Massachusetts Chart Audit

There needs to be the appropriate directions for use here. What ID to mark, etc. This will depend upon how the form will be coded.

For this chart audit, use the following codes:
[1] for **Yes**
[2] for **No**
[3] for **Not Applicable**

For each item, determine if MBC Massachusetts services standards were met and within the appropriate time frame ...

Assessment Services

1.	**Initial Evaluation:** provided by senior licensed clinicians (includes participants, Hx, MSE, diagnostic & biosoc formu, prim/sec impair)
2.	**Psychiatric Evaluation:** provided within appropriate timeframe for biopsych assess, diagnostic clarification, treatment planning and psychopharm
3.	**Nursing Evaluation:** provided upon admission as needed
4.	**Psychosocial/Systems Assessment:** effort made to involve all avail signif others in assessment within appropriate timeframe
5.	**Biomedical Assessment:** physical/lab evaluation provided or arranged as needed for diagnostic clarificaton and biomed stabilization accord to stand
6.	**Other:** other assessments provided as needed for crisis eval and stabilization and to clarify differential diagnoses and formulate treatment plans
7.	**Treatment Planning and Implementation:** Development of primary and secondary objectives, timeframes, targeted service profile within timeframe
8.	**Care Coordination:** Documented attempts to contact and involve in treatment all current caregivers within timeframe according to standards
9.	**Care Coordination:** Senior consultation sought and provided to current caregivers in situations involving treatment failure, impasse, or ext high risk
10.	**Treatment Services Biomedical:** provided directly or via consultation as needed for crisis stabilization or treatment of active medical problems
11.	**Psychiatric:** treatment and/or consultation provided as needed to address biopsychiatric problems
12.	**Nursing:** monitoring and/or nursing management provided as needed to address biopsychiatric problems
13.	**Individual Psychotherapy/Case Management:** provided by licensed clinicians within appropriate timeframes and frequencies
14.	**Family/Systems Therapy:** provided by licensed clinicians within appropriate timeframes and frequencies
15.	**Group Psychotherapy:** provided within appropriate timeframes and frequencies
16.	**Discharge/Transition Service:** planning and implementation; pts meet with continuing care providers; active recruitment of community support
17.	**Is Risk Assessment Present?** [1] for Yes [2] for No
18.	**Safety and Liability Review: was there appropriate ...** Red flag procedures

© 1992 Response Technologies, Inc. East Greenwich, RI 02818

24   CHAPTER 2   USING PERFORMANCE MEASUREMENT AS A QUALITY IMPROVEMENT TOOL

FIGURE 2-5 *Continued*

For this chart audit, use the following codes:
[1] for **Yes**
[2] for **No**
[3] for **Not Applicable**

19. Supervisory/Mandatory Referral/Producures
20. Scheduling
21. Referral for psychiatric/medical evaluation/treatment
22. Intensity/frequency of treatment and level of care
23. Medication(s) prescribed with associated lab tests
24. Master treatment plan completed
25. Request for prior clinical records
26. Differential diagnosis considered
27. Diagnosis supported by clinical information
28.
29.
30.
31.
32.
33.
34.
35.

© 1992 Response Technologies, Inc. East Greenwich, RI 02818

Source: Reprinted, with permission, from HCIA Response, copyright 1992.

Data analysis issues were also considered at this juncture in the project. For example, data collection systems for gathering patient demographics (for example, patient sex and age) had to be designed. The eventual performance "report cards" would need to be adjusted to account for differences in the facilities' patient mixes and available levels of care.

Provider Input

A task force was convened and met regularly for 5 weeks to design the measurement processes. It comprised MBC project leaders and representatives from the facilities who were participating in the pilot project. The group identified data collection methods that would be easy to administer at the provider level and would allow for timely transfer of data to MBC. Several important measurement processes were established:

- To ensure confidentiality of satisfaction survey responses, patients are provided with a envelope in which they seal their completed survey.
- A log (figure 2-6) was designed for providers' use in tracking and reporting administration of the BASIS-32 questionnaire and the distribution of satisfaction surveys. Providers are also encouraged to use the form to document any difficulties encountered in survey administration as well as patient inability or refusal to participate.
- A chart audit process was established in which MBC case managers make appointments with each provider site to review up to 30 charts in a 4-hour period. Providers agree to have the charts ready when the case manager arrives for the appointment. At the completion of the audit the case manager leaves a copy of the review form with the clinicians to further their awareness of the audit criteria.
- A letter was developed by the task group and distributed to provider staff outlining the objectives of the performance management project and the performance measurements to be included in the pilot phase. The letter was signed by both MBC and facility leadership. Each provider agreed to discuss the project at staff meetings prior to the project start date.
- An MBC hot line was established to enable providers' staff to phone with questions regarding data collection, questionnaire administration, and so on.
- A patient information sheet (figure 2-7) was developed for distribution by the providers to all patients asked to participate in the project.
- All data-gathering tools (BASIS-32, patient satisfaction survey, chart audit tool) were designed as scannable forms using technology available from HCIA Response Technologies.[29] HCIA Response is capable of printing the BASIS-32 and other chosen measurement tools onto scannable forms that are completed by paper and pencil and then scanned into the database. Because only some providers chose to purchase scanners, MBC assumed the responsibility of scanning forms from all project participants.

Measurement Procedure

The flowchart in figure 2-8 outlines the major steps of the performance measurement process used for the pilot project:

1. MBC sends each provider a packet containing BASIS-32 forms, provider log sheets, and patient satisfaction surveys. The BASIS-32 and patient satisfaction forms are all prestamped with the provider's system identification number for ease of identification and data entry on their return to MBC.

FIGURE 2-6 Provider Log

MBC Performance Management Pilot Program Log

Site: _____ Site#: _____ Date Sent to MBC: _____ Follow-up sent _____

ID#		For Intensive Treatment providers only:		Readmit Information (circle one) No prior Treatment		
Last Name		1-30 days	31-60 days	61-90 days	91-365 days	365+ days
First Name		*Please Indicate all levels of care provided (circle):*				
DOB		*Outpatient: Indiv. Group Family Couple Psychopharm*				
Primary Therapist		*Intensive: Inpatient Partial/Day Subacute Resid. IOP*				
Initial Basis 32 Date (within 24 hrs)	DATE:	Session #				
Second Basis 32 Date (before 5th visit or Discharge)	DATE:	Session #				
Patient Satisfaction Survey Date	DATE:	Session #				
Refused Survey	Initial	Second	Notes:			
Drop out	AMA	Eloped	Notes:			
Unable to administer (Clinical Reason)	Sub. Abuse Other:	Psychosis	Notes:			
Unable to administer (Administrative reason)	I forgot Snow day	Dog ate it Other	Notes:			

Notes: _____

Send on Fridays to MBC, attach the full sheet Basis 32 or Patient Satisfaction

Readmit = to an intensive level of care with any provider

Drop out = more than 30 days from last missed scheduled appointment with no reschedule.

Intensive Levels of Care Providers have 24 hours to administer initial Basis 32 (IOP"s and PHP's may administer at the next session). When discharged, patient must complete before leaving care. Patients moving from intensive levels of care to outpatient will complete two sets of surveys.

Outpatient providers must administer initial Basis 32 before or during the first session. Second Basis 32 and Patient Satisfaction must be before the 5th session. (Please *mark the session number [completed] next to the administration date*)

PLEASE VERIFY THE ID# BEFORE SENDING TO MBC -- CALL 800-753-8827 IF QUESTIONS (Ask for Meg Anzalone, Ph.D. or Jim Kimberly, LCSW)

White Copy = Initial copy after 1st Basis 32   Yellow Copy = Final Copy after 2nd Basis 32   Pink Copy = Provider File Copy

Source: Reprinted, with permission, from Merit Behavioral Care Corporation.

FIGURE 2-7 Patient Information Sheet

MBC Provider Performance Management Program
Patient Information Sheet

You are being asked to participate in a joint project with your treatment provider and your managed care company in which certain information will be collected about your care and your satisfaction during your treatment. This project will be used to measure overall treatment with your provider and will be used to enhance and improve services. In some instances, your treatment provider is also conducting satisfaction studies. We appreciate your help and participation in working to improve the quality of care for all. Participation in this pilot program is completely voluntary. *Your care and treatment will not be affected in any way if you decline or accept participation.*

You will be asked to describe the symptoms which brought you into treatment. If you are in an intensive level of care, you will be asked again at the time of discharge to describe your symptoms and complete a satisfaction survey, sealing it in a self-addressed envelope. If you are in outpatient treatment, you will be asked to complete these forms again at the beginning of the 5th session or at discharge from treatment, whichever comes first. These instruments are easily completed in a few minutes.

Your information is confidential and will be protected like other confidential medical records. You will **not** be able to be identified from the information contained in any report.

Although not all questions will be applicable to you and your situation, please answer them to the best of your ability.

For further information or help in answering your questions, please speak with your provider.

MBC manages the use of your mental health benefit offered by Blue Cross Blue Shield of Massachusetts.

Source: Reprinted, with permission, from Merit Behavioral Care Corporation.

---

2. The providers are responsible for administering the BASIS-32 to each new patient at the time of admission or by the second outpatient session. For all new patients, the providers enter patient data on the provider log and answer the last question on the BASIS-32 form.

3. All patients receiving intensive treatment (inpatient or structured acute outpatient) are given the BASIS-32 again at discharge along with the patient satisfaction survey. For patients receiving routine outpatient treatment, the BASIS-32 is administered again just before the fifth session or the last session, whichever comes first. The patient satisfaction survey is also given at this time.

4. Patients completing the satisfaction survey are asked to seal it in an envelope to protect confidentiality.

5. Each week providers mail to MBC all completed BASIS-32 forms and patient satisfaction surveys along with their updated provider logs.

After data collection began in January 1995, MBC maintained regular contact with participating providers. This communication was helpful in resolving unforeseen data collection problems. Performance measurement processes were refined as the pilot progressed. Because MBC was not able to anticipate all of the operational concerns of the line staff responsible for survey administration and data collection, the hot line proved to be an important communication tool between MBC and providers.

TRANSFORM DATA INTO INFORMATION

Providers viewed the calculation and feedback of patients' BASIS-32 scores as one of the most important aspects of the MBC performance management system. It was MBC's goal to provide real-time feedback of patient-specific BASIS-32 scores to individual facilities. It anticipated that these scores would be communicated to providers within a day or two of questionnaire completion for inpatients and within a week for outpatients. The intent was to have the results available to caregivers for treatment-

FIGURE 2-8 Provider Performance Measurement Process

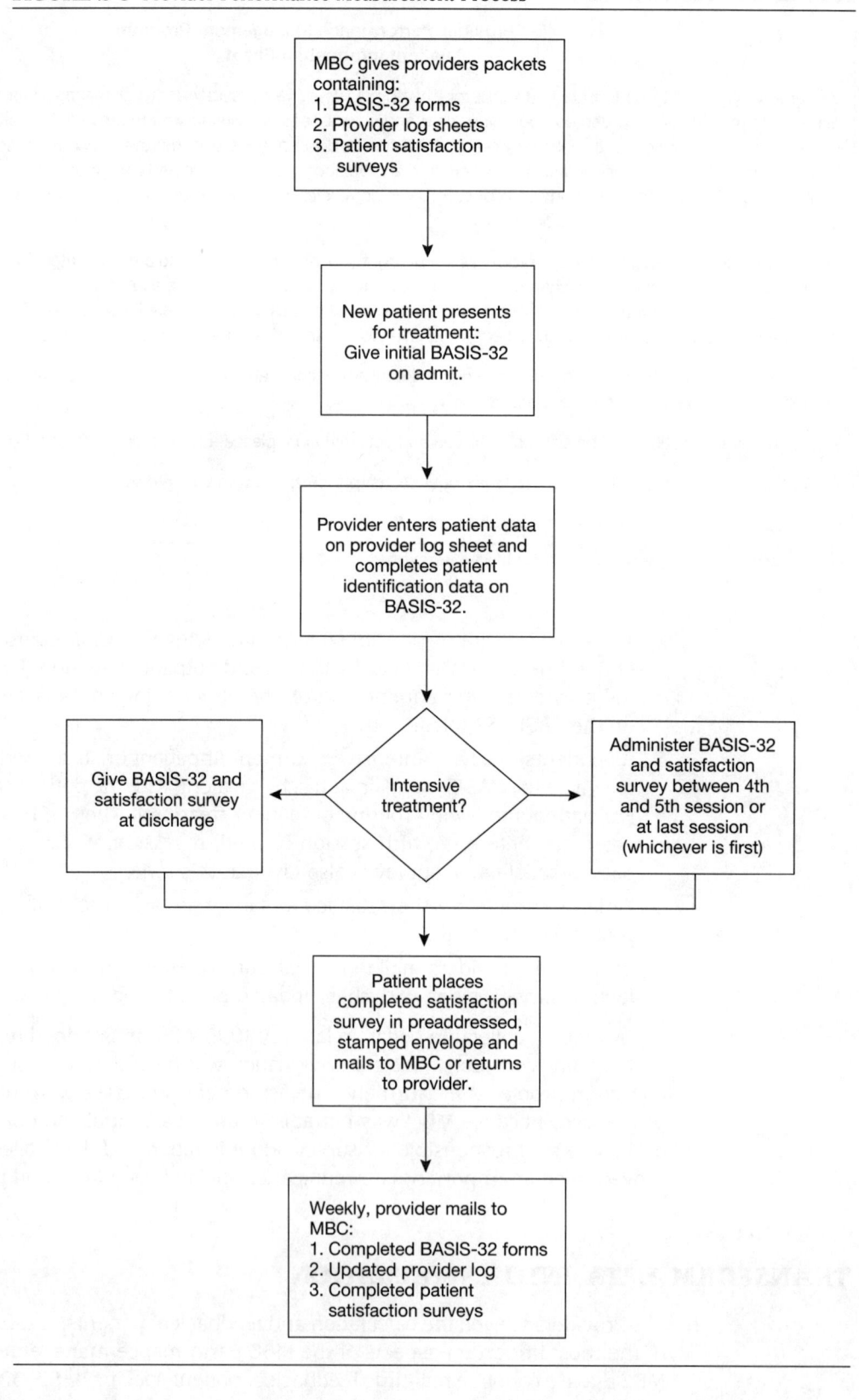

```
┌─────────────────────────┐
│ MBC gives providers     │
│ packets containing:     │
│ 1. BASIS-32 forms       │
│ 2. Provider log sheets  │
│ 3. Patient satisfaction │
│    surveys              │
└───────────┬─────────────┘
            ▼
┌─────────────────────────┐
│ New patient presents    │
│ for treatment:          │
│ Give initial BASIS-32   │
│ on admit.               │
└───────────┬─────────────┘
            ▼
┌─────────────────────────┐
│ Provider enters patient │
│ data on provider log    │
│ sheet and completes     │
│ patient identification  │
│ data on BASIS-32.       │
└───────────┬─────────────┘
            ▼
                    ◇ Intensive treatment? ◇
        ┌───────────┘           └───────────┐
        ▼                                   ▼
┌──────────────────┐              ┌──────────────────────┐
│ Give BASIS-32    │              │ Administer BASIS-32  │
│ and satisfaction │              │ and satisfaction     │
│ survey at        │              │ survey between 4th   │
│ discharge        │              │ and 5th session or   │
│                  │              │ at last session      │
│                  │              │ (whichever is first) │
└────────┬─────────┘              └──────────┬───────────┘
         └──────────────┬──────────────────────┘
                        ▼
┌──────────────────────────────┐
│ Patient places completed     │
│ satisfaction survey in       │
│ preaddressed, stamped        │
│ envelope and mails to MBC    │
│ or returns to provider.      │
└──────────────┬───────────────┘
               ▼
┌──────────────────────────────┐
│ Weekly, provider mails to    │
│ MBC:                         │
│ 1. Completed BASIS-32 forms  │
│ 2. Updated provider log      │
│ 3. Completed patient         │
│    satisfaction surveys      │
└──────────────────────────────┘
```

FIGURE 2-9 Sample Aggregate Performance Report for One Provider Facility

Report Date:	8/15/96		
Report Range:	From: 1/1/96	To: 6/31/96	
Facility/Site:	Facility 3		
Site Type:	Intensive Treatment		

Performance Dimension		Network Average	Facility Average
Utilization			
	Average days or sessions per patient	4.37	5.73
	Standard deviation	5.18	
Patient Satisfaction			
	Aggregate average score	81.49	75.22
	Standard deviation	13.04	
	Compliance	26%	
Chart Audit			
	Aggregate average scores	82.94	82.47
	Standard deviation	13.49	
Clinical Outcome			
	Initial BASIS-32 aggregate average score	1.53	2.94
	Change in BASIS-32 aggregate average score (higher indicates greater change)	−0.60	−0.28
	Standard deviation of change	1.00	
	Follow-up compliance	41%	

Note: Fictitious data for presentation purposes only.

planning purposes. However, unanticipated difficulties with the HCIA Response software and its compatibility with the MBC information system made this goal impossible to achieve early on.

Aggregate performance analysis required the design of a performance management information system. From May through December 1995, MBC worked with HCIA Response to design an information system that would support the production of aggregate performance measurement data. HCIA Response's Starting Line™ database was configured to include fields for all data elements in the BASIS-32, the chart audit, and the satisfaction survey and all utilization data. The first three components would be input from the scannable forms; utilization data would be downloaded from the MBC claims database.

Once the Starting Line™ database was configured, information from the scannable forms and the MBC claims database was entered into the system. The first performance measurement report was produced for the study time period of January 1 to June 1, 1996. A sample of this report is shown in figure 2-9. The information contained in the report allowed MBC to compare each facility's performance with the network average.

A ranking system that MBC had previously defined for its outpatient provider performance project was used to assess performance. This ranking system was developed and refined during 1995 and 1996 by the corporate provider-profiling task force. In the interest of consistency, the MBC Massachusetts medical director and the quality

TABLE 2-3 Performance Management Profile Ranking Categories and Criteria

Category	Criteria
Exceptional achievement in a performance dimension	1. Performance within 1 standard deviation of network norm for utilization 2. Score above 30th percentile 3. Meets MBC credentialing criteria
Prime	1. Exceptional performance in a minimum of three out of the four performance dimensions 2. Meets MBC credentialing criteria
Preferred	1. Exceptional performance in a minimum of two out of the four performance dimensions 2. Meets MBC credentialing criteria
Participating	1. Provider participates in data collection for a minimum of two out of the four performance dimensions 2. Meets MBC credentialing criteria

director who participated in these task force discussions agreed to adopt this profiling ranking system for the pilot project.

The goal of facility profiling is to furnish feedback to providers about their performance relative to the network as a whole. MBC wished to acknowledge in developing this system that all network providers maintain credentials accepted among their peers as qualifying them to practice behavioral health care within their discipline. Provider performance measurement is a systematic assessment of patterns in the delivery of health care in which the focus is on patterns of care within two contexts:

1. Facility performance as compared with a network aggregate of similar practitioners or, where available, an acknowledged standard of care
2. Facility performance as compared with the provider or facility's own practice patterns

Facilities that fell within 1/2 standard deviation of the network average for utilization or within 1/4 standard deviation of the mean in any of the other performance dimensions were considered to meet standards in that dimension. Facilities were also categorized as prime, preferred, or participating, according to the ranking criteria shown in table 2-3. In addition, the provider's compliance with MBC credentialing criteria was required for all categories. Three ranking categories were considered necessary to differentiate facilities. Facilities are provided their own ranking as compared with the network aggregate for their use in internal quality improvement initiatives.

Noncompliance reports (figure 2-10) are also produced to identify reasons that survey tools are not administered to patients. These reports help MBC and its providers to continually improve the survey administration process.

As of this writing, MBC is in the final stages of the data analysis and report phase. It is working on constructing rank reports for each performance dimension and detailed reports for each measurement tool. These reports will show network and facility averages for each item on each tool as well as averages on each performance dimension. Once completed, the information will be used to optimize the quality improvement system. MBC will collaborate with providers to identify improvement opportunities, design action plans for improvement, and evaluate the results of action plans. As previously mentioned, MBC has no intention of using the data to blackball individual caregivers or facilities. Providers will use the patient-specific and aggregate comparison data to examine their systems and processes and determine quality improvement actions. By moving away from the micromanagement of individual cases and focusing

FIGURE 2-10 Noncompliance Report

Report Range:		From: 1/1/96 To: 12/31/96		Report Date: December 18, 1996
Site Name	No. Episodes of Care	No. Surveys Unable to Administer	Noncompliance, %	Reason:
Facility 1	6	1	16.67	1 - Patient no-show for appointment
Facility 2	57	80	35.09	8 - Reason not available 1 - "Dog ate survey tool" 8 - Patient forgot 1 - Human error 1 - Patient not offered survey 1 - Other
Facility 3	38	1	2.63	1 - Patient forgot to complete first BASIS-32
Facility 4	2	1	50.00	1 - Patient forgot
Facility 5	20	4	20.00	2 - Paperwork not given to patient 1 - Patient forgot 1 - Staff did not administer second BASIS-32

on systems data, network providers will have complete ownership of their own quality processes.

CONCLUSION

Successful managed care initiatives must balance financial and clinical quality outcomes. In this environment networkwide performance management systems have become increasingly important. In 1995 the Massachusetts Division of Merit Behavioral Care began to develop a performance management system to gather reliable performance data across four health care dimensions: clinical outcomes, utilization, technical performance, and patient satisfaction.

Rather than develop new measurement tools, MBC chose already validated or widely tested process and outcome behavioral health measures. MBC service standards were incorporated into the chart audit criteria, the BASIS-32 served as foundation for clinical outcome measurements, and the MBC Corporate Patient Satisfaction Survey was used to gather satisfaction data.

Performance measurements from the pilot project were formatted into provider "report cards." These measurements were statistically analyzed, and criteria were developed to rate providers as *prime, preferred,* or *participating.* The assumptions underlying the performance ratings will continue to be analyzed for statistical significance and adjusted accordingly as the project progresses.

The pilot performance measurement project is only the first step in MBC's performance management initiative. Still to be resolved are issues related to differing population norms based on initial patient illness severity scores and other demographic scores. The MBC chart audit tool will likely need further refinement as MBC continues to align the criteria with its service standards.

Lessons Learned

Provider participation was the most important component in the success of the performance measurement project. Facility input regarding data collection procedures was invaluable in creating a user-friendly system. Providers helped draft the communications that went out to facility staff, the people ultimately responsible for data collection. Providers also helped draft the notice given to patients who were being asked to participate in the process at a vulnerable and difficult time in their lives. Insightful recommendations from providers helped MBC create practical systems, including:

- Methods to assure patients of the confidentiality of their responses
- Techniques for securing wholehearted participation and meaningful feedback from facility staff
- Simple methods for facilities to use for logging and tracking data collection activities

Unfortunately, formal provider input was limited to 5 weeks of the implementation phase of the performance management system. Instead of creating a short-lived implementation task group, continued regular meetings would have been useful throughout the entire pilot phase. A consumer focus group also would have been valuable for gathering information about consumers' experiences in completing the BASIS-32 and patient satisfaction survey. This feedback could have been used to improve the process and the satisfaction tool.

One of the biggest project challenges was the information system component. Although MBC purchased a predesigned database product, the software had to be modified to produce reports of aggregate data for each facility. These difficulties were compounded by the usual internal waiting list for information system support and by software operation problems. Hindsight suggests that a more realistic budget for information system support would have been extremely useful, as would the expectation that ironing out difficulties would take much longer than anticipated. It also would have been helpful if MBC had realized that even the best proprietary software system is likely to need modifications to enable interfaces with existing corporate software and hardware systems.

A workable performance management system requires sound and practical measurement tools, reliable processes for data collection, and a database for analysis and reporting. The ideal performance management database would include the following elements:

- A relational database architecture that allows for coordination and integration of information from multiple files
- Ease of programming for novice computer users
- Capability to run on a network
- Capacity to upload and download information easily from other database platforms
- Ability to generate facility-wide and patient-specific performance measurement reports

Sufficient financial resources must be allocated for data collection, analysis, and reporting. Without these resources the Check component of the performance improvement process (table 2-1) is not possible. The human resources necessary for a successful performance management system include in-house managed care organization performance measurement expertise and adequate staff dedicated to data tracking, collection, analysis, and reporting. The managed care organization staff also needs to spend a considerable amount of time at provider sites to assist with office staff education and support two-way communication opportunities.

Next Steps

The three next steps for the MBC provider performance management system will be to:

1. Expand the pilot project to encompass all facilities in Massachusetts
2. Work with providers to improve compliance with performance standards and with measurement processes
3. Implement fax and fax-back systems for real-time data collection and feedback of patients' BASIS-32 scores

In addition to provider-related improvements, MBC will be conducting patient focus groups to gather customers' suggestions for improving the performance management system.

Summary

The pilot project described in this chapter has helped focus MBC Massachusetts and its providers on the importance of performance measurement as a performance management tool. Rather than design clinical paths or guidelines to micromanage health care processes, MBC and its providers strongly believe that valid and reliable performance management strategies, such as performance measurements, will enhance the clinician's decision-making ability. As Donald Berwick suggests, "All learners need some form of measurement."[30] It is MBC's hope that its performance management system will play an important role in advancing the art and science of behavioral health care in the state of Massachusetts.

References

1. Schyve, P. M. Outcomes as performance measures. In: *Using Clinical Practice Guidelines to Evaluate Quality of Care,* vol. 1, *Issues.* Rockville, MD: U.S. Department of Public Health and Human Services, Public Health Service, Agency for Health Care Policy and Research, Mar. 1995.
2. Eisen, S. V., Dill, D. L., and Grob, M. C. Reliability and validity of a brief patient-instrument for psychiatric outcome evaluation. *Hospital and Community Psychiatry* 45(3):242–47, 1994.
3. Walton, M. *The Deming Management Method.* New York City: Dodd, Mead, 1986.
4. Quoted in Spath, P. L., *AIMing for Quality Results: An Improvement Primer for Healthcare Organizations.* Forest Grove, OR: Brown-Spath and Associates, 1994.
5. Conte, H., Ratto, R., Clutz, K., and others. Determinants of outpatients' satisfaction with therapists: relation to outcome. *Journal of Psychotherapy Practice and Research* 4(1):43–51, winter 1995.
6. Spath, P. L. The evolution of medical effectiveness and outcomes management initiatives. In: P. Spath, editor. *Medical Effectiveness and Outcomes Management: Issues, Methods and Case Studies.* Chicago: American Hospital Publishing, 1996, pp. 3–7.
7. Vibbert, S., editor. *The 1996 Behavioral Outcomes and Guidelines Sourcebook.* New York City: Faulkner and Gray's Healthcare Information Center, 1995, p. A16.
8. Rubin, H. M. D. Patient evaluations of hospital care: a review of the literature. *Medical Care* 28 (suppl. to no. 9):S3–S10, 1990.
9. Beck, A. T. *Beck Depression Inventory Manual.* Revised edition. San Antonio, TX: Psychological Corporation, 1987.
10. Parikh, R. M., Eden, D. T., Price, T. R., and Robinson, R. G. The sensitivity and specificity of the Center for Epidemiologic Studies Depression Scale in screening for post-stroke depression. *International Journal of Psychiatry and Medicine* 18(2):169–81, 1988.
11. Ware, J. E., Kosinski, M. L., and Keller, S. D. *SF-36 Physical and Mental Component Summary Measures: A User's Manual.* Boston: The Health Institute, New England Medical Center, 1994.

12. Bilodeau, A. InterMountain offers a new psych assessment tool. *Clinical Data Management* 1(5):5, 1994.
13. Deroghis, L. R., and Melisaratos, N. The Brief Symptom Inventory: an introductory report. *Psychological Medicine* 13:595–605, 1983.
14. Eisen, Dill, and Grob.
15. Goldman, H. H., Skodol, A. E., and Lave, T. R. Revising Axis V for DSM-IV: a review of measures of social functioning. *American Journal of Psychiatry* 149(9):1148–56, Sept. 1992.
16. Further information is available from Hal Mark at Psych Sentinel, Department of Community Medicine, University of Connecticut Medical School, Farmington, CT 06030-1910; (203) 679-3276.
17. Bigelo, B., and Berthot, B. The Psychiatric Symptom Assessment Scale (PSAS). *Psychopharmacology Bulletin* 25(2):168–79, 1989.
18. MacLellan, A. T., Luborsky, L., Woody, G. E., and others. An improved diagnostic evaluation instrument for substance abuse patients: the Addiction Severity Index. *Journal of Nervous and Mental Disorders* 168:26–33, 1980.
19. Health Outcomes Institute. *User's Manual: Depression TyPE Specification.* Bloomington, MN: Health Outcomes Institute, 1994.
20. Joint Commission on Accreditation of Healthcare Organizations. *Forms, Charts, and Other Tools for Performance Improvement.* Oakbrook Terrace, IL: JCAHO, 1994, pp. 83–103.
21. Palmer, R. H., and Banks, N. J. Designing and testing medical review criteria and performance measures. In: *Using Clinical Practice Guidelines to Evaluate Quality of Care,* vol. 2, *Methods.* Rockville, MD: U.S. Department of Public Health and Human Services, Public Health Service, Agency for Health Care Policy and Research, 1995, pp. 53–54.
22. International Society for the Study of Dissociation. *Guidelines for Treating Dissociative Identity Disorder in Adults.* Skokie, IL: ISSD, 1994.
23. Tenne, A. R., and DeToro, I. J. *Total Quality Management: Three Steps to Continuous Improvement.* Reading, MA: Addison-Wesley, 1992, p. 84.
24. Rubiu.
25. Kibbee, P. Considerations for the survey process. In: *Quality Management in Ambulatory Care.* Chicago: American Hospital Publishing, 1992, p. 156.
26. Ware, J. E., and Hays, R. D. Methods for measuring patient satisfaction with specific medical encounters. *Medical Care* 26(4): 393–402, Apr. 1988.
27. Lambert, M. Conceptualizing and selecting measures of treatment outcome: Implications for drug abuse outcome studies. In: L. S. Onken, editor. *Psychotherapy and Counseling in the Treatment of Drug Abuse.* Rockville, MD: National Institute on Drug Abuse, 1990.
28. Eisen, Dill, and Grob.
29. Further information may be obtained directly from HCAI Response Technologies, 1485 South County Trail, East Greenwich, RI 02818; (800) 522-1440.
30. Berwick, D. M. A primer on leading the improvement of systems. Presented at the First Annual European Forum on Quality Improvement in Health Care, London, Mar. 9, 1996.

CHAPTER 3

Improving Outpatient Care with Clinical Practice Guidelines

Gail O'Mahaney VanZyl and Gary Goby

FirstCare Health (FCH), a physician-driven integrated health network formed in 1992, comprises a 45-member primary care medical group (FirstCare Physicians) and Albany General Hospital (AGH), a 68-bed, acute care hospital. The network serves a population of 125,000 people living in and around Albany, OR, which is located 40 miles north of Eugene in the mid-Willamette valley. Outpatient care in the community health network is provided by family practice, internal medicine, pediatrics, and OB-GYN primary care medical practices located in nine clinics. Other outpatient services include home health, urgent care, outpatient surgery, and hospice care. Inpatient services include critical care, general medical and surgical acute care, dialysis, labor and delivery, nursery, level 3 trauma emergency services, and pediatrics.

FCH was formed to enable the hospital and primary care physicians to bid for fully capitated health plan contracts. Concurrent with the organization of FCH, the state of Oregon was introducing the Oregon Health Plan, a capitated reimbursement insurance program for poverty-level residents. In addition, several commercial health plans were offering full-risk-sharing capitated products to local employers and seniors.

To survive successfully as a health care network, FCH had to deliver the right patient care at the right time and create a structure that could respond to the accreditation requirements of the National Committee for Quality Assurance (NCQA). These demands required the hospital staff and primary care physicians to change the way they had traditionally done business. To support its partners during this time of change, FCH had to enact a strategy that would allow professional and personal growth. For this reason the development and implementation of clinical practice guidelines (CPGs) became a high-priority initiative. This chapter describes the quality-focused environment that lays the groundwork for all improvement initiatives within FCH, the process of CPG design and implementation, and the lessons learned from the guideline experience.

WHY CLINICAL PRACTICE GUIDELINES?

Clinical practice guidelines are systematically developed statements designed to assist practitioner and patient decisions about appropriate health care for specific clinical circumstances.[1] CPGs tend to focus on those aspects of diagnosis and treatment for which evidence is required.[2] Research is an important first step in guideline development, whereas clinical pathways include many intervention recommendations that are not evidence based. Consequently, FCH chose CPGs as the foundation of its continuous quality improvement (CQI) efforts.

The development and implementation of CPGs within the integrated health network was influenced by two factors:

1. Desire to reduce costs and maintain quality
2. Need to measure and improve important aspects of patient care delivery

FCH realized that financial success in a managed care environment could only be achieved if providers delivered cost-efficient, clinically effective care to all health plan participants. The success of these managed care endeavors depended on the appropriate use of diagnostic and therapeutic resources (testing, treatment, specialist referrals, surgery, and drugs) and the control of high-cost services (emergency care and inpatient stays). Because primary care providers direct the use of these resources, those providers choosing less effective treatment strategies can increase costs unnecessarily. By persuading physicians and other caregivers to follow the most efficient practices, measuring the results, and informing the clinicians of those results, FCH hoped to reduce variation in care and produce better outcomes.

Another factor impacting guideline development at FCH was the accreditation standards of the NCQA. Many of the commercial health plans associated with FCH were pursuing NCQA accreditation and therefore had to measure and improve important aspects of service, such as patient access, preventive health interventions, medical record documentation, patient satisfaction, and resource utilization. FCH had not routinely measured these aspects of care, nor had providers enacted community-wide improvement efforts. CPGs were viewed as a solution, for they could provide a framework for performance measurement and ultimately enhance patient care outcomes.

THE QUALITY-FOCUSED ENVIRONMENT

The FCH organization is distinctly quality oriented, as evidenced by its ongoing commitment to CQI. Starting in 1990, the entire hospital staff (from the chief executive officer to the housekeepers) was trained in the key concepts of CQI, modeled after the teachings of Joseph Juran[3] and W. Edwards Deming.[4] The core principles of the CQI philosophy at AGH include fact-based decision making, teamwork, systems thinking, and customer awareness. By 1991 the hospital staff had successfully institutionalized the concepts of CQI in the clinical services and administrative areas.

The Dawn of Managed Care

As the era of managed care neared, hospital leaders were well prepared to use CQI tools to assist in the planning and formation of an integrated health care organization.[5] Thirty-six local primary care providers joined the newly formed FirstCare Physicians organization in 1992. The new focus on primary care and the alliance with FirstCare Physicians brought many changes to AGH. The governing board and chief executive

FIGURE 3-1 Clinical Practice Guideline Development Process Applied to the Shewhart Cycle

"Drilldown" analysis of outcomes or significant variation

Measure variation in achieving predetermined outcome measurements (clinical, cost, functional)

ACT — CHECK — PLAN — DO

Identify an opportunity to improve practice

Gather a team of key stakeholders and experts

Conduct research; identify benchmark if available

Define expected outcomes in clinical, cost, and fuctional outcomes

Develop draft gain feedback from users

Implement guideline via educational program and handout materials

Note: The cycle has been modified to reflect the time commitment of each component in the cycle; the plan component is by far the most important and time consuming of the overall process.

officer agreed that FCH had to be a physician-driven organization, so strategic planning and operations were modified to achieve this vision. Collaboration between the hospital and the primary care clinics became the focus of many of the CQI efforts.

The hospital's CQI training efforts had occurred prior to the formation of FirstCare Physicians; therefore, the medical groups did not receive formal CQI education. However, leaders agreed that CQI teams would receive "just in time" training in CQI tools and techniques throughout the life of each project.

The Clinical Practice Guideline Initiative

To kick off the CPG initiative, an operational definition of "clinical practice guideline" was formulated. Rather than create a unique definition, FCH chose to adopt Harvard Community Health Plan's definition: "A (clinical practice guideline) sets forth a stepwise procedure for making decisions about the diagnosis and treatment of clinical problems."[6]

This definition influenced the decision to use clinical algorithms for presenting the CPGs. *Clinical algorithms* are written guides to stepwise evaluation and management strategies that include:

- Explicit descriptions of an ordered sequence of steps to be taken in patient care under specific circumstances
- Required observations to be made
- Decisions to be considered
- Actions to be taken

A CPG development model was drafted based on the hospital's CQI process. This relationship was not widely advertised because it was feared that physicians might be uncomfortable using a hospital-based method for office practice process improvements. The key components of guideline development and implementation were outlined according to the plan-do-check-act cycle. (See figure 3-1.) The model for creating guidelines formulated by the Agency for Health Care Policy and Research was considered in defining the steps in the plan phase.[7]

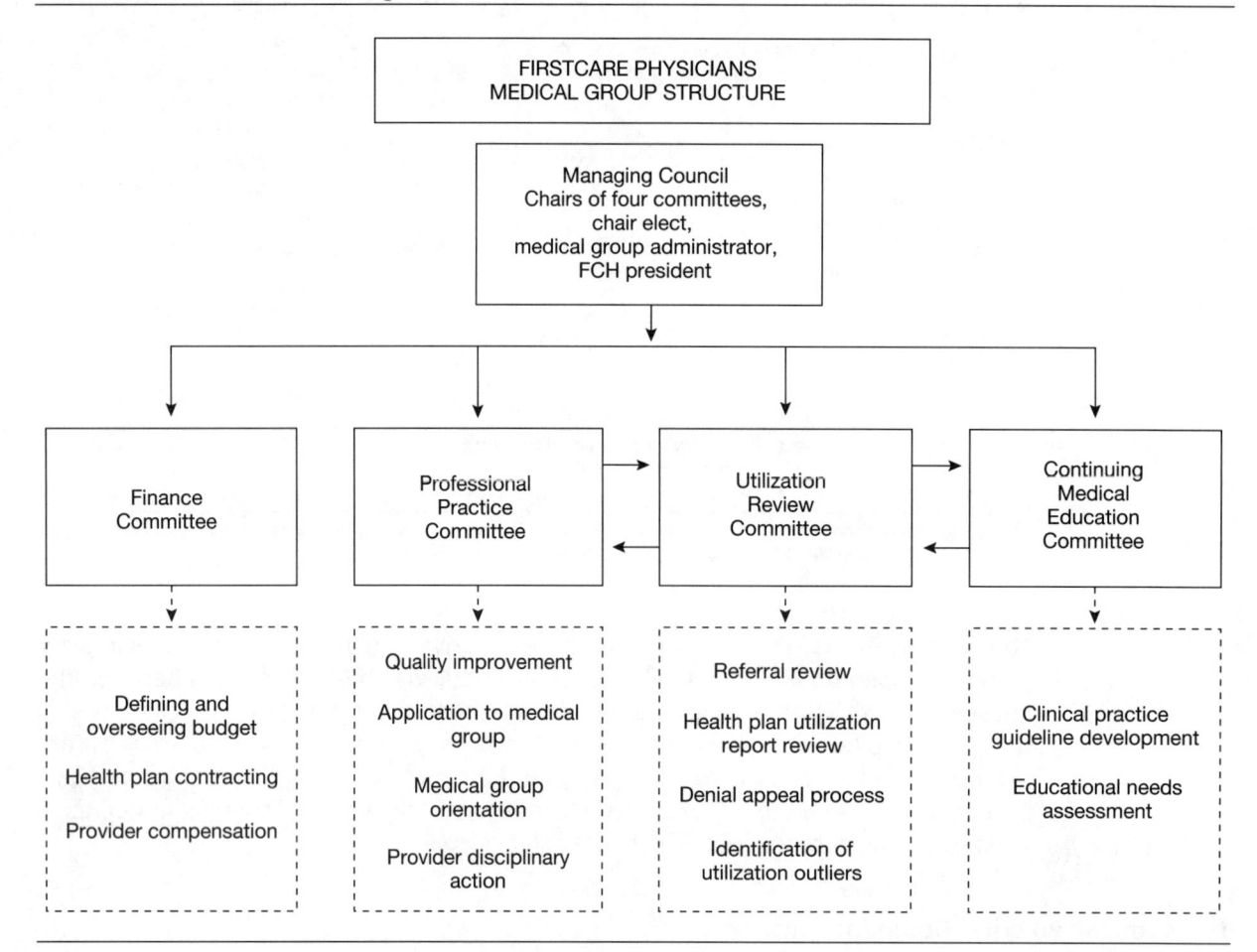

FIGURE 3-2 FirstCare Health Organizational Structure, 1993

```
                    FIRSTCARE PHYSICIANS
                    MEDICAL GROUP STRUCTURE

                         Managing Council
                    Chairs of four committees,
                           chair elect,
                    medical group administrator,
                          FCH president

      ┌──────────────┬──────────────┬──────────────┐
      ▼              ▼              ▼              ▼
   Finance      Professional    Utilization     Continuing
  Committee       Practice        Review          Medical
                 Committee      Committee        Education
                                                 Committee
```

Finance Committee	Professional Practice Committee	Utilization Review Committee	Continuing Medical Education Committee
Defining and overseeing budget	Quality improvement	Referral review	Clinical practice guideline development
Health plan contracting	Application to medical group	Health plan utilization report review	Educational needs assessment
Provider compensation	Medical group orientation	Denial appeal process	
	Provider disciplinary action	Identification of utilization outliers	

ISSUES THAT STYMIED THE FIRST CLINICAL PRACTICE GUIDELINE EFFORT

In 1993 FCH began its CPG development initiative. The initial motivation came from the need to control the cost of care. However, these first efforts were less than successful for a variety of reasons. An ineffective organizational structure based on traditional peer review thinking and a lack of appreciation of the financial incentives of capitated reimbursement caused FCH to rethink its original CPG initiative.

Organizational Structure Based on Traditional Peer Review

The original organizational structure (figure 3-2) of FCH consisted of four committees that reported to the medical staff executive committee, called the "managing council." Members of these committees were almost exclusively medical staff members, with the exception of the medical group administrator and the quality management resource person. An important drawback to this structure was the lack of clear responsibility for CPG development. All of the committees in the initial structure had monitoring and reporting responsibilities, but none were specifically charged with developing CPGs to improve patient care processes. Two barriers needed to be overcome to resolve this problem:

1. For years the medical staff peer review had used the "bad apples" approach reported by Donald Berwick, MD, in his landmark *New England Journal of Medicine* editorial of 1989.[8] The historical purpose of peer review was to find outliers and inform these physicians of their outlier status, on the assumption that the individual providers would then seek education or set a benchmark with peers to improve their own practice. There were two inherent problems with this philosophy.
   — Because the physician was viewed as the cause of process variation, little attention was paid to the significant variation within the health care system itself.
   — It was assumed that the outlier physicians recognized their contribution to process variation. However, most physicians reacted to the "bad apple" approach by defending their practices and casting blame on other providers or at the delivery system. This response threw peer review committees into a whirlpool of finger pointing rather than promoting patient care improvements.
2. Physicians practicing at AGH, like most physicians, took substantial pride in their patient management skills. They viewed CPGs as a slap in the face, a suggestion that "you're not good enough, and that's why guidelines are needed." In addition, the current health care environment was so filled with financial and operational change that the imposition of a personal change in practice was not welcomed by the physicians.

These two key issues forced FCH to recognize that significant medical staff leadership was necessary to support CPG development. CPGs had to be seen as an important mechanism for improving quality of care and reducing costs, rather than as a threat to physician autonomy. Aware that changing physicians' personal practice would not be easy, FCH set out to identify "champion physicians" who were respected in their peer communities. These champions were found within the medical-group-based committees. Educational resources were committed to these champions, although one basic program sponsored by the Institute for Healthcare Quality Improvement was enough to train and energize them.[9]

Focus on Outpatient Care

Another hindrance to early CPG development efforts was the decision to focus on decreasing hospital costs rather than improving primary care services. The first initiatives were directed at high-cost, high-volume, or high-risk diagnoses for hospitalized patients, such as chronic obstructive pulmonary disease and congestive heart failure (CHF).

The first CPG development effort had been directed at improving inpatient care for patients with CHF. After a work group was formed to develop the CHF guideline, it was realized that this decision had many drawbacks:

- Patients with CHF are not a homogeneous group. They have many comorbidities and other contributing factors that influence treatment decisions.
- Practice variations are often caused by patient diversities, not necessarily inappropriate treatment choices.

The work group members were not able to define clearly the patient population to whom the CPG guideline would apply, nor could they agree on one treatment regimen. The CHF project was shelved after three unproductive meetings when it became evident that, although a basic standard of practice for inpatient CHF management existed in the community, variations in diagnosis and treatment were too complex to study adequately.

Managed Care Learning Curve

Another drawback to selecting inpatient diagnoses for CPG development was that the medical group did not initially see the value of reducing hospital expenditures because they did not yet perceive themselves as an integrated health care organization. This reaction was largely due to the managed care learning curve: it takes time for independent physicians to recognize that their success in a capitated reimbursement environment is greatly influenced by their ability to manage costs throughout the continuum of care. The physicians had not yet recognized that controlling expensive hospital costs could benefit their reimbursement. This reality was the opposite of physicians' traditional financial incentives, which rewarded them for more office visits.

Rather than try to overcome this learning deficit quickly, FCH leaders chose to refocus their CPG efforts on outpatient services. During the turbulent times of change it was easier for physicians to focus on their comfort zone: their office practice.

These issues overwhelmed the first CPG design efforts. As a result FCH reevaluated its start-up decisions.

THE REDESIGNED GUIDELINE DEVELOPMENT PROCESS

In 1995 FCH began its second and *renewed* CPG design and implementation process. The first step was to redesign the FCH organizational structure and redefine the committee functions. (See figure 3-3.) Included in this process was a clear understanding that any or all of the committees could identify the need for a CPG. An ad hoc committee of local experts would develop the draft CPG. The professional practice committee would be the oversight committee responsible for ensuring that the key components of care were addressed by the CPG. The original continuing medical education committee was dissolved due to lack of participation, and a single physician, identified as the quality champion, was given the authority to facilitate CPG development at the ad hoc committee level.

The new CPG development process focused on high-volume primary care diagnoses. The goal was to gain the physicians' confidence in CPGs as a helpful, nonthreatening tool for fairly nonchallenging diagnoses. Once this support was garnered the CPG initiative could then be expanded to more complex and costly conditions.

Selection of Outpatient Clinical Practice Guideline Topics

The managing council charged the professional practice and utilization review committees with reexamining the CPG initiative from an office-based viewpoint. The committees recognized that if outpatient management could be stabilized and outcomes improved, FCH would reap the benefits of reduced office visits and improved access to the already congested primary care practices.

With an outpatient focus in mind, the financial database was accessed to identify high-volume outpatient clinic diagnoses. The professional practice and utilization review committees jointly recommended starting with three CPG topics:

1. Acute sinusitis
2. Acute pharyngitis-tonsillitis
3. Otitis media

The managing council approved the recommendation and began to form ad hoc teams to develop CPGs for these diagnoses. The acute pharyngitis-tonsillitis team, the first group formed, consisted of two local otolaryngologists who agreed to participate,

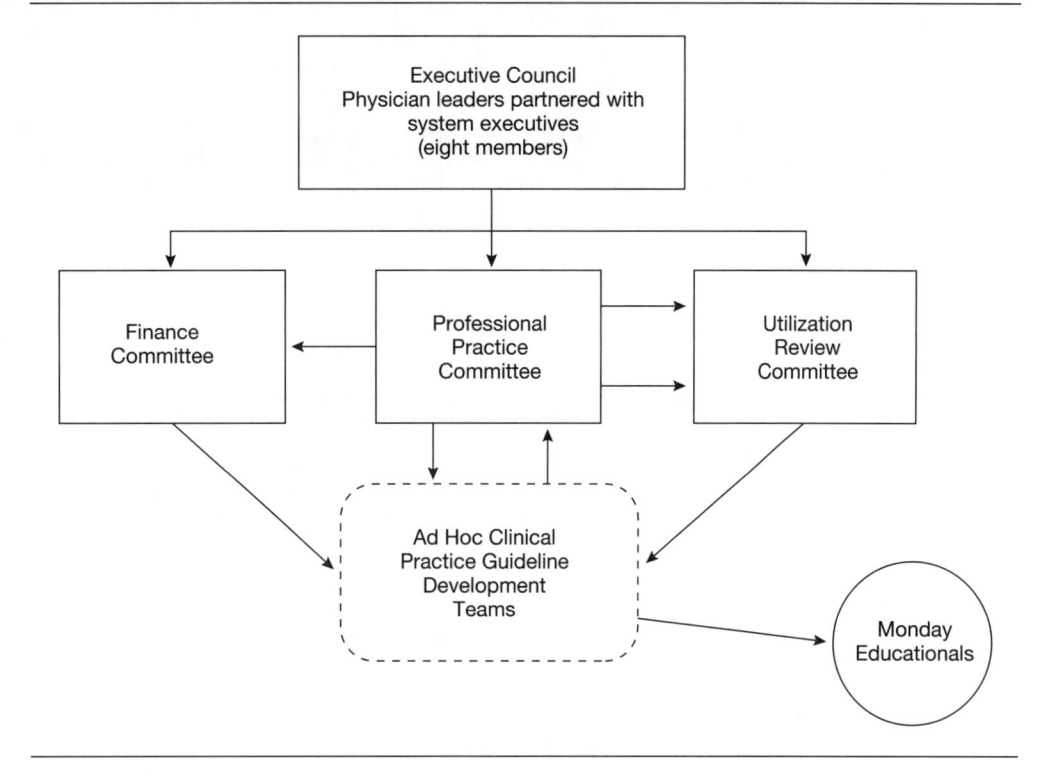

FIGURE 3-3 FirstCare Health Organizational Structure, 1995

```
                    Executive Council
                Physician leaders partnered with
                      system executives
                       (eight members)
       ┌───────────────────┬───────────────────┐
       ▼                   ▼                   ▼
   Finance            Professional         Utilization
  Committee   ◄────    Practice    ────►     Review
              ────►   Committee    ◄────   Committee
       │                   │                   │
       │                   ▼                   │
       │           Ad Hoc Clinical             │
       └─────►     Practice Guideline    ◄─────┘
                    Development
                       Teams
                         │
                         ▼
                      Monday
                    Educationals
```

two family practice physicians, one internal medicine physician, and one pediatrician. Consistent with the organization's quality improvement plan, the team was given a 100-day time line for completion of the project.

A literature search was conducted to identify recently published studies on the topic of pharyngitis-tonsillitis. The ad hoc team looked specifically for studies containing enough patients that the researchers had come to statistically significant conclusions. In addition, the availability of nationally developed, evidence-based guidelines was researched. Local and regional providers were asked whether they had developed CPGs for acute pharyngitis-tonsillitis.

The research findings were reviewed by the "quality champion" physician, who evaluated the evidence underlying the practice recommendations. Those articles and resources considered valid and reliable served as the basis for developing the first draft of FCH's pharyngitis-tonsillitis CPG. This draft CPG and the associated research articles on which it was based were distributed to all ad hoc team members for their review and approval. Minimal changes were recommended by the membership of the ad hoc team.

Clinical Practice Guideline Presentation Format

Guideline presentation is an important component of the development process. Those organizations that have operationalized CPGs successfully have designed tools that clearly state the treatment recommendations and the patient population to whom the recommendations apply.[10] When FCH physicians were asked what would gain their cooperation in using CPGs, their overwhelming response was that the CPGs must be quick to read, easy to access, and as specific as possible.

To meet these needs FCH chose to display its CPGs in a clinical algorithm format. A *clinical algorithm* is a set of rules for solving a problem in a finite number of steps.

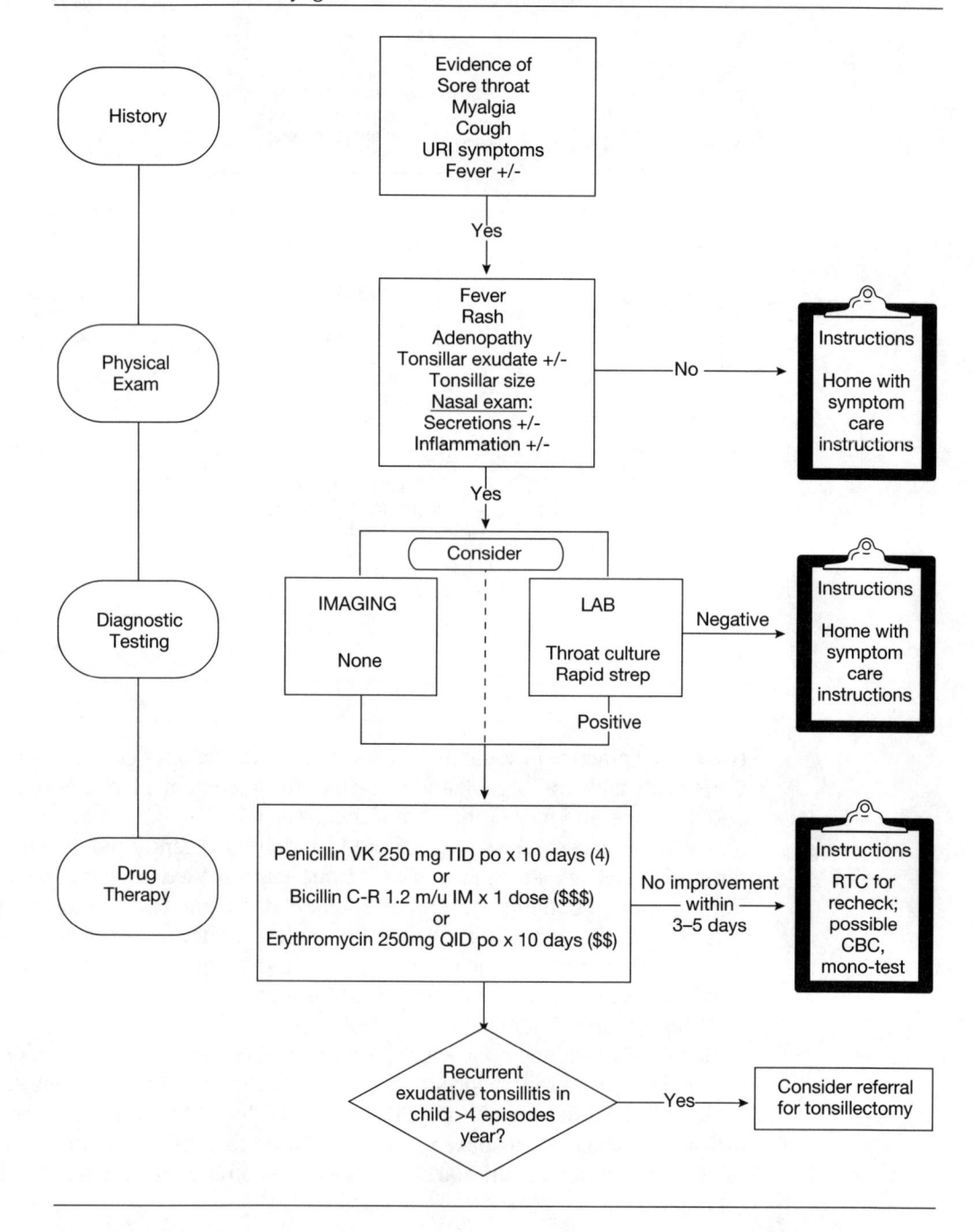

FIGURE 3-4 Acute Pharyngitis-Tonsillitis Clinical Practice Guideline

```
History ──► Evidence of
            Sore throat
            Myalgia
            Cough
            URI symptoms
            Fever +/-
                │
               Yes
                ▼
Physical ──► Fever
Exam         Rash
             Adenopathy
             Tonsillar exudate +/-
             Tonsillar size           ──No──► Instructions
             Nasal exam:                       Home with
             Secretions +/-                    symptom care
             Inflammation +/-                  instructions
                │
               Yes
                ▼
             Consider
Diagnostic   ┌─────────┬─────────┐
Testing ──► IMAGING    LAB        ──Negative──► Instructions
            None       Throat culture            Home with
                       Rapid strep               symptom care
                           │                     instructions
                        Positive
                           ▼
Drug ──► Penicillin VK 250 mg TID po x 10 days (4)
Therapy    or
         Bicillin C-R 1.2 m/u IM x 1 dose ($$$)    ──No improvement──► Instructions
           or                                        within 3-5 days    RTC for recheck;
         Erythromycin 250mg QID po x 10 days ($$)                        possible CBC,
                │                                                        mono-test
                ▼
         Recurrent
         exudative tonsillitis in  ──Yes──► Consider referral
         child >4 episodes                  for tonsillectomy
         year?
```

It diagrams a CPG into a step-by-step decision tree.[11] The acute pharyngitis-tonsillitis CPG is illustrated in figure 3-4.

Next the guideline needed to be reproduced in a medium that could be readily accessed by outpatient caregivers. The ideal medium would be electronic; however, computerized patient records are a goal for the future, not today's reality. Therefore, another presentation tool had to be designed. After reviewing several possible display instruments, the professional practice committee decided to print the CPGs on laminated 7-by-9-inch card stock and provide clinics with three-ring binders for storing all the guidelines. This provider resource manual is made available to all primary care providers, the emergency room, and the local community health clinic.

GUIDELINE DISSEMINATION

Securing conformance to guidelines is not an easy task. As Haines and Feder suggest, "Writing them is easier than making them work."[12] To encourage caregivers to adopt CPGs, FCH returned to its core philosophy: Guidelines are an educational tool and a guide to effective clinical management. Existing mechanisms for professional education were used to operationalize the first CPG. The development team recommended that the acute pharyngitis-tonsillitis CPG be presented as part of the "Monday educationals," a weekly medical-staff-sponsored program that helps physicians earn their continuing medical education credits locally. By presenting the guideline at this regularly held educational program, FCH reinforced the idea that CPGs are educational, not punitive.

The CPG work group recommended that a local ENT specialist and a primary care physician jointly conduct the educational session that focused on the effective treatment of acute pharyngitis-tonsillitis. During the session the presenting physicians discussed theory, physiology, treatment, and evaluation. To summarize the concepts program attendees received a copy of the CPG at the end of the session. However, following the wisdom of David M. Eddy, MD, the guideline was offered as "advice," not as an order.[13] This model for educating physicians has proved successful, and the Monday educationals continue to be used to familiarize caregivers with new CPGs.

Because the goal of CPGs was to reduce variation in the system of patient care, physicians' office staff needed education also. This education was provided either by videotaping the educational presentation made to the physicians or by repeating the presentation at an office staff meeting. Ideally, physicians and their office staff would attend the Monday educationals together; however, these sessions are so well attended by physicians that there is not enough space for additional participants.

MINIMIZING GUIDELINE LIABILITY CONCERNS

Investigations have shown that CPGs are used nearly equally in defending and prosecuting medical malpractice cases.[14] To minimize the threat of increased liability related to CPGs, risk management and recordkeeping are important factors in deployment. The following recommendations for reducing liability concerns, suggested by the FCH risk management department, are enforced during CPG development and implementation:

- The organization-wide purpose and role of CPGs are defined in a clearly worded policy statement to the effect that CPG recommendations are considered advisory and are not intended to create a standard of care. CPGs may be modified based on an individual patient's need.
- A bibliography of all resources used in the development of each CPG is maintained. This includes literature sources, benchmarking data, and names of individuals who contributed recommendations.
- In the development of guidelines, terminology and phrasing are used that emphasize their advisory nature. Alternative treatment options are also stated. Whenever possible, the guideline is written in specific terms because research has suggested that vague guideline statements are unlikely to influence provider behavior.[15]
- The CPG development team verifies that the CPG recommendations are based on evidence, not personal preferences. Guidelines developed by medical professional organizations are used as the keystone when evaluating local practices. Variations from nationally developed guidelines are investigated as possible local quality-of-care concerns.

- Effective data for each guideline, and for subsequent updates, are clearly noted on the guideline.
- A schedule for regular review and updating of distributed guidelines is established. At FCH, CPGs are formally reviewed by the professional practice committee at least every 3 years.
- Archival copies of each CPG and revision, including the date of each revision, are maintained for at least 7 years. Pediatric guidelines are stored indefinitely.

MEASURING VARIATION

During CPG development each ad hoc team defines expected clinical, cost, and functional outcomes as part of the plan step of the development process. These expected outcomes are measured prior to CPG development and deployment to provide a baseline from which improvements are measured. For example the pharyngitis-tonsillitis CPG recommends that the patient's history include documentation of five elements: sore throat, myalgia, cough, upper respiratory symptoms, and presence or absence of fever. A study was conducted to determine if at least three of these five elements were present in patients' clinic records. The percentage of records in compliance with this measure steadily increased after the pharyngitis-tonsillitis CPG was implemented. (See figure 3-5.)

The most challenging outcome data to collect are functional and health status measurement data. Functional status measurement systems assess the patient's physical, mental, and social functioning. More than 100 measures of functional and health status now exist.[16] Prior to the CPG initiative, FCH had already chosen to use the SF-36, a 36-item questionnaire that measures nine health concepts: physical function; role function, physical; bodily pain; general health; vitality; social function; role func-

FIGURE 3-5 Acute Pharyngitis-Tonsillitis Clinical Outcome Measurement

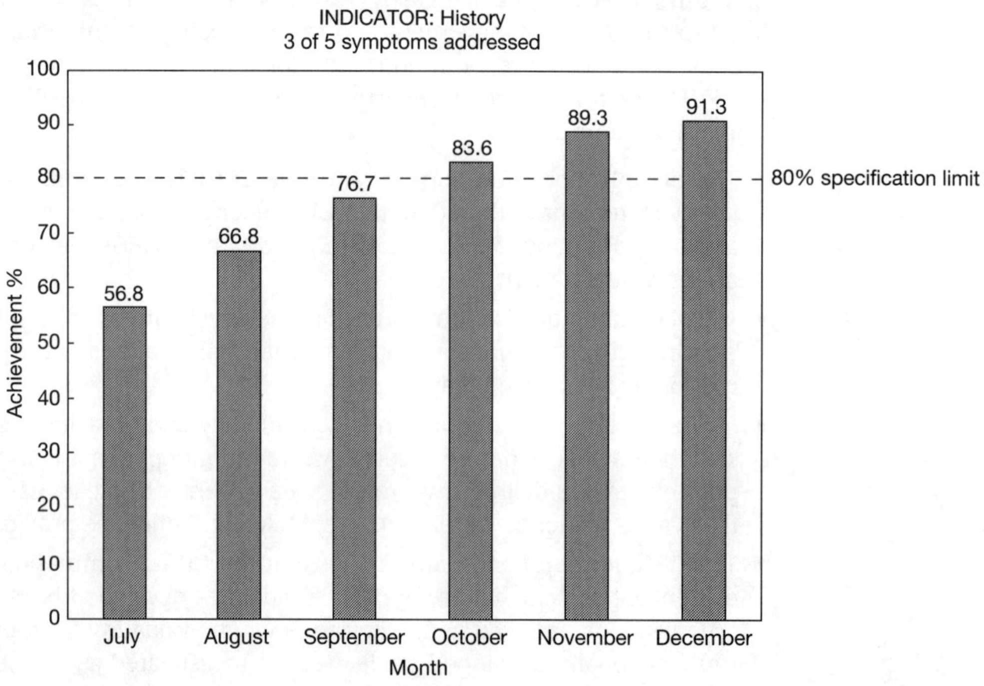

INDICATOR: History
3 of 5 symptoms addressed

Month	Achievement %
July	56.8
August	66.8
September	76.7
October	83.6
November	89.3
December	91.3

80% specification limit

FIGURE 3-6 FirstCare Health Organizational Performance Improvement Report Elements, 1997

Base Data
- Inpatient admissions
- Average hospital length of stay
- Number of surgical procedures by month (inpatient and outpatient)

Clinical Measures
- Incidence of cardiac or respiratory arrests
- Hospital readmission rate
- Hospital complication rate
- Wound infection rate
- C-section rate
- Incidence of C-section decision to incision time of 30 minutes or less
- Mortality rate
- Average door to needle time for thrombolytic therapy
- Clinical practice guideline measures
  - Clinical outcomes
  - Patient satisfaction with service
  - Long-term patient functional status

Financial Measures
- Operating margin
- Receivable days
- Number of delinquent medical records

Customer Satisfaction Measures
- Patient satisfaction survey results
- Incidence of patient falls
- Incidence of medication errors

Risk Management Measures
- Number of pending claims
- Incidence of patient falls
- Compliance with COBRA regulations

tion, emotional; mental health; and reported health transition.[17] Plans are under way to administer the SF-36 to CPG patient populations. The information gleaned from this functional status measurement methodology will be used to determine whether long-term patient outcomes vary by service provider.

REPORTING GUIDELINE PERFORMANCE MEASUREMENT DATA

Although the CPG program is just getting off the ground, there are plans to incorporate the CPG deployment and measurement process into FCH organization-wide performance improvement reports. These reports include measures of clinical, cost, and patent satisfaction outcomes. (See figure 3-6.) The specificity of reports ranges from very detailed at the departmental level to a broader report of measurement results at the governance level. The measurements chosen for reporting are based on the organization's strategic and operational plan as well as key clinical initiatives, such as the CPG development and implementation process. FCH uses the "dashboard" format as its report model.[18]

The CPG initiative provides a new framework for collecting performance measurement data to report to network leadership and the governing board, the groups responsible for overseeing the quality of care received by health care delivery system customers. The guideline design and implementation model is easily understood by laypersons:

- Define the most effective process for providing care to a patient with a specific disease
- Measure how well caregivers are doing it

Measurement of variation and outcomes related to a specific CPG provides leadership with fact-based performance improvement reports. As shown in figure 3-6, CPG-related measures will eventually be included as a subcategory of the "clinical" component of the dashboard report. The entire detailed CPG development process, starting with topic identification and ending with CPG revisions based on outcome measures, is shown in figure 3-7.

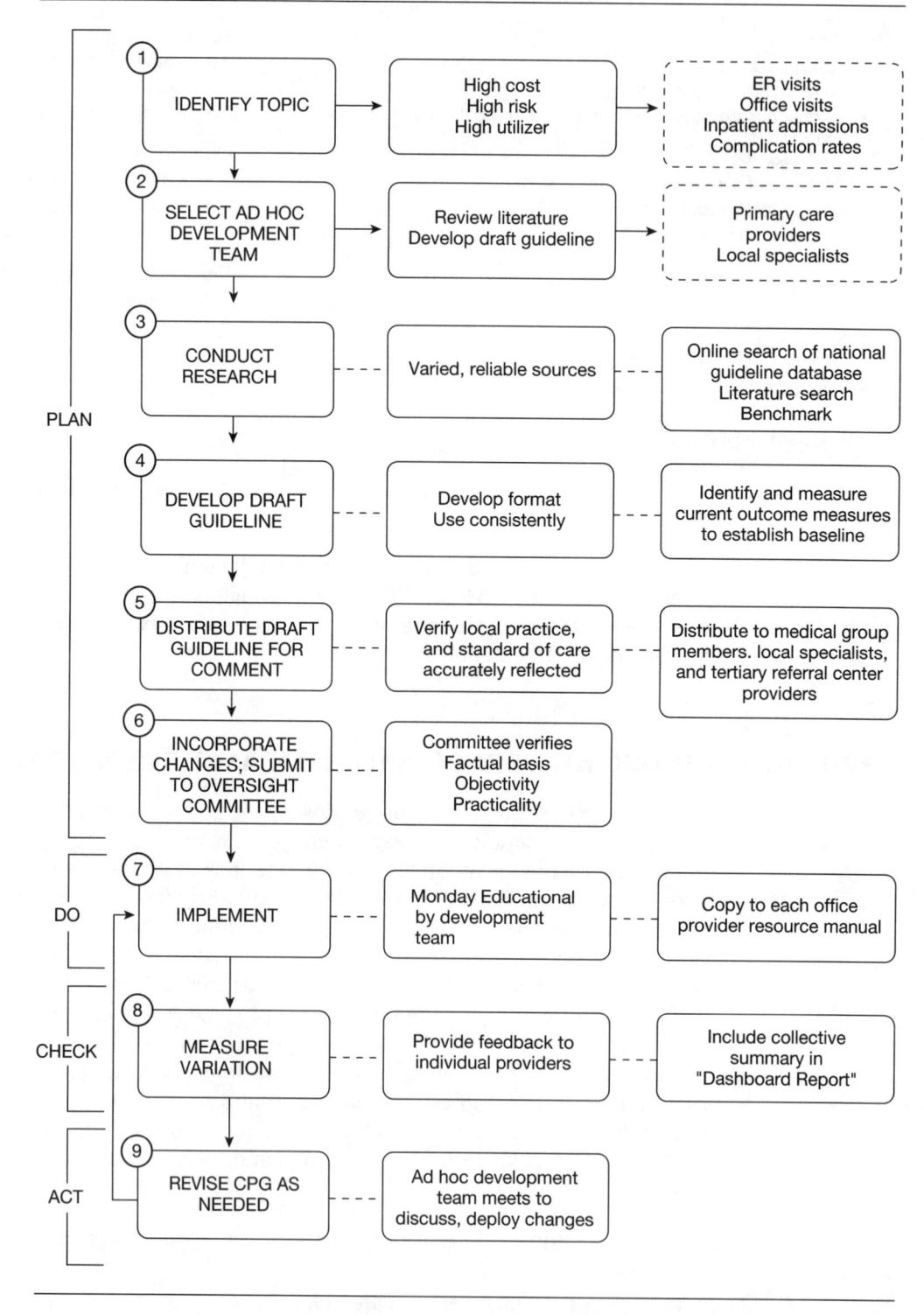

FIGURE 3-7 Clinical Practice Guideline Development Process

```
PLAN
  1. IDENTIFY TOPIC → High cost / High risk / High utilizer → ER visits / Office visits / Inpatient admissions / Complication rates
  2. SELECT AD HOC DEVELOPMENT TEAM → Review literature / Develop draft guideline → Primary care providers / Local specialists
  3. CONDUCT RESEARCH --- Varied, reliable sources --- Online search of national guideline database / Literature search / Benchmark
  4. DEVELOP DRAFT GUIDELINE --- Develop format / Use consistently --- Identify and measure current outcome measures to establish baseline
  5. DISTRIBUTE DRAFT GUIDELINE FOR COMMENT --- Verify local practice, and standard of care accurately reflected --- Distribute to medical group members, local specialists, and tertiary referral center providers
  6. INCORPORATE CHANGES; SUBMIT TO OVERSIGHT COMMITTEE --- Committee verifies Factual basis / Objectivity / Practicality

DO
  7. IMPLEMENT --- Monday Educational by development team --- Copy to each office provider resource manual

CHECK
  8. MEASURE VARIATION --- Provide feedback to individual providers --- Include collective summary in "Dashboard Report"

ACT
  9. REVISE CPG AS NEEDED --- Ad hoc development team meets to discuss, deploy changes
```

CONCLUSION

FirstCare Health has been pursuing its CPG initiative for 3 years. During this short time caregivers and administrative leaders have overcome significant hurdles and improved on the design and implementation process. Significant realizations are listed below.

Lessons Learned

- *CPGs are an outcomes improvement tool.* Do not use CPGs for utilization review or provider credentialing purposes, at least in the early phases of the project. Demonstrate this commitment by only involving the quality improvement committee in the CPG design and implementation process. If CPGs will eventually be used to detect performance problems, wait until the CPGs are widely accepted by practitioners and measurement data are established as reliable and valid.

- *CPGs were welcomed by borderline providers, but were insulting to exceptional providers.* FCH's primary reason for implementing CPGs was to reduce variation causing both overutilization and underutilization. Borderline providers are represented at both ends of this spectrum. CPGs help these providers reduce their variation and improve the overall quality of care provided by the network. To address the concerns expressed by exceptional providers, the importance of CPGs in improving the network's aggregate performance should be emphasized.

- *Application of CPGs to practice should be a matter of choice.* Physicians are fact based and research oriented in their education and usually welcome the provision of fact-based research to improve their own practice. A few providers have disregarded the CPGs published thus far by FCH, although most providers have expressed appreciation and requested additional copies. The goal of the FCH CPG initiative was to provide CPGs as a service, not a mandate, to providers. Like many organizations, FCH has chosen to make participation voluntary.[19]

- *Keep a local focus.* Physicians have confidence in guidelines that they or their peers take part in developing or that are developed by their professional organization. Therefore, guidelines adopted by a consensus of local physicians are more likely to be accepted.[20] Externally derived CPGs are a valuable benchmark; however, it is important to demonstrate a commitment to local focus by developing and using your own format.

- *Keep it simple.* Start CPG development with simple, clinic-based diagnosis topics (for example, a high-volume diagnosis such as pharyngitis) rather than hospital-based or high-cost cases. By starting with uncomplicated topics you will gain experience in the development process and encourage use of the CPG. FCH found that when it chose uncomplicated outpatient diagnoses for CPG development, the work group process went smoothly. The successes of the first projects improved everyone's confidence, making CPG development for more complex, high-cost diagnoses much easier.

- *Involve the specialists.* Although many patient conditions are managed by primary care physicians, it is important to involve specialists in the CPG development process. Specialists should help in formulating CPG recommendations and provide input in defining clinical situations in which a specialty referral is appropriate. For example, the clinical situation in which pediatric patients should be referred for myringotomy is clearly illustrated in the otitis media CPG (figure 3-8). By involving specialists, the FCH primary care group realized another benefit: the specialists learned about the expertise of family medicine and internal medicine practitioners. Most important, the collaboration that occurred with CPG development helped restore primary care—specialist relationships that had been disrupted during the formation of the network. The CPG design process reminded all caregivers of the importance of maintaining a patient-focused attitude during times of change in the health care delivery system.

- *Determine your CPG investment-to-benefit ratio.* Ideally, the outcome improvements resulting from CPG design and implementation outweigh the resources allocated to

FIGURE 3-8 Serous Otitis in Pediatrics Clinical Practice Guidelines

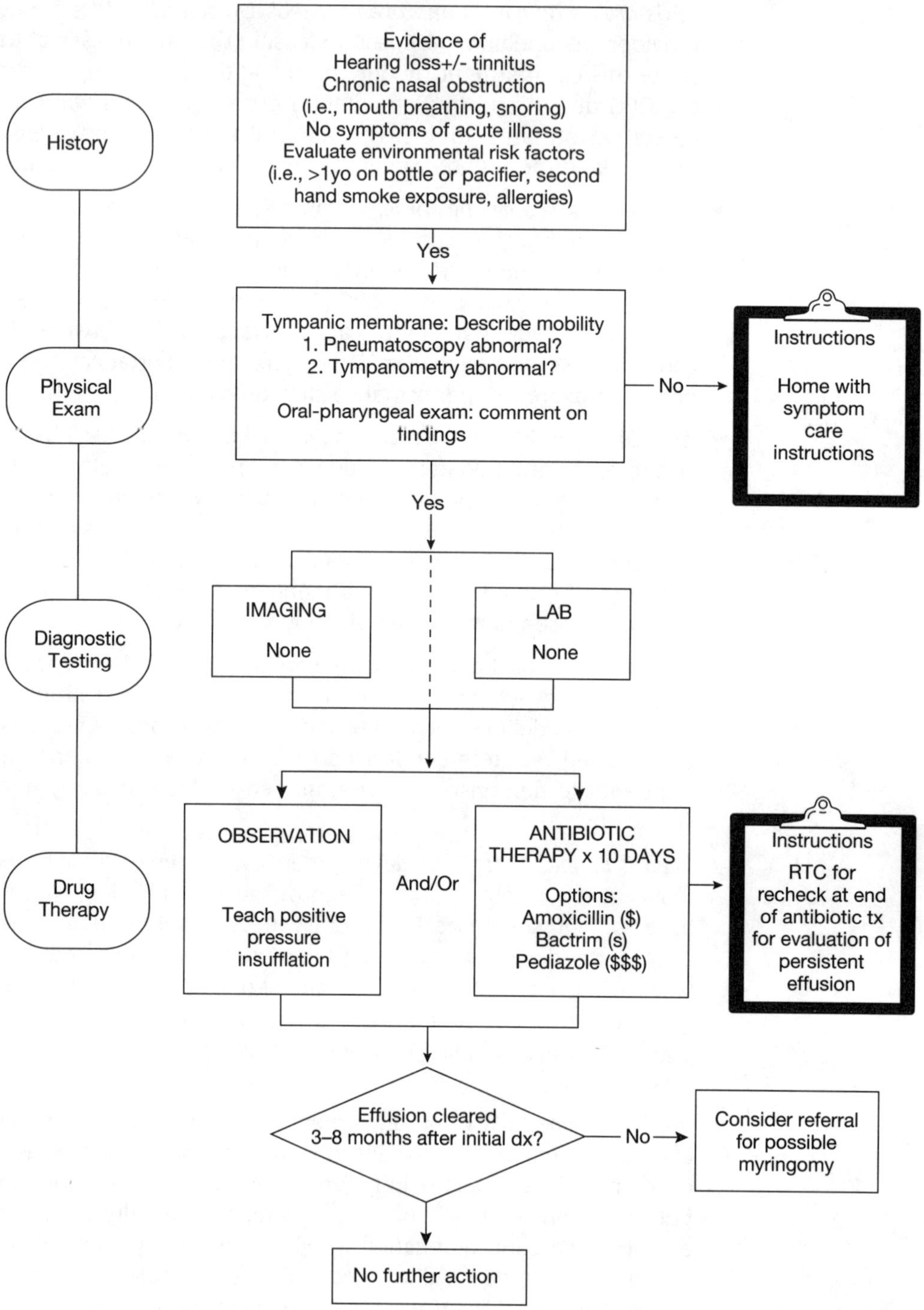

Note: Population is age group more than 6 weeks old.

the project. Because FCH has only begun to gather post–CPG implementation outcome data, this important ratio has yet to be determined.

- *Access to performance data may be restricted by the network's many nonintegrated databases.* As in many newly formed integrated health care delivery systems, FCH information systems are fragmented. The medical group has a separate information system from that of the hospital. Gathering data about treatments and outcomes across the spectrum of care is difficult and time consuming, although not impossible.

Once outcome measurement data elements are defined, the most efficient information sources must be identified. Whenever possible, use existing information systems to gain the information. When faced with nonintegrated databases, work with the individual system managers to define the data elements needed from their information systems. Once the data elements from the various systems are downloaded into a central database, the necessary reports can be produced. This type of electronic data collection is complex, so it may be more efficient to acquire information manually through patient record reviews. For example, the information necessary to evaluate compliance with the history component of the pharyngitis-tonsillitis CPG (figure 3-5) was manually abstracted from patient records at each of the nine physician offices. The data were then entered into a spreadsheet program using a laptop computer. While such manual data collection is costly, a much more costly choice would be to implement CPGs and never provide feedback to practitioners. Groups who have been successful at implementing guidelines stress the importance of providing caregivers with immediate feedback on their compliance.[21]

- *It is important to standardize performance measurement formulas.* Identify and consistently use a standard denominator whenever possible to convert subjective data to normative data. FCH uses the following formula for all performance measures:

    No. of positive results ÷ Study sample size × 100.

This formula yields a performance measure that indicates the rate of compliance per 100 visits, patients, and so on. Use of this standardized formula allows some normalization of data findings, although statistical significance depends on sample size. The formula is consistently used for performance measurement reporting to ensure that today's results will be comparable with tomorrow's study findings.

When making outcome data comparisons with other facilities, it will be important to standardize the operational definitions and methods of calculation so that data comparisons will be valid. This type of benchmarking data will become more available as regulatory agencies such as NCQA and the Joint Commission on Accreditation of Healthcare Organizations mandate the use of recognized databases.

Summary

Three years after starting the initial CPG development process, FCH's providers are committed to the concept of patient care improvement through variation reduction. The primary vehicle for accomplishing this task is the CPG, a constructive response to the changing health care reimbursement environment.

The network helps to keep all provider groups financially viable to ensure that the people in the Albany community can continue to have their health care needs met locally. CPGs reinforce this goal by ensuring effective and efficient health care services that improve the health of the community. FCH does not plan to develop CPGs for every diagnosis; however, it will continue to develop CPGs for high-volume, high-cost, or high-risk diagnoses that are believed to have an impact on community health. As of this writing, work groups are developing CPGs for the diagnosis of diabetes, perinatal care, and clinical preventive health. These more complex initiatives are made easier by the work groups' previous experience with simpler projects.

The final step in the CPG implementation model is about to be taken. Comprehensive data are being gathered about compliance with the pharyngitis-tonsillitis, sinusitis, and otitis media guidelines along with relevant outcome measures. Considerable practice variations in assessment, treatment, follow-up, and outcomes were discovered prior to the CPG development process. FCH is confident that post–CPG implementation data will show clinical effectiveness and patient satisfaction improvements, as well as cost reductions.

Although FCH is finally on the road to acceptance of CPGs by the medical group providers, considerable work lies ahead. The education of the governing body in the use of outcome measurement data and the acquisition of reliable performance measurement data remains. However, FCH leaders are encouraged that the attitude of providers toward CPGs has changed from threatened to appreciative. The organization's overriding goal is to become the community's health care choice. By providing clinically proven, standardized, and cost-effective mechanisms of patient care designed to meet community needs, FCH expects to achieve this goal.

References

1. Field, M. J., and Lohr, K. N., editors. *Clinical Practice Guidelines: Directions for a New Program.* Washington, DC: National Academy, 1990.
2. Woolf, S. H. *Interim Manual for Clinical Practice Guideline Development: A Protocol for Expert Panels Convened by the Office of the Forum for Quality and Effectiveness in Health Care* (publication no. AHCPR-91-19). Rockville, MD: U.S. Department of Pulbic Health and Human Services, Public Health Service, Agency for Health Care Policy and Research, 1991, p. 13.
3. Juran, J. M. *Juran on Leadership for Quality: An Executive Handbook.* New York City: Free Press, 1989.
4. Deming, W. E. *Out of the Crisis.* Cambridge, MA: Massachusetts Institute of Technology Center for Advanced Engineering Study, 1986.
5. For more information about the FCH strategic quality planning initiative, see Melvin, M., and Collett, C., editors. *Breakthrough Leadership: Achieving Organizational Alignment through Hoshin Planning.* Chicago: American Hospital Publishing, 1995, pp. 73–93.
6. Gottlieb, L., and others. Clinical practice guidelines at an HMO: development and implementation in a quality improvement model. *Quality Review Bulletin* 16(2):80, 1990.
7. U.S. Department of Public Health and Human Services, Public Health Service, Agency for Health Care Policy and Research. *Using Clinical Practice Guidelines to Evaluate Quality of Care.* Vol. 1, Issues. Rockville, MD: AHCPR, Mar. 1995, p. 6.
8. Berwick, D. M. Continuous improvement as an ideal in health care. *New England Journal of Medicine* 320:53–55, 1989.
9. For information about this programs call (617) 754-4800.
10. Hayward, R. S. A., and others. Implementing preventive care guidelines: information tools for the clinician. *Mayo Clinic Visit,* July 1992.
11. Spath, P. L. VHA looks at clinical practice guidelines, pathways, and algorithms. *Journal of the American Health Information Management Association* 67(6):44–46, 1996.
12. Haines, A., and Feder, G. Guidance on guidelines: writing them is easier than making them work. *British Medical Journal* 305:785–86, 1992.
13. Eddy, D. M. Three battles to watch in the 1990s. *JAMA* 270(4):520–26, 1993.
14. Hyams, A. L., Brandenburg, J. A., Lipsitz, S. R., and others. Practice guidelines and malpractice litigation: a two-way street. *Annals of Internal Medicine* 122(6):451–55, Mar. 1995.
15. McDonald, C. J., and Overhage, J. M. Guidelines you can follow and trust: an ideal and an example. *JAMA* 271(11):872–73, Mar. 16, 1994.
16. DeLuca, J. M., and Cagan, R. E. Controlling for patient variables in medical effectiveness/outcomes management studies. In: P. Spath, editor. *Medical Effectiveness and Outcomes Management: Issues, Methods, and Case Studies.* Chicago: American Hospital Publishing, 1996, pp. 35–37.
17. Ware, J. E., Snow, K. K., Kosinski, M., and others. *SF-36 Health Survey: Manual and Interpretation Guide.* Boston: Health Institute, New England Medical Center, 1993.

18. O'Rourke, L., and others. Principles for developing governance reports on quality and performance. *The Quality Letter* 6(3):2–28, 1993.
19. Reinertsen, J. L. Living guidelines. *Healthcare Forum Journal* 37(6):56–61, 1994.
20. U.S. Government Accounting Office. *Practice Guidelines: Managed Care Plans Customize Guidelines to Meet Local Interests* (publication no. GAO/HEHS-96-95). Washington, DC: USGAO. Letter report, May 30, 1996.
21. Veterans Health Administration Quality Management Institute and Education Center's Clinical Practice Guideline Panel. *Clinical Decision Making Aids: Clinical Practice Guidelines/Clinical Pathways/Clinical Algorithms, Version 1*. Durham, NC: Department of Veterans Affairs, Veterans Health Administration. Unpublished report, Aug. 1995.

CHAPTER 4

Reducing Practice Variation in Open Heart Surgeries

Mary Lu Gerke

Lutheran Hospital in LaCrosse, WI, began developing a clinical path in 1993 for patients undergoing open heart surgery. The path was intended as a tool to assure that all patients were cared for in the same standard way. Although the concept of standards was not new to caregivers at Lutheran Hospital, developing an integrated care plan for patients over a delineated time frame was. Caregivers involved with open heart surgery were asked to be part of a clinical path steering committee cochaired by the nursing and medical directors of the intensive care unit (ICU). Through group discussion the committee was quickly able to identify the interventions that were expected to occur each day. However, when the process it had defined was compared with actual practices, many variations were found. These variations seemed primarily related to the care provider's preferences. It became apparent that the open heart surgery path would not be successful unless clinicians could tackle the issue of practice pattern variation. Therefore, path implementation plans were put on hold.

This chapter describes how Lutheran Hospital used a continuous quality improvement (CQI) approach to overcome the challenges of practice pattern analysis and variation reduction. The end result was an open heart surgery process improvement initiative that integrated "best practice" standards into patient care to enhance outcomes and promote better health care team communication.

CONTINUOUS QUALITY IMPROVEMENT APPROACH TO PRACTICE PATTERN ANALYSIS

The first hurdle in addressing practice pattern variation was determining where to begin the practice pattern analysis. Open heart surgery patients undergo many different interventions throughout their hospitalization. Caregivers wanted to focus on stabilizing those processes having the greatest impact on costs and outcomes. Using benchmarking and other CQI methods, the committee studied the current process and identified those activities that seemed to be most important.

Next the committee realized that a large amount of data would be needed to study the consequence of variation in significant processes. For example, to answer the questions, How much sedation is necessary for open heart surgery patients? and What is the impact of prolonged sedation on patients' ICU length of stay? would require abstraction of data from 30 to 50 records of discharged patients. Just locating all the necessary records could take several weeks because patient records are regularly moved from the hospital to the affiliated ambulatory center and back to the hospital again. To address these information management concerns, Lutheran Hospital used automated technologies and sophisticated evaluation techniques.

The Lutheran Hospital ICU implemented the Hewlett Packard (HP) CAREVUE™ clinical information system in June 1990 to document patient care. Although the system had data collection capabilities for internal performance measurement activities, this capacity had not been fully utilized. In 1993 Lutheran Hospital received notice from HP that it was offering a limited number of fellowships to CAREVUE™ users interested in utilizing the CAREVUE™ system for their CQI efforts. This notice came at an opportune time, as cardiac caregivers were in the midst of discussing practice pattern variations in open heart surgery patients. Lutheran Hospital submitted an application for one of the scholarships, proposing that a study be done to determine the relationship between postoperative sedation and the time required for coronary artery bypass graft (CABG) patients to return to their preoperative cognitive and mobility statuses. This topic was chosen because earlier evaluations by the open heart surgery path steering committee had shown this to be an area of significant variation. The committee members had suspected that this variation impacted several different outcomes, including:

- Length of time patients are on a ventilator
- Patients' ICU length of stay and their total hospital length of stay
- Number of patient falls
- Time required for patients to return to their preoperative cognitive and mental states

In April 1994 Lutheran Hospital was notified that its CABG patient sedation project had been selected for HP funding. Fellowship winners received 3 days of CQI process training for all team members at the HP headquarters in Boston, coaching from HP quality process engineers, a technical assistance package for the CAREVUE™ 9000 system, and a personal computer with data analysis software.

Lutheran Hospital's CQI team for the CABG patient postoperative sedation project included the medical and nursing directors of the ICU, two ICU nurses, the information systems director, the respiratory care supervisor, and the quality improvement services director. At the 3-day CQI seminar the team was taught the FOCUS-PDCA model of continuous improvement:[1]

- *F*ind a process for improvement
- *O*rganize a group that knows the process
- *C*larify the current knowledge of the process
- *U*nderstand the causes of process variation
- *S*elect the process improvement
- *P*lan . . . develop an overall plan

- *Do* . . . implement a process change
- *Check* . . . measure the effect of the change
- *Act* . . . implement the best practice and system changes

FOCUS-PDCA APPLIED TO CORONARY ARTERY BYPASS PATIENT SEDATION PRACTICES

The CQI team first clarified the objective for the CABG patient postoperative sedation project. It agreed that inconsistencies existed in sedation practices which in turn contributed to patients':

- Prolonged intubation and mechanical ventilation
- Decreased ability to participate in activities of daily living
- Decreased ability to participate in cardiac rehabilitation

The project objective was followed by the formulation of an issue statement, which clearly described the objective of the study: "To reduce the time required for the CABG patients to return to their preoperative cognitive and mobility status."

The team also established the following measures to determine project success:

- Decrease in patient intubation times
- Decrease in the number of days between a patient's ICU admission and return to preoperative falls risk score (as measured by Lutheran Hospital's Falls Risk Scoring System)
- Decrease in the number of days between a patient's ICU admission and their return to preoperative cognitive and mental statuses (as measured by the Mayo Mini-Mental score)[2]
- Improved assessment and documentation of patients' mental status
- Decrease in number of hours patient is sedated
- Improved cognition and mobility status for patients (as measured by the Ramsey score)[3]
- Decrease in ICU and hospital lengths of stay
- Decrease in total hospital charges

To determine current performance, baseline data were collected manually from records of discharged patients seen over a 3-month period in late 1993. The data collection form is shown in figure 4-1. The study included 58 patients undergoing CABG, excluding reexploration, resternotomy, open chest, and intraaortic balloon pump procedures. The results, shown in table 4-1, would be compared with postproject data to judge the success of the initiative.

Clarifying Current Process Knowledge

Next the CABG CQI team clarified its current knowledge of the process, asking the questions, What is our current sedation practice? and How do all the events relate to one another? Using a process map, the team diagrammed the sedation management practices for CABG patients from the preoperative period to the time they are ready for transfer from the ICU. (See figure 4-2.)

FIGURE 4-1 Manual Data Collection Worksheet

		ICU admit date		/ /
		ICU admit time		

	Recorder	
	Patient ID	

Date (MM/DD/YY)		/ /	/ /	/ /	/ /	/ /	/ /	/ /	/ /	/ /
Time	Preop									
Falls risk score										
Mayo Mini-Mental score										
Sedation score										

Total length of stay (days)		→	Comments:

Total hospital bill	$	→	

Fall incident?	Yes No	→	

Readmitted within 30 days?	Yes No	→	

Smoking history		→	Currently smoking?	Yes No
			Pack years	
			Quit < 2 months prior to admission?	Yes No

Alcohol history?	Yes No	→	Alcohol comments:

Anesthesiologist(s)	→	Intraoperative medications

Pulmonologist: ....
ASA score: ....
Extubation time: ....

ICU bolus medications	Date and time of last dose
Ativan	
Midazolam	
Propofol	
Morphine sulfate	
Demerol	
Other	

→ Continuous __   PCA __
   PCA/Continuous __

TABLE 4-1 Preproject Baseline Performance Data (58 coronary artery bypass graft patients)

Performance Measure	Study Results
Average intubation time	13.8 hours
Days between ICU admission and return to preop and falls risk score	4.36 days
Days between ICU admission and return to preop Mayo Mini-Mental score	2.4 days
Total number of sedation hours in ICU	8.43 hours
Average Ramsey score at initiation of weaning from ventilator	2.69
Hospital average length of stay	9.3 days
ICU average length of stay	1.55 days
Average hospital charges	$29,270
Readmissions within 30 days	12.28%

Understanding Causes of Process Variation

To understand the causes of variations in processes, the team discussed the origins of current sedation practices. It discovered that sedation is administered to patients during the postoperative, ICU phase of care for two main reasons:

1. The patient undergoing CABG is especially vulnerable to myocardial ischemia during the first 2 hours following revascularization.
2. Delirium is the most commonly encountered mental disturbance in the critically ill patient.[4,5]

After reviewing the course of treatment for CABG patients at Lutheran Hospital, the team found several issues of interest related to sedation practices:

- The three sedation agents used at Lutheran Hospital were Versed, Propofol, and, on a limited basis, Ativan. The agent selection in the 1993 baseline data (58 patients) was distributed as follows:
  — Versed 26 (44 percent)
  — Propofol 8 (14 percent)
  — Propofol and Ativan 12 (21 percent)
  — None 12 (21 percent)
- Use of sedation for CABG patients had been increasing steadily.
- The level of patients' sedation was not being assessed consistently by the nursing staff.

It was theorized by the CABG CQI team members that ventilator weaning delays could be attributed to increased use of patient sedation. Team members were also concerned that some patients were still somnolent at the time they were transferred out of the ICU, causing an increased risk of falls.

Selecting Process Improvements

Taking these findings into consideration, the CABG CQI team created a cause-and-effect diagram (figure 4-3) to identify all possible causes of patients' decreased mental and mobility statuses. The team identified two major cause categories over which it believed caregivers had little control at the present time: *patient factors* and *surgery department practice issues*. It concentrated its efforts on the cause categories of *staff* and *methods*, focusing specifically on the improvement of opportunities related to

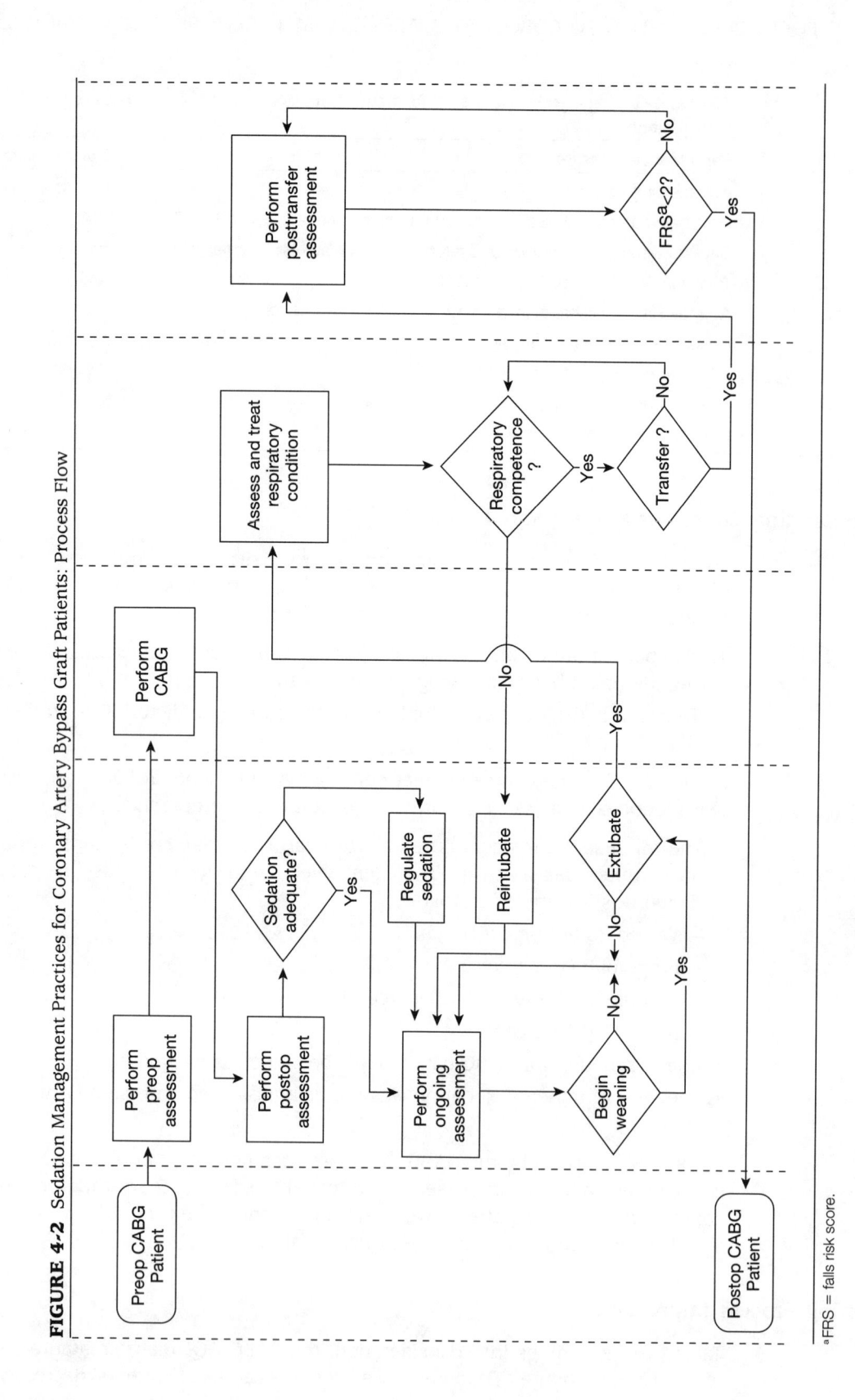

FIGURE 4-2 Sedation Management Practices for Coronary Artery Bypass Graft Patients: Process Flow

[a]FRS = falls risk score.

FIGURE 4-3 Cause-and-Effect Diagram Used to Determine the Cause of Decreased Mental and Mobility Statuses in Coronary Artery Bypass Graft Patients

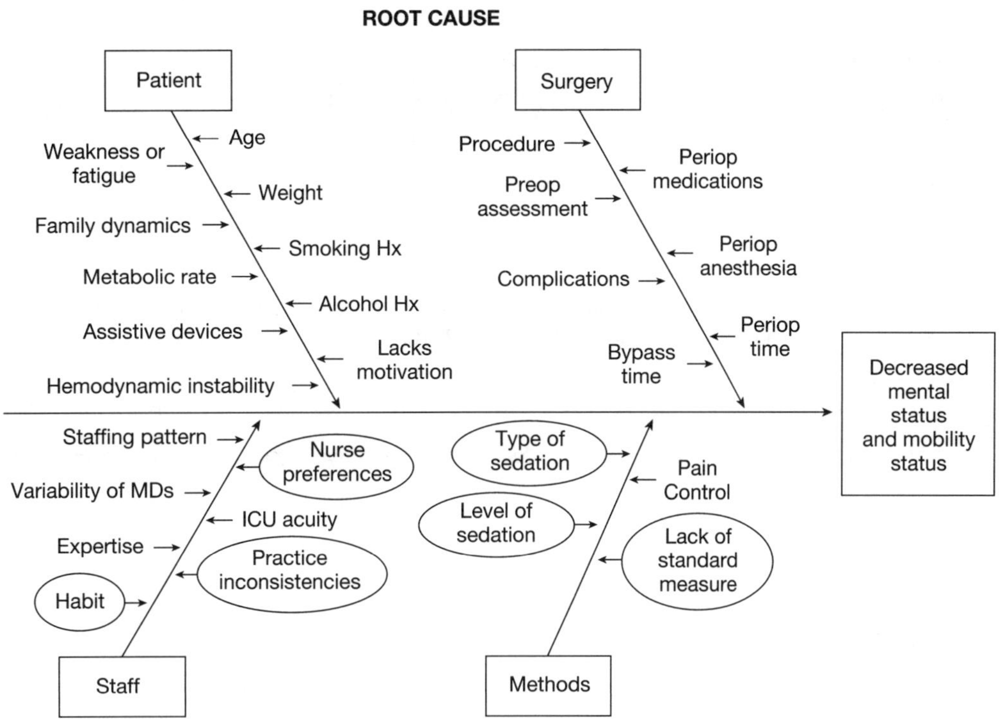

habit, practice inconsistencies, nurse preferences, type of sedation, level of sedation, and *lack of standard measure.*

Developing an Overall Plan

Process improvements were to be implemented that were most likely to achieve the CQI team's objectives for the CABG patient postoperative sedation project. The system changes that the team designed and implemented included the following:

1. The medical staff approved the use of the Mayo Mini-Mental Status (figure 4-4), the Ramsey Sedation Scale (figure 4-5), and the Lutheran Hospital Falls Risk Scoring System (figure 4-6) for cardiovascular patient assessments in the ICU and cardiovascular step-down unit. By using standardized patient scoring systems, the variation in patient assessments would be reduced.

2. A sedation protocol (figure 4-7) for cardiovascular patients was developed by the team and approved by all involved physicians. Recommendations in the protocol were derived from current literature sources.[6-9] The Ramsey Sedation Scale was incorporated into the protocol and the nursing staff directed to use the measure at regular intervals to assess patients' sedation levels. The 1993 retrospective study of patient sedation scores and start of ventilator weaning had shown that patients had an average Ramsey score of 2.69 when weaning was initiated. For this reason the desired level of patient sedation was set at 2–3 to facilitate timely weaning from the ventilator.

3. The nurses in the ICU and cardiac step-down unit would use the Falls Risk Standard/Treatment Flowsheet (figure 4-8) to determine each patient's falls risk score and monitor progress.

FIGURE 4-4 Mayo Mini-Mental Status Worksheet

1. Orientation (maximum score = 8)

How many of the following can the patient recall? One point for each correct answer.

    A. Full name   E. State

    B. Current address   F. Current day of week or month

    C. Current locale   G. Current month

    D. City   H. Year

Total: _____

2. Attention (maximum score = 7)

I will give you a series of seven (7) numbers. Please pay close attention to them. Wait until I am finished, then repeat the numbers back to me in the same order as I have given them. (2, 4, 6, 8, 10, 12, 14)

Total: _____

3. Learning (maximum score = 4)

I will give you four (4) words. I would like you to learn them, keep them in mind, and repeat them from time to time when I ask you.

    1. apple   3. tunnel

    2. Mr. Johnson   4. charity

Total: _____

4. Calculations (maximum score = 4)

How many of the following calculations can the patient correctly answer? Give one point for each correct answer.

    A. 5 × 13 (five times thirteen)   C. 58 ÷ 2 (fifty-eight divided by two)

    B. 65 − 7 (sixty-five minus seven)   D. 29 + 11 (twenty-nine plus eleven)

Total: _____

5. Abstraction (maximum score = 3)

I will give you two (2) words. Tell me the similarities between them.

    1. orange / banana

    2. horse / dog

    3. table / bookcase

Total: _____

6. Information (maximum score = 4)

    A. Draw a clock face showing 11:15.

    B. Copy a cube.

        (adequate representation = 2 points)
        (incomplete = 1 point)
        (inability to perform = 0 points)

Total: _____

7. Recall (maximum score = 4)

Recall the four (4) words given in no. 3—the Learning section.

    1. apple   3. tunnel

    2. Mr. Johnson   4. charity

Total: _____

Daily Total: _____

Source: Reprinted, with permission, from Folstein, M. F., Folstein, S. E., and McHugh, P. R. Mini-Mental State: a practical method for grading the cognitive state of patients for the clinician. *Journal of Psychiatric Research* 12:189–98, 1975, Elsevier Science Ltd, Oxford, England.

FIGURE 4-5 Ramsey Sedation Scale

Levels	Degree of Sedation
1	Anxious, agitated, or restless
2	Cooperative, accepting of therapy, oriented
3	Asleep, brisk response to verbal stimuli
4	Asleep, sluggish response to verbal stimuli
5	No response to loud verbal stimuli
6	No response to painful stimuli

Source: Reprinted, with permission, from Ramsey, M. A. E. Controlled sedation with alphaxalone-alphadolone. *British Medical Journal* 2(6):656–59, June 1974.

FIGURE 4-6 Lutheran Hospital Falls Risk Scoring System

Patient risk factors to be assessed each shift:

- Confusion or disorientation
- Elimination (incontinence, nocturia, frequency)
- History of falls in past 3 months (not slip or trip)
- Nonadaptive mobility or generalized weakness
- Dizziness or vertigo
- Medical diagnosis of cancer
- Medical diagnosis of depression

If two or more risk factors are present, implement interventions. In some patient situations one risk factor warrants implementation of interventions.

4. To improve the efficiency of nursing documentation, the Mayo Mini-Mental Status, Ramsey Sedation Scale, and the Lutheran Hospital Falls Risk Scoring System were formatted and programmed into the HP CAREVUE™ information system.

To ensure that the data needed for measuring the action plans' effectiveness would be readily available, all necessary data elements had to be prospectively identified. In many instances the CAREVUE™ system could be modified to meet the data collection requirements, although some data would still need to be gathered manually, as shown in figure 4-9. Configuration of the CAREVUE™ system required considerable involvement of CABG CQI team members from the quality improvement and information systems departments. HP supplied technical support to help modify the CAREVUE™ database to accommodate postimplementation evaluation activities. Using the database export function of CAREVUE™, the information necessary for measuring performance could be downloaded into a PC-based spreadsheet program for more detailed analysis.

Implementing Process Changes

The first priority of the CABG patient postoperative sedation project was to standardize the assessment of sedation levels and the administration of sedative agents. Therefore, the action plans were phased in, beginning with the introduction of the Ramsey

FIGURE 4-7 Sedation Protocol for Open Heart Surgery Patients

Sedation Agent:
1. Propofol
2. Versed

When to Sedate:
1. Open chest
2. Multiple inotropic drugs or
   >0.1 mcg/kg/min norepinephrine
   >0.1 mcg/kg/min epinephrine
   >10 mcg/kg/min dopamine
3. Unstable hemodynamics (persistent CI less than 1.8)
4. Over 5 cm PEEP
5. PaO_2/FiO_2 ratio less than 200
6. Metabolic acidosis with B.E. greater than −5
7. Excessive bleeding (greater than 200 cc/hr)
8. Paralytic agents currently being utilized
9. Restlessness or anxiety causing:
   Unsafe conditions for patient or staff
   Pulmonary or hemodynamic compromise

How to Sedate:
1. Initiate Propofol at 5 mcg/kg/min.
2. Increase by 5 mcg/kg/min every 15 minutes until desired level of sedation attained. Maximum dose = 50 mcg/kg/min.
3. If unable to attain desired level of sedation, bolus with 1–2 mg Versed and initiate drip at 1–4 mg.

Level of Sedation:
1. Ramsey Sedation Scale rating of 3–4

Weaning Assessment:
1. Wean sedation as soon as possible to a level of 2–3 on the Ramsey Sedation Scale.
2. Anticipate weaning from ventilator within 4 hours postop.

Sedation Assessment:
1. Conduct assessment using Ramsey Sedation Scale every 1 hour for 4 hours, then every 2 hours until extubated, then every 4 hours with other routine ICU assessments.

Sedation Scale. Education was provided for the nursing and medical staffs regarding the purpose and use of the Ramsey scoring system. Random audits were conducted to assure that the staff understood the assessment process and used the tool appropriately.

The next step was to implement the Mayo Mini-Mental Status assessment to test the cognitive status of open heart patients. A small group of ICU nurses were instructed in the use of this tool. These nurses were responsible for surveying patients prior to their open heart surgery and again at the time of their discharge from the hospital. The survey data were entered into a database for analysis. To assure interrater reliability, the assessment tool was tested on five patients.

Because the falls risk assessment was already being used successfully by the cardiovascular nursing staff, education was not needed. The tool had been validated prior to the CABG patient postoperative sedation project, so further testing was not necessary. The sedation protocol orders were approved by the medical staff and implemented. Physicians and nurses in the ICU were educated in the purpose and use of the protocol orders.

Measuring the Effect of the Changes

The first postimplementation study occurred after all the process improvements had been put in place on June 1, 1994. Once 15 patients who met study criteria were seen in the ICU, data were extracted from the CAREVUE™ system to determine the effectiveness of the new assessments and interventions. The first postimplementation data results are shown in table 4-2.

FIGURE 4-8 Falls Risk Standard/Treatment Flowsheet

LUTHERAN HOSPITAL - LACROSSE
LA CROSSE, WISCONSIN 54601

FALL RISK STANDARD/TREATMENT FLOWSHEET
MED/SURG

DATE SHIFT	0700-1500	1500-2300	2300-0700	0700-1500	1500-2300	2300-0700	0700-1500	1500-2300	2300-0700	0700-1500	1500-2300	2300-0700	0700-1500	1500-2300	2300-0700
ASSESS RISK FACTORS q SHIFT: D/B: + / -															
Confusion/disorientation															
Elimination (incontinence, nocturia, frequency)															
Hx falls in last 3 mos. (not slip/trip)															
Non-adaptive mobility/ generalized weakness															
Dizziness/vertigo															
Med Dx Cancer															
Med Dx Depression															
Other:															
Number of risk factors/total															

IF 2 OR MORE RISK FACTORS - IMPLEMENT INTERVENTIONS
IN SOME PT SITUATIONS 1 RISK FACTOR WARRANTS IMPLEMENTING INTERVENTIONS

INTERVENTIONS - FALL RISK

Fall Prevention Ed. and/or Brochure delivered to: D/B: P = Patient F = Family O = Other															
Re-orient to person/place/time DBI															
Assess elimination needs q 2 h while awake: DBI															
Assist c elim: D/B: U = urinal placed B = bedpan/urinal in reach C = commode at bedside D = assist to BR F = foley															
(OVER)															

40-929A 4/93

FALL RISK STANDARD/TREATMENT FLOWSHEET - MED/SURG.

Source: Reprinted, with permission, from Gundersen Lutheran.

FIGURE 4-9 Data Elements

Captured in the HP CAREVUE™ 9000 System
- Patient name
- Age
- Gender
- Height and weight
- Clinic number
- Dates of admission to ICU and transfer out of ICU
- Diagnosis
- Alcohol and smoking history
- Surgical procedure
- Postop time returned to ICU
- Preadmission medications
- Ejection fraction
- Intubation date and time
- Extubation date and time
- Date and time weaning initiated and completed

- Reason weaning not initiated or weaning terminated
- FiO_2 and PEEP levels
- Pulmonary mechanics
- RSB index
- Hemodynamics/vital signs/ABGs/SaO_2 pre-, during, and postweaning
- Concurrent drug titration during weaning
- Date and time of last sedation dose prior to weaning
- Assessments pre- and postweaning and upon transfer:
  — Sedation rating
  — Mental status
- APACHE score
- Risk management factors, e.g., restraints, bed position, Falls Risk score

Captured manually
- Total hospital length of stay
- Risk management factors posttransfer to cardiac rehab
- Pre-ICU and post-ICU transfer mental status assessment

- Post-ICU transfer Falls Risk score
- Discharge mental status and mobility status

TABLE 4-2 First Postimplementation Study Results Compared with Baseline Data

Performance Measure	Baseline Study Results N = 58	Study 1 Results N = 15
Average intubation time	13.8 hours	14.2 hours
Days between ICU admission and return to preop falls risk score	4.36 days	3.42 days
Days between ICU admission and return to preop Mayo Mini-Metal score	2.4 days	1.67 days
Total number of sedation hours in ICU	8.43 hours	8.36 hours
Average Ramsey score at initiation of weaning from ventilator	2.69	2.15
Hospital average length of stay	9.3 days	8.8 days
ICU average length of stay	1.55 days	1.42 days
Average hospital charges	$29,270	$26,282
Readmissions within 30 days	12.28%	6.67%
Sedation Used		
Versed	26 (44%)	4 (26.6%)
Propofol	8 (14%)	1 (6.6%)
Propofol and Versed	12 (21%)	3 (20%)
None	12 (21%)	6 (40%)

The CABG CQI team analyzed the data and found that after implementing standardized assessment tools and the sedation protocol, the number of days between the patients' ICU admission and return to their preoperative mental status dropped from preintervention level of 2.4 days to 1.67 days. Other significant changes, such as a decrease in sedation time from 8.43 hours to 8.36 hours and reduction of ICU length of stay, were noted. It was also gratifying for the project team to discover that the process changes did not increase patients' risk of readmission, which actually decreased after the changes were introduced. Now it was time to implement the open heart surgery clinical path, which included these new assessment tools and the sedation protocol. (See figure 4-10.)

Implementing the Clinical Path

Following physician and staff education in the purpose and use of the clinical path, in September 1994 the path was entered into the CAREVUE™ system. After 15 CABG patients who met study criteria were treated using the path as a guide, performance data were extracted from the CAREVUE™ system. The findings from this second postimplementation study are shown in table 4-3.

The CABG CQI team analyzed the data, comparing the baseline data and results from the two postimplementation studies. It was easy to measure the progress that had been obtained by first implementing the assessment tools and then the clinical path. The results showed a significant decrease in sedation time from a baseline of 8.43 hours to 3.77 hours; intubation time decreased from 13.8 hours to 10.0 hours; and ICU length of stay decreased from 1.55 days to less than 24 hours. Data on the use of sedation agents showed that the clinical path had accomplished the goal of reducing variation in ordering practices.

Patients' total hospital charges decreased from $29,270 preproject to $22,622 postproject. This reduction was due to many factors, including decreases in ICU length of stay, sedation time, and total hospital length of stay.

CONCLUSION

By embracing the CQI philosophy, caregivers at Lutheran Hospital were able to improve patient management practices for open heart surgery patients.

Lessons Learned

During the initial stages of the CQI project in open heart surgery, many important lessons were learned. Insights gained are listed below.

Reduction of Significant Process Variation Must Precede Path Implementation If the open heart surgery clinical path steering committee had implemented the CABG path in 1993, when it was first developed, many patients would have "fallen off" the path. Although everyone could agree on the ideal plan of care, it was apparent that physician and nurse practice differences were causing unintended variations. Instead of moving ahead with path implementation anyway, the steering committee retreated from its original charge and initiated a practice pattern analysis study. Using data derived from closed record reviews, the CABG CQI team selected key practice issues that appeared to be influencing patient outcomes. Out of this analysis came the development and implementation of:

- Standardized nursing assessments of patient sedation levels
- A sedation protocol

These actions resulted in documented process improvements.

Once significant variations in practices had been reduced, the clinical path was implemented. As shown by the data from the second postimplementation study, introduction of the path led to even greater improvements. It is unlikely these path-related improvements would have been possible without the sedation project

FIGURE 4-10 Coronary Artery Bypass Graft Clinical Path

Gundersen Lutheran
Care Path - Coronary Artery Bypass
Target LOS 5 Days

	Pre-Op	Post-op Day #1	Post-op Day #2
PROGRESS TOWARD DISCHARGE (✓ if met, circle if not met and explain in progress note)	☐ Admission protocol completed ☐ Nursing and discharge data base completed ☐ Pt/family verbalize understanding of care path progression and post-op routines	☐ Pt extubated w/adequate SpO$_2$ on nasal O$_2$ ☐ Hemodynamically stable s̄ IV meds ☐ Tolerates ambulation to chair ☐ Pt responds to prn diuretic therapy ☐ Weight gain < 7 kg ☐ Pt/family state CP expectations for POD 1	☐ Oxygenation WNL - weaning O$_2$ ☐ Heart rhythm/BP stable for pt. ☐ Tolerate ambulation in room ☐ Pain relieved c̄ po meds ☐ Tolerates po intake without N/V ☐ Weight decreasing to pre-op ☐ Pt/family state CP expectations for POD 2
CONSULT	Cardiac rehabilitaion Oral surgery clearance if valve		
TESTS/DIAGNOSTICS	- CXR within 60 days - Hgb, plt, wbc, UA, PT/INR, PTT, fibriogen, lytes, Cr., glucose - T & C 4 units prbc's 5u platelets - 12 lead EKG	Hgb, K, CPK, EKG, CXR	Hgb, K
MEDICATIONS/IV/BLOOD	Allopurinol as directed DC heparin as per Cardiology Pre-op meds per anesthesia Hold Coumadin 4 days pre-op	Wean off IV to po.analgesics K replacement protocol/diuresis DC NTG, vasoactive meds as tolerated. Restart pre-op meds as needed	Po pain med Percocet/Ibuprofen Pre-op meds resumed as needed Iron supplement if Hgb < 10 Peripheral heplock
TREATMENTS/INTERVENTIONS	Hibiclens shower Shave/prep Pre-op height & weight Surgical consent signed	DC CVP/PA/A lines once stable off gtts. VS q 1° - 2°----> q 4° p̄ transfer Weigh a.m. I & O q 1°----> q 8 p̄ transfer Change dressings before transfer DC NG tube & foley O$_2$ per NC to keep SpO$_2$ > 90% IS q 1°, CDB q2° WA Cap pacer wires if not in use Initiate diabetic, anticoag, pain flowsheets if applicable DC CT	VS q 4° Daily weight, I & O q shift Remove dressing if not draining Cap pacer wires RT - wean O$_2$/NP to keep SpO$_2$ > 90%
ACTIVITY/MOBILITY	Ad lib, as tolerated	OOB tid for meals c̄ LE elevated. Bath at bedside, BRP c̄ assist walk in room c̄ assist	OOB for meals Bathe at sink c̄ assist BPR c̄ assist Ambulate tid distance as tolerated
NUTRITION	General diet Carbohydrate controlled if DM NPO p̄ MN	Clear liquid - advance as tolerated	Advance to General diet/carbohydrate controlled if DM
PATIENT/FAMILY EDUCATION KEY: Initial = Patient demonstrates/verbalizes understanding	☐ Review pre-op video c pt/family ☐ Review info re:/Advance Directive ☐ Review Care Path - post-op expectations. ☐ PCA use/pain scale ☐ C & DB return demo ☐ Incentive spirometry return demo ☐ Foot circles return demo ☐ Pre-op checklist completed ☐ Pre-op medication teaching	**ICU** ☐ Prepare pt/family for transfer ☐ Reinforce activity, pulmonary care **TELEMETRY** ☐ 6W orientation/routines ☐ Reinforce pain management ☐ Sternal precautions ☐ Transfer techniques/activity ☐ Use of incentive spirometry ☐ Review care path c̄ pt/family	☐ Reinforce pulmonary care ☐ Provide pt care updates, progress ☐ OHS homegoing binder review ☐ Homegoing video ☐ Homegoing activity guideline ☐ Pulse taking demo ☐ Energy conservation ☐ Stop smoking ☐ Anticoagulant therapy ☐ Incision care ☐ Weight ☐ Pain Rx ☐ Risk factors ☐ Lifting ☐ Driving ☐ Emotions ☐ Sexuality ☐ Phase II C. rehab ☐ ADL's ☐ Appetite ☐ Medications/home
DISCHARGE PLANNING	Discharge assessment completed. Consult Social Service if needed CM assess support system & home situation. ☐ Discuss pt. care path		CM/CVS APN reviews CP expectations c̄ pt. & family Notify CM if anticipated DC planning needs
DAILY REVIEW BY	_____ RN _____ RN _____ RN	_____ RN _____ RN _____ RN	_____ RN _____ RN _____ RN

#40-1062 Page #1 2/96

FIGURE 4-10 *Continued*

Gundersen Lutheran
Care Path - Open Heart Surgery
Target LOS 5 Days

	POD #3	POD #4	POD #5	POD #6
Progress toward discharge	☐ Oxygenation WNL for pt. on RA ☐ Cardiac Rhythm/BP WNL for pt. ☐ Pt. tolerates ambulation >5min tid ☐ Pain relieved c̄ po meds ☐ Tolerates diet s̄ N/V ☐ Pt/family state CP expectations for POD 3	☐ Cardiac & resp. status off telemetry ☐ Pt tolerates ambulation in hall > 5 min qid ☐ Pain relieved by po meds ☐ Dietary intake & elimination normal for pt. ☐ Pt/family finalize plans for discharge ☐	☐ Cardiac & respiratory status stable ☐ Independent c ADL's & activity ☐ Pain relieved c̄ po meds ☐ Nutrition & elimination normal for patient ☐ Pt/family homegoing education completed ☐	☐ Cardiac & respiratory status stable ☐ Independent c ADL's & activity ☐ Pain relieved c̄ po meds ☐ Nutrition & elimination normal for patient ☐ Pt/family homegoing education completed ☐
Consults	Diabetic education if appropriate Social Services prn Smoking cessation prn			
Tests/diagnostics		CXR if needed		
Medications/IV/Blood	Percocet-----> Lor tabs ECASA, bid Colace Ibuprofen, LOC prn Diuretics/K+ prn weight > pre-op Iron for Hgb < 10 prn	Percocet ---> Lor tabs ECASA, Colace bid Iron if Hgb < 10 MD/PA write discharge prescriptions	Nursing D/C heplock IV Home c̄ discharge prescriptions & instructions	Nursing D/C heplock IV Home c̄ discharge prescriptions & instructions
Treatments/Interventions	Nursing: Monitor VS q 8° Daily weight, I & O q shift Remove dressing if not draining Wean/DC O₂ if SpO₂ > 90% on RA Encourage independence c̄ IS q 1-2° Offer LOC if needed	Nursing: Monitor VS q shift Daily weight, d/c I & O unless diuresing Wound open to air, contain drainage Encourage independent IS q 1-2 WA MD/PA: DC pacing wire if not used x 24 hrs. DC telemetry if no significant arrhythmias x 24 hrs.	Nursing: VS q shift Weigh daily Wound open to air Encourage IS use Assure all lines/suture removed prior to DC'd Remove CT suture - replace c̄ steristrips MD/PA DC pacer wires DC telemetry	Nursing: VS q shift Weigh daily Wound open to air Encourage IS use Assure all lines/suture removed prior to DC'd Remove CT suture - replace c̄ steristrips MD/PA DC pacer wires DC telemetry
Activity/Mobility	OOB for meals Bathe unassisted or chair shower c̄ assist BRP unassisted Assist to ambulate > 5min tid Distance as tolerated	Nursing: OOB tid (4hrs/day) Independent self care - chair shower c̄ assist Ambulate independently qid ↑ distance as tolerated	Walk 5-10 min. 4-5 x/day unassisted Independent c̄ ADL's	Walk 5-10 min. 4-5 x/day unassisted Independent c̄ ADL's
Nutrition	As tolerated General	General	General	General
Patient/Family Education	☐ Reinforce pulmonary care ☐ Provide pt care updates, progress ☐ OHS homegoing binder ☐ Home going video ☐ Home going activity guidelines ☐ Pulse taking demo ☐ Energy conservation ☐ Stop smoking ☐ Anticoagulant therapy ☐ Incision care ☐Weight ☐ Pain Rx ☐Risk factors ☐ Lifting ☐Driving ☐ Emotions ☐Sexuality ☐ Phase II C. rehab ☐ ADL's ☐ Nutrition ☐ Medications/home ☐ Appetite ☐	☐ Reinforce pulmonary care ☐ Provide pt care updates, progress ☐ OHS homegoing binder ☐ Home going video ☐ Home going activity guidelines ☐ Pulse taking demo ☐ Energy conservation ☐ Stop smoking ☐ Anticoagulant therapy ☐ Incision care ☐Weight ☐ Pain Rx ☐Risk factors ☐ Lifting ☐Driving ☐ Emotions ☐Sexuality ☐ Phase II C. rehab ☐ ADL's ☐ Nutrition ☐ Medications/home ☐ Appetite ☐	☐ Reinforce pulmonary care ☐ Provide pt care updates, progress ☐ OHS homegoing binder ☐ Home going video ☐ Home going activity guidelines ☐ Pulse taking demo ☐ Energy conservation ☐ Stop smoking ☐ Anticoagulant therapy ☐ Incision care ☐Weight ☐ Pain Rx ☐Risk factors ☐ Lifting ☐Driving ☐ Emotions ☐Sexuality ☐ Phase II C. rehab ☐ ADL's ☐ Appetite ☐ Medications/home	☐ Reinforce pulmonary care ☐ Provide pt care updates, progress ☐ OHS homegoing binder ☐ Home going video ☐ Home going activity guidelines ☐ Pulse taking demo ☐ Energy conservation ☐ Stop smoking ☐ Anticoagulant therapy ☐ Incision care ☐Weight ☐ Pain Rx ☐Risk factors ☐ Lifting ☐Driving ☐ Emotions ☐Sexuality ☐ Phase II C. rehab ☐ ADL's ☐ Appetite ☐ Medications/home
Discharge Planning	CM discuss plan for discharge c̄ pt/family Assess DC needs, DME, HH referral Social Service Consult prn	Finalize plans for discharge c̄ pt/family	MD write DC orders Arrange outpatient followup c̄ MD DC by 1200	MD write DC orders Arrange outpatient followup c̄ MD DC by 1200
Daily review by	_____RN _____RN _____RN	_____RN _____RN _____RN	07-15_____RN 15-23_____RN 03-07_____RN	_____RN _____RN _____RN

Expected outcomes for discharge   Initial
                                                                                                                                  Yes   No

1. Patient/family understand self care instructions for ADL's, meds, diet, activity, medical followup and emergency notification procedures.
2. Pain controlled at level acceptable to patient
3. Patient is free from symptomatic arrhythmias and is hemodynamically stable. SBP 90-160 and HR 60-100.
4. Weight at or below pre-op with therapeutic K+ level.
5. Patient is free from dyspnea c̄ SpO₂ > 90% on RA or at baseline.
6. Wound edges approximated and sternum stable, afebrile without signs and symptoms of infection.
7. Tolerates 5-10 min. unassisted ambulation qid or prescribed level s̄ symptoms.

#40-1062 Page #2   2/96

Source: Reprinted, with permission, from Gundersen Lutheran.

TABLE 4-3 Second Postimplementation Study Results Compared with Baseline Data and First Study Results

Performance Measure	Baseline Study Results N = 58	Study 1 Results N = 15	Study 2 Results N = 15
Average intubation time	13.8 hours	14.2 hours	10.0 hours
Days between ICU admission and return to preop falls risk score	4.36 days	3.42 days	2.1 days
Days between ICU admission and return to preop Mayo Mini-Mental score	2.4 days	1.67 days	1.87 days
Total number of sedation hours in ICU	8.43 hours	8.36 hours	3.77* hours
Average Ramsey score at initiation of weaning from ventilator	2.69	2.15	2.6
Hospital average length of stay	9.3 days	8.8 days	8.5 days
ICU average length of stay	1.55 days	1.42 days	.94** days
Average hospital charges	$29,270	$26,282	$22,622***
Readmissions within 30 days	12.28%	6.67%	6.67%
Sedation Used			
Versed	26 (44%)	4 (26.6%)	0
Propofol	8 (14%)	1 (6.6%)	9 (60%)
Propofol and Versed	12 (21%)	3 (20%)	0
None	12 (21%)	6 (40%)	6 (40%)

*Significant difference between baseline and study 2 results at $p < 0.05$.
**Significant difference between baseline and study 1 and study 2 and between study 1 and study 2 at $p > 0.05$.
***Significant difference between baseline and study 2 at $p < 0.05$.

that preceded path implementation. During this project the cardiovascular caregivers learned to work together as a team and discovered how to use data to solve problems. This collaborative effort greatly improved the likelihood that the open heart surgery path would be successful. Caregivers will continue to use the study model established by the CABG CQI team to evaluate other practice pattern variations, such as pain medication administration, differences in anesthesia practices, and so on.

Automated Data Collection Is a Vital Component of Process Improvement The CQI project in open heart surgery would not have been as successful without an automated information system. Data retrieval and analysis is the most labor-intensive component of any CQI project. Without the ability of Lutheran Hospital caregivers to document the study data elements concurrently in the CAREVUE™ system, each of the three sedation studies would have required manual review of closed records at a staff cost of approximately $10,000 per study. This expenditure is hard to justify in today's cost-conscious environment. Although the eventual patient management improvement gains might outweigh the study costs, the resources must be expended *long before* cost savings are realized.

What did the HP CAREVUE™ clinical information system component of the CQI project cost? Fortunately, the system had been in place at Lutheran Hospital for 4 years before the project was conducted. Organizations that do not have a bedside clinical information system would find that adding one is a major expense. Moreover, as was the case at Lutheran, having a bedside clinical information system in place does not mean it is being used to its full potential. This situation is perhaps the costliest of all: monies had been spent for automated data collection, yet caregivers were continuing to gather data manually.

By working with HP technicians, Lutheran Hospital caregivers learned how to modify the CAREVUE™ system to gather study data, thereby reducing the actual work of study data retrieval and analysis by 33 percent. Now that the information system has been reconfigured to capture performance measurement data, the same or similar patient outcome studies can be conducted easily. For example, ICU caregivers are currently using the CAREVUE™ system to capture data necessary for a study on pain medication administration for open heart surgery patients.

Teams Must Be Trained in CQI Methods Team training in CQI methods is an important element of success. For Lutheran Hospital, the costs of the 3-day CQI training conference and some of the initial CQI learning was covered through the HP fellowship grant. However, future CQI project teams also need education. For this reason Lutheran Hospital has committed to training an internal CQI resource team whose members will serve as facilitators for all interdisciplinary projects throughout the facility.

Summary

Organizations across the country are working hard to respond to the demands of a new health care environment. Clinical paths have become a familiar tool for stabilizing the patient care process. However, the path tool by itself does not effect change. Reducing significant practice variation requires a CQI approach to practice pattern analysis. When the cardiovascular caregivers at Lutheran Hospital realized that their goal was CQI rather than design and implementation of a clinical path, genuine progress was made. Through collaboration and knowledge-based decision making the clinicians identified "best practices" and implemented process changes that increased the efficiency of services and improved patient outcomes.

References

1. Walton, M. *Deming Management at Work*. New York City: Putnam, 1990.
2. Kokmen, E., Naessens, J. M., and Offord, K. P. A short test of mental status: descriptions and preliminary results. *Mayo Clinic Proceedings* 62(4):281–88, Apr. 1987.
3. Ramsey, M. A. E. Controlled sedation with alphaxalone-alphadolone. *British Medical Journal* 2(6):656–59, June 1974.
4. Fish, D. Treatment of delirium in the critically ill patient. *Clinical Pharmacy* 10(6):456–66, June 1991.
5. Roekaerts, P., Huygen, F., and de Lange, S. Infusion of propofol versus midazolam for sedation in the intensive care unit following coronary artery surgery. *Journal of Cardiothoracic and Vascular Anesthesia* 7(2):142–47, Apr. 1993.
6. McMurray, T. J., Collier, P. S., Carson, I. W., and others. Propofol sedation after open heart surgery: a clinical and pharmacokinetic study. *Anaesthesia* 45(4):322–26, 1990.
7. Aikinhead, A. R., Willatts, S., Park, G. R., and others. Comparison of propofol and midazolam for sedation in critically ill patients. *Lancet* 2(8665):704–9, 1989.
8. Doherty, M. Benzodiazepine sedation in critically ill patients. *AACN Clinical Issues* 2(4):748–63, 1991.
9. Westphal, L. M., Cheng, E. Y., White, P. F., and others. Use of midazolam infusion for sedation following cardiac surgery. *Anesthesiology* 67(2):257–62, 1987.

CHAPTER 5

Creating a Multidisciplinary Disease Management Initiative

Lisa M. Zavorski and Barbara Taptich

St. Francis Medical Center, a 426-bed acute care facility in Trenton, NJ, first introduced clinical pathways in 1990. The impetus for pathway development was the state's issuance of the Nursing Incentive Reimbursement Award (NIRA) to the medical center. The goal of this grant was to improve the professional practice of nurses by increasing their accountability for the quality of patient care, providing them with increased responsibility and autonomy for care, and enhancing interdisciplinary collaboration in executing the patient plan of care. St. Francis Medical Center adopted a traditional clinical path model as its strategy for meeting the grant's objectives.[1] In addition to supporting the professional development of nurses, clinical paths were viewed as a mechanism for improving interdisciplinary collaboration, enhancing patient outcomes, and achieving more effective utilization management.

HISTORICAL PERSPECTIVE

Clinical pathway evolution at St. Francis Medical Center has occurred in stages. Minimal progress was made in streamlining physician practices; pathway content was reflective of current physician ordering practices. Various approaches were operationalized as the program matured. The *nursing development model* was used in the early stage of the program and focused primarily on nursing processes to meet the goals of the NIRA grant. Over a 3-year period, 10 nursing-oriented pathways were developed. Also developed was the position of care manager to assure the coordination of care for patients on a particular patient unit. The manager's role was to facilitate communication between care providers and to coordinate medical center services in order to decrease lengths of stay and improve patient outcomes.

These early pathway and care management activities demonstrated the effectiveness of the program. In 1993 administrative and medical staff leaders agreed that the clinical pathway process should be expanded beyond nursing to encourage greater interdisciplinary participation and increase physician acceptance. Physicians concluded that they were more likely to refer to a pathway if they were a part of the initial development.

During this transition clinical pathways evolved into an important patient care management tool for all caregivers at the medical center. Pathway recommendations, developed through a multidisciplinary process, helped to assure that services and resources were appropriately used. Pathways also provided the synergy in necessary care processes for effective patient care management.

This chapter details the experiences and challenges encountered by St. Francis Medical Center as it designed and implemented its *interdisciplinary development model* of care management, a structured approach to developing interdisciplinary protocols, including physician and caregiver practice guidelines. Described herein is the development of clinical pathways, pathway content and variance reporting, the evolution of case management strategies, and the role of the pathways and case management in performance improvement projects. To illustrate the interdisciplinary development model in action, readers will learn how medical center caregivers developed a continuum-of-care program for patients with congestive heart failure (CHF).

DEVELOPING INTERDISCIPLINARY PATHWAYS

With the advent of the interdisciplinary development model, the clinical pathway format had to change. The nursing-oriented paths developed at St. Francis Medical Center had been illustrated in a traditional horizontal matrix format, with the major functions listed down the left side of the path and day progression steps shown across the top. This standard format was used for all pathways developed for the nursing development model.

Pathway Development Teams

Since practice guidelines, protocols, and individualized patient outcomes were to be incorporated into the interdisciplinary pathways, clinicians agreed that the previous format was too constraining. For this reason pathway development teams were formed, with members determined by the director of utilization management and physician leaders. These teams were allowed to customize the path format to meet the needs of targeted populations. The one element that had to be included on each pathway was a disclaimer: "This pathway is a 'Tool' to facilitate multidisciplinary patient care. Patient care will be tailored to the individual patient and may differ from the pathway. The care pathway does not replace clinical judgement of the professional health care team, including the physician's order." This disclaimer was felt to be important, since physician-related practice guidelines would be included in the interdisciplinary pathways.

Pathway content could also vary from one patient population to the next. The pathway development teams were allowed to define care processes unique to the specific patient group being studied. In addition, they established the start and stop boundaries for that path because some pathways begin prior to hospitalization and continue beyond discharge.

Interdisciplinary Pathway Design Teams

Once the format issues were resolved, interdisciplinary path design teams were established for each pathway to be developed. The teams were originally chartered by the utilization management oversight group, but the medical center's quality council has taken over this responsibility. Members on each design team included a medical staff team leader, a quality department representative, the nursing standards director, and a representative from pastoral care and nursing education, respectively. Members were also chosen from relevant ancillary service areas.

Physician Subgroups

Because the pathway recommendations required medical staff input, the design teams formed physician subgroups to create the practice guidelines to be incorporated into the pathway. Members of the physician subgroup were selected by the path design team. Physician participation was critical in examining the efficiency of physician practices and the impact of practice variations on the medical center's resource management goals. Practice guidelines were developed by utilizing information from a variety of resources. Literature searches were conducted to identify practice guidelines developed by national medical organizations as well as demonstrated "best practice" examples from other hospitals. It was also important to understand current practice behaviors, so retrospective chart reviews were conducted to identify variations in ordering practices among St. Francis physicians.

Discipline-Specific Requirements

The new pathways complemented the patient plan of care, making it relatively easy to make the transition from the nursing elements defined in the nursing development model to the interdisciplinary paths. Ancillary service representatives served as active path design team participants to ensure that their discipline-specific requirements were included in the paths.

Peer-to-Peer Presentations

As the pathways were completed, they were presented at all medical staff department and section meetings for approval prior to implementation. Probably one of the most important factors in the success of the interdisciplinary pathways was the presentation process. Physician leaders in each division introduced the pathways to their colleagues. These peer-to-peer presentations produced the support necessary for medical staff buy-in and implementation approval.

Since 1993, 51 interdisciplinary pathways have been developed and approved for use. For example, several pathways have been developed for patients with CHF. These pathways correspond to patients' varying acuity levels—acute complicated patients (figure 5-1), acute uncomplicated patients, and patients capable of rapid diuresis or early discharge. This stratification has helped to minimize pathway variances and streamline the plan of care to meet the unique needs of CHF population subgroups.

Generic Medical and Surgical Pathways

To ensure that all patients benefit from a well-coordinated care experience, generic medical and surgical pathways have been designed and implemented for those patients who do not have a disease- or procedure-specific pathway. The generic medical

FIGURE 5-1 Congestive Heart Failure Pathway

St. Francis Medical Center **CONGESTIVE HEART FAILURE**
Trenton, New Jersey

Date Developed: 3/93 Date Initiated: 5/93 Date Revised: _____

Admission Date: __/__/__ Discharge Date: __/__/__
Final DRG: _____
Estimated Length of Stay: _____
PMH: _____
_____

This pathway is a "Tool" to facilitate multidisciplinary patient care. Patient care will be tailored to the individual patient and may differ from the pathway. The care pathway does not replace clinical judgement of the professional health care team, including the physician's order.

Page 1 of 2

Shaded boxes represent the goal day

Key Indicators are Bolded and Asterisked

Category	Item	ED	AD	1	2	3	4 (DC)	5
PATIENT OUTCOME	Patient verbalizes understanding of lifestyle, activity & medication education*						▓	
DISCHARGE PLANNING	Nursing assessment for Discharge Planning**	▓						
	Coordinate discharge planning needs (ICC)*		▓					
	Finalize D/C planning arrangements*						▓	
	Discharge assessment*				▓	▓		
	Discharge if lungs clear, edema < or =2+, patient ambulatory and on PO meds*						▓	
CONSULTS/ REFERRALS	Medical if indicated							
	Cardiology if indicated							
	Nutrition							
	Physical Therapy		▓					
	Pastoral Care							
TESTS/ PROCEDURES	Admission Chem Screen	▓						
	Cardiac Profile	▓						
	CBC with auto diff	▓						
	PT/APTT	▓						
	ABG or Pulse Oximetry	▓						
	Magnesium	▓						
	FBS	▓						
	Chem 6/K+			▓				
	EKG*	▓						
	CXR	▓						
	Echocardiogram*		▓					
	Stress test							
	Cardiac cath if indicated							
TREATMENT/ ASSESSMENTS/ ELIMINATION	Cardiac Monitor	▓						
	Telemetry							
	VS Q 1 hour							
	VS Q 2 hours							
	VS Q 4 hours							
	Assess lung sounds, neck vein dist. and edema*		▓	▓	▓	▓		
	Height and Weight assessment*	▓						
	I&O*	▓	▓	▓	▓	▓	▓	
	KVO							
	Heplock							
	Heart/lung sounds Q 2 hour							
	Heart/lung sounds Q 4 hour							
	Assess pulse oximetry on O2 and RA and prn*		▓					
MEDICATION/ PAIN MNGT	Review patient's pre-admission meds*	▓						
	IV diuretics ordered*	▓						
	PO diuretics*				▓			
	Vasodilators							
	Oxygen PRN							
	Assessment to D/C oxygen*				▓			
NUTRITION	Sodium/fluid restriction as indicated							
ACTIVITY	Bedrest							
	OOB to chair*			▓				
	Ambulate in room*				▓			
	Ambulate in hall*					▓	▓	

PATHWAY CONTINUED ON NEXT PAGE

FIGURE 5-1 *Continued*

St. Francis Medical Center Trenton, New Jersey		CONGESTIVE HEART FAILURE										
Admission Date: _/_/_ Discharge Date:_/_/_ Final DRG: _____ Estimated Length of Stay:_____ PMH: _____		This pathway is a "Tool" to facilitate multidisciplinary patient care. Patient care will be tailored to the individual patient and may differ from the pathway. The care pathway does not replace clinical judgement of the professional health care team, including the physician's order.										
			DATE					Shaded boxes represent the goal day				
Page 2 of 2	*Key Indicators are Bolded and Asterisk*		DAY	ED	AD	1	2	3	4	DC 5		
PATIENT/ FAMILY EDUCATION	Orientation to hospital											
	Lifestyle, activity and medication education*											
	Reinforce education*											
	Review Discharge Instructions											
	Check patient has prescriptions											
COMORBID CARE Dx:_____												
UTILIZATION	Admission Review											
	Continued Stay Review											
	Discharge Review											
NURSING	7:00 AM to 3:30 P.M.	Place Initials in the appropriate box										
	3:00 PM to 11:30 P.M.											
	11:00 PM to 7:00 AM											

Place Initials in the box alongside the standard when completed (Team Coordinator)
Provide a variance explanation code if key indicator completed on a day other than the target day (Team Coordinator or ICC)

Source: Reprinted, with permission, from St. Francis Medical Center.

pathway (figure 5-2) is not time specific but provides checkpoints at critical phases of care that affect the patient's transition to the next appropriate level of care. Pathway content focuses on processes, providing an additional tool for the health care team to use in making decisions about the timing and appropriateness of care. The generic pathways are also used for those patients who "fall off" their diagnosis- or procedure-specific path during hospitalization.

Documentation Integration

As the pathway program evolved, so did the need to integrate it with the interdisciplinary care plan. Integration has minimized duplicative documentation by the nursing staff and has centralized patient care parameters in a single document. An initiative is under way to develop exception-based preprinted physician orders that correspond to the daily pathway recommendations. This initiative has prompted physician groups to become more involved in evaluating, and in many instances reevaluating, the patient care guidelines previously established and approved by the medical staff.

INTERDISCIPLINARY PATHWAY VARIANCES

The inclusion of physician practice guidelines in the pathways resulted in more clinically relevant pathway content. It soon became apparent that pathways should focus on the outcomes of care rather than the tasks, so the pathway variance-reporting process was revised.

Initially, any deviation from a pathway recommendation was identified as a variance, resulting in volumes of data that proved to be of minimal value. With the new focus on patient outcomes, clinicians acknowledged that not every element on the

CHAPTER 5 CREATING A MULTIDISCIPLINARY DISEASE MANAGEMENT INITIATIVE

FIGURE 5-2 Generic Medical Pathway

St. Francis Medical Center, Trenton, New Jersey — GENERIC MEDICAL

Admission Date: _/_/_ Discharge Date: _/_/_
Final DRG: _____
Estimated Length of Stay: _____

Collaboration Key:
- PF = Patient/Family
- R = Resident
- PAT = Preadmit
- P = Physician
- A = Ancillary Dept.
- PC = Pastoral Care
- TC = Team Coor.
- ICC = Int. Case Coor.

This pathway is a "Tool" to facilitate multidisciplinary patient care. Patient care will be tailored to the individual patient and may differ from the pathway. The care pathway does not replace clinical judgement of the professional health care team, including the physician's order.

Shaded boxes represent the goal day

Phases: Diagnostic (24 hrs, 48 hrs) | Recovery | Transition (Pre-D/C, D/C 24 hrs)

Key Indicators are Bolded and Asterisked
SHADED GUIDELINE REPRESENTS GERIATRIC FOCUS

Page 1 of 2

Category	Collaboration	Item
PATIENT OUTCOME	P,R,TC,IC,A	1. Pt. tolerating adequate nutritional intake
	P,R,TC,IC,A	2. Pts. activity appropriate for specific D/C setting
	P,R,TC,IC,A	3. Pt./Caretaker verbalizes understanding and/or demonstrates understanding of D/C teaching*
	P,R,TC,ICC	Pt. discharged if D/C criteria met*
DISCHARGE PLANNING	TC,ICC	Assessment completed for D/C Planning intervention*
	TC,ICC	Assess home environment*
	P,R,TC	Eval. for D/C readiness and coordinate D/C order*
	P,R,TC	Coordinate D/C plan*
	P,R,TC	Assess for treatment or testing in alternate setting if indicated*
	ICC,TC	Finalize continued care arrangements including needed paperwork and DME arrangements*
	P,R,TC,ICC	Patient discharged*
ASSESSMENTS	P,R,TC	Assess appropriateness of preadmission medications*
	P,R,TC,IC,A	Patient risk assessment (Falls, ADL's, infection, etc)
	TC	Assess skin integrity
	P,R,TC	Assess cognition
	P,R,TC	Assess nutritional/fluid status*
	P,R,TC	Assess to D/C O2 if indicated
	P,R,TC	Assess to switch to PO antibiotics if indicated*
	P,R,TC	Advanced directive
	P,R,TC	Code status
CONSULTS/ REFERRALS	P,R,TC,A	Nutrition if indicated
	P,R,TC,ICC	Discharge Planning if indicated
	P,R,TC,A	PT if indicated
	PC	Pastoral Care
	P,R,TC	Consult for feeding tube placement if indicated*
	P,R,TC,IC,A	Other
TESTS/ PROCEDURES	P,R,TC,A	Admission Chem Screen
	P,R,TC,A	Chem 6 if indicated
	P,R,TC,A	CBC
	P,R,TC,A	Urinalysis
	P,R,TC,A	Cultures as indicated/Other diagnostic lab procedures
	P,R,TC,A	Diagnostic Radiology as indicated
	P,R,TC,A	Diagnostic Cardiology as indicated
	P,R,TC,A	Consider thyroid studies if geriatric patient
	P,R,TC	Check study/testing results and coordinate plan of care or D/C based on results*
	P,R,TC,A	Minor diagnostic procedure if indicated*
TREATMENTS/ INTERVENTIONS ELIMINATION	TC	VS Q 8 AM and 8 PM or as ordered
	TC	VS prior to D/C*
	TC	Skin care
	P,R,TC	Assess bowel function
	TC	Tube/drain care if indicated
	TC	Weight*
	P,R,TC	D/C Foley cath if indicated*
	P,R,TC	D/C IV if indicated*

PATHWAY CONTINUED ON NEXT PAGE

KEY PROCESSES:
1. Mobilization
2. Patient/Family/SO teaching
3. Test/procedure turnaround
4. Pain management
5. Discharge planning
6. Nutrition

FIGURE 5-2 Continued

					Shaded boxes represent the goal day	
St. Francis Medical Center, Trenton, New Jersey		**GENERIC MEDICAL**				

Admission Date: _/_/_ Discharge Date: _/_/_
Final DRG: _____
Estimated Length of Stay: _____
PMH: _____

This pathway is a "Tool" to facilitate multidisciplinary patient care. Patient care will be tailored to the individual patient and may differ from the pathway. The care pathway does not replace clinical judgement of the professional health care team, including the physician's order.

				Diagnostic	Recovery	Transition
			DATE			Pre-D/C | D/C
		Key Indicators are Bolded and Asterisked	DAY	24 hrs. | 48 hrs.		24 hrs.
Page 2 of 2	Collaboration	*SHADED GUIDELINE REPRESENTS GERIATRIC FOCUS				
MEDICATION/ PAIN MNGT	P,R,TC	Switch to PO Antibiotics if indicated*				
	P,R,TC	Stool softener/Laxative if indicated				
	P,R,TC	Nightime sedation if indicated				
	P,R,TC	Pain medication if indicated				
ACTIVITY	P,R,TC,A	OOB or progressive activity as indicated*				
	TC	Turn Q 2 hrs. if on bedrest				
	TC,A	Range of motion as indicated				
	A	Departmental PT if indicated				
NUTRITION	P,R,TC,A	Diet as ordered/assess for progression				
	P,R,TC,A	Supplementation as indicated				
	P,R,TC,A	Assess for disease specific diet as indicated				
PATIENT/ FAMILY EDUCATION	R,TC,A,PF	Orientation to hospital routine and environment				
	P,R,TC,A,PF	Explain all studies				
	P,R,TC,PF	Medications				
	P,R,TC,PF	Disease specific teaching*				
	P,R,TC,PF	D/C teaching				
	P,R,TC,PF	Review Discharge Instructions				
	P,R,TC	Check patient has prescriptions				
COMORBID CARE Dr._____						
UTILIZATION	ICC	Admission Review				
	ICC	Continued Stay Review				
	ICC	Discharge Review*				
NURSING	7:00 AM to 3:30 P.M.	Place Initials in the appropriate box				
	3:00 PM to 11:30 P.M.					
	11:00 PM to 7:00 AM					

Place Initials in the box alongside the standard when completed (Team Coordinator)
Provide a variance explanation code if key indicator completed on a day other than the target day (Team Coordinator or ICC)

Source: Reprinted, with permission, from St. Francis Medical Center.

---

pathway had an impact on patient outcome. For this reason the variance-reporting process was modified so that data were collected only for those interventions considered to have a significant impact on patient outcomes or appropriateness of care (that is, the evidence-based recommendations). These interventions, termed *key indicators* (see, for example, figure 5-1), are selected by the pathway design team during the initial pathway development process. Key indicators have two purposes:

1. Provide the health care team with several critical aspects of care to be evaluated concurrently to maximize patient outcomes
2. Provide the basis for variance collection, as data are gathered only for these indicators

Early attempts at managing large volumes of pathway variance data proved to be cumbersome and time consuming. This problem has been eliminated through automation. St. Francis Medical Center, a part of the Catholic Healthcare Initiatives (CHI) system, recently installed the CHI-selected decision support system entitled Transition Systems, Inc. (TSI). The system's quality management module, Transition for Quality, integrates pathway data with quality, utilization, and financial information. TSI functions as a data repository and provides automated reports that support many of the performance improvement initiatives within the medical center.

CASE MANAGEMENT EVOLUTION

With the launching of the clinical pathway program in 1990, nurse care coordinators were designated for each patient unit. As liaisons between the caregivers to promote coordinated patient care, they were also responsible for overseeing patients' progress on the pathways and for reporting variances. With the advent of the interdisciplinary development model, the care coordinators became service line focused.

One advantage of the previous unit-based model of care management was that the coordinator developed a rapport with the nursing staff on a particular unit. A significant disadvantage was the coordinator's inability to support patient care continuity as patients moved from unit to unit. The unit-based model also precluded the care coordinator from developing expertise in a particular clinical area, resulting in a generalized approach to care coordination.

The service-line model of care management offered the care coordinator an opportunity to develop specific clinical expertise and provide specialized, condition-unique case management. In this model the care coordinator followed patients wherever they were receiving care, which improved continuity of care. As for rapport with the health care team, service-line care coordinators seemed to have no difficulties collaborating with caregivers within a specialty or unit. An added advantage to the service-line approach was that patients became more familiar with their care coordinators because the same person oversaw their progress on subsequent hospital admissions.

Further, the service-line model proved to enhance pathway variance data collection and interpretation. Aggregated variance data became more reliable once care coordinators having specific clinical expertise were involved in the reporting process. Patterns of care that emerged in the analysis of variance data were more likely to be statistically significant.

In 1994 St. Francis Medical Center implemented a *patient-focused care model* of service delivery. In this model patients having similar resource and service needs are cared for on the same nursing unit. Patient care coordination became the responsibility of the bedside nurse, the team coordinator. Key to the success of the model implementation was the clinical pathway system. Coordinating care using pathways as a guide had become part of the culture of the medical center and was therefore easily assimilated into the bedside nurse's role. During the transition care coordinators served as one-on-one resources for the unit staff members to reinforce their team coordinator role and assist them in learning new skills. In addition, each patient's pathway status was included in the shift report and became an integral component of the patient interdisciplinary care-planning rounds.

In 1995 the care coordinator's function was again redesigned and redefined. These individuals were retrained to provide support for utilization review, social services, discharge planning, and outcomes management functions. This was a milestone in the development of the program. It provided the transition from a care management model, focusing solely on coordination of care in the acute setting, to a case management model, in which one person coordinates care and links services across the continuum.

Today the original care coordinators, along with other staff, serve as integrated case coordinators (ICCs). They support care management efforts by collaborating with the team coordinator and the patient's physician to identify and collect pathway variance data, while also performing their other duties.

PERFORMANCE IMPROVEMENT

St. Francis Medical Center has incorporated clinical pathways into its performance improvement initiatives. Mechanisms aimed at improving patient outcomes include:

- Monitoring of key indicators
- Management of resource consumption
- Education of patients and their families to improve their understanding of disease and care processes and encourage participation in achieving improved outcomes

The key indicators identified by pathway design teams complement other quality initiatives under way within the medical center. The goal is to eliminate duplicative data collection and provide valuable information to support the performance improvement initiatives. A quality management representative works with the pathway design teams to identify critical outcome measures and refine study parameters. The ICCs collect utilization data (that is, level of care, necessity of care, utilization of resources, and efficacy of care) and enter these data into the quality management module of the TSI system.

Trended data are forwarded to service-line teams composed of interdisciplinary representatives, including a physician leader and a quality department representative. These teams analyze the data, identify improvement opportunities, and coordinate the implementation of activities aimed at refining care processes. The service-line teams are also responsible for recommending, implementing, and monitoring pathway processes, including revisions, when necessary. Team structure allows for centralized accountability, monitoring, and oversight for service-line performance.

CARE CONNECTION: THE CONGESTIVE HEART FAILURE DISEASE MANAGEMENT INITIATIVE

As St. Francis Medical Center entered into more managed care contracts, it became apparent that patient care needed to be coordinated across the continuum. If resource consumption, length of stay, and quality goals were to be achieved, a disease management initiative was necessary. More than half (62.5 percent) of employee benefits managers of major corporations view disease management programs as an important service from HMOs.[2] To manage patients who have chronic diseases, necessary support systems and services must be made available to physicians, as well as to patients and their families. As a first step toward achieving these goals, clinicians worked together to develop a disease management model for patients with CHF.

Disease management is an approach to controlling a defined illness or injury by integrating all components of health care to provide the best total patient outcomes at the most reasonable or effective cost.[3] By introducing interventions throughout the life cycles of acute and chronic diseases, disease management aims to improve patient outcomes. This approach also blends patient care with systematic measurement, data analysis, and proactive patient intervention techniques.[4] *Care Connection* is the term used by St. Francis Medical Center to describe its disease management initiative.

FIGURE 5-3 Development Model

Establishing the diagnosis or condition to be managed
⬇
Defining measurable goals for the disease management intervention
⬇
Identifying optimal treatments and interventions for achieving goals
⬇
Providing education and continued support for physicians, patients, and allied health professionals
⬇
Measuring outcomes and providing feedback to caregivers

The interdisciplinary development model of care management, which had previously been applied only to inpatients, played an integral role in the development and implementation of the disease management program. In addition, the CHF disease management project provided an opportunity for clinicians to develop a program template that would be used to design additional disease management programs for other patient populations.

A continuous quality improvement approach (figure 5-3) was used to develop and implement the Care Connection program. These steps are detailed in the remainder of this chapter.

ESTABLISHING THE DIAGNOSIS OR CONDITION TO BE MANAGED

Prior to the implementation of the disease management program, data were collected to support project need. The following information from the U.S. Department of Health and Human Services was included in the analysis:[5]

- During this century chronic diseases have replaced infectious diseases as the leading causes of death.
- Three chronic diseases—heart disease, cancer, and stroke—account for more than 70 percent of the deaths in the age 65+ population.
- More than 80 percent of Americans aged 65 and older suffer from one or more chronic diseases.

CHF is the highest volume diagnosis for inpatient care in the United States, with approximately $10 billion in health care dollars being spent annually for this patient population.[6] The St. Francis experience was typical of these national trends. For several years patients with CHF (DRG 127) have constituted the highest volume of hospital admissions. The majority of inpatient admissions at St. Francis originate in the emergency department. Very few patients with CHF have a single admission. In fact, data indicated that 60 percent of patients seen at St. Francis for treatment of CHF had at least two admissions each year, 22 percent had three admissions, and 18 percent had more than four admissions. Dialogue with patients suggested that they perceived their quality of life to be diminished by their dependence on inpatient care. Based on these data, the medical center's quality council elected to make the heart failure population the focus of the first disease management program, entitled *Care Connection: CHF.*

DEFINING MEASURABLE GOALS

The goal of disease management is to provide an alternative to traditional inpatient care for patients with chronic disease by managing their care across the continuum. The objectives of the CHF pilot program as established by the quality council included the following:

- Improve the perceived quality of life of the patient with chronic CHF.
- Decrease emergency department visits.
- Decrease inpatient admissions.
- Decrease length of stay for admitted patients.

IDENTIFYING OPTIMAL TREATMENTS AND INTERVENTIONS

A multidisciplinary project team, which included all providers identified as contributors to the care of this patient population, was assembled. (See figure 5-4.) To identify the disease management interventions necessary for achieving the program goals, the CHF project team reviewed several research studies on CHF. The team found that the typical patient with chronic CHF has an interesting health profile that contributes to and explains his or her high use of health care resources, for example:[7]

- Approximately 82 percent of patients with chronic CHF are over age 65.
- More than 50 percent of the age 65+ population has three or more comorbidities that affect treatment and prognosis. On average, this population takes six different medications daily to manage disease process or comorbid condition.
- It is not uncommon for patients with CHF to survive 5–10 years after their initial diagnosis.

The bulk of the U.S. health care dollar typically has been utilized for managing acute episodes of CHF in emergency and inpatient settings. Historically, very few resources have been invested in disease prevention or alternative disease management strategies. The CHF patient's traditional cycle of dependence on acute services appeared to be influenced by the following four factors:[8]

FIGURE 5-4 Multidisciplinary Team Members

Team leader	Physician sponsor	Team facilitator
Director of Heart Institute	Cardiologist	Director of utilization management

Team members
  Care coordinator from cardiology
  Director of ambulatory services
  Nurse practitioner
  Director of noninvasive cardiology
  Cardiac rehab nurse
  Nurse manager from cardiac care unit or step-down unit
  Cardiopulmonary clinical specialist
  Nurse manager from outreach services
  Outreach social worker
  Community health nurse

Advisory team
  Director of quality improvement or risk management
  Medical director of emergency department
  Medical residency director
  Medical resident
  Medical director of community outreach
  Director of medical records
  Director of patient services
  Director of utilization review
  Manager of clinic
  Nursing or patient education coordinator

FIGURE 5-5 Cause-and-Effect Diagram for the Management of Congestive Heart Failure

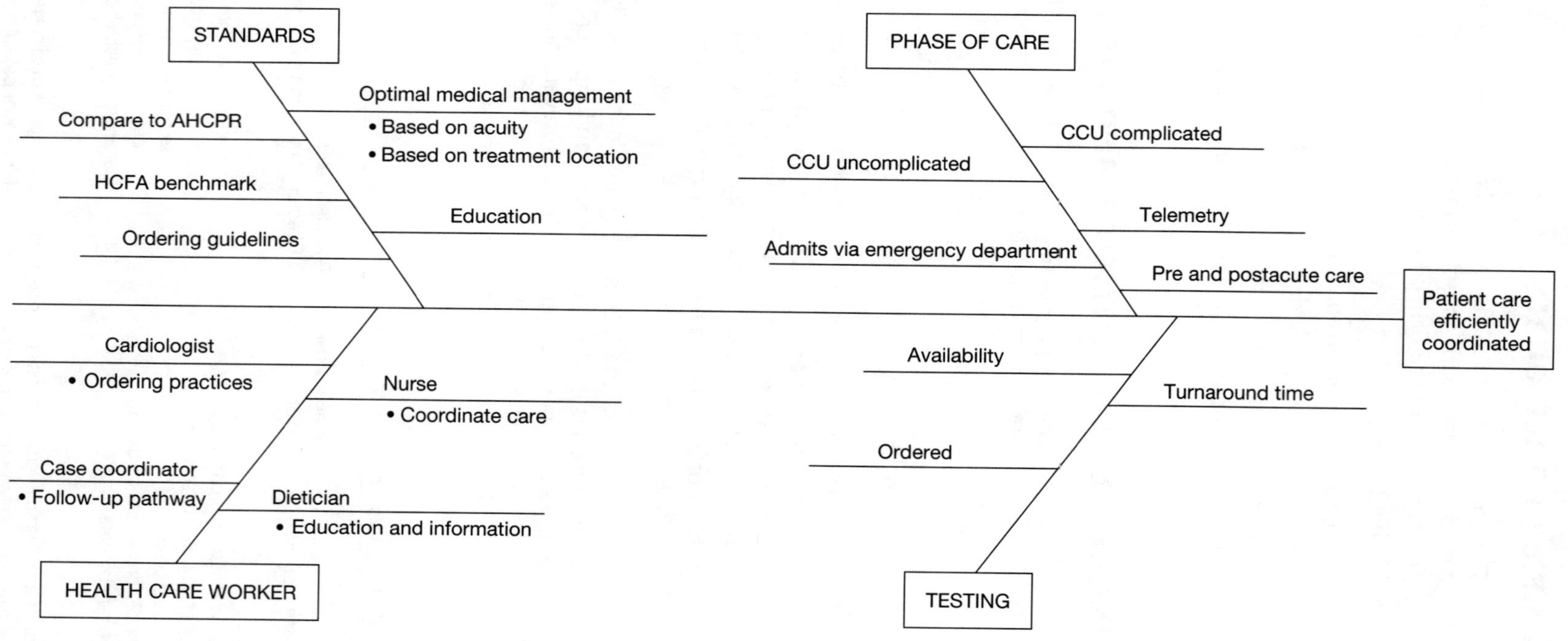

1. Patients and their families typically have not been educated to detect and manage early CHF symptoms.
2. This lack of knowledge causes delays in managing early CHF symptoms, and by the time patients present for treatment, their situation exceeds the capability of physician office management.
3. Patients are then directed to the emergency department, where more than 90 percent of those seen are admitted to the hospital.
4. Reimbursement methodologies encourage caregivers to focus on decreasing CHF patients' length of stay. This results in earlier discharge, which increases the patients' risk of hospital readmission.

The CHF project team members used information they gleaned from the literature to select the key factors that needed to be in place to break the CHF patient's cycle of acute care dependence. The team developed a cause-and-effect diagram, a problem-solving tool indicating effects and causes and how they interrelate.[9] The team analyzed the strengths and weakness of the current CHF patient care system and identified high-priority factors, such as emergency department visits and lack of postdischarge support, that appear to be causing unnecessary hospital admissions. (See figure 5-5.)

The cause-and-effect diagramming exercise helped the team select the important issues that needed to be addressed by the Care Connection: CHF program. Based on the team's brainstorming exercise, these issues included:

- Physician support for referral into the program, approval of protocols, and assistance with patient management
- Mechanisms to provide opportunities to interact with patients and monitor progress
- A care coordinator to oversee the program, coordinate multiple components, and identify and resolve issues as they develop
- A multidisciplinary team having knowledge and experience in the management of patients with CHF
- Methods of communicating with patients to assure prompt contact with team members and timely management of clinical issues
- Patient and family empowerment to facilitate active participation in the program and shift locus of control
- Resources required for patient management, such as scales, appropriate food, medications, and telephones

A variety of strategies for addressing these issues were discussed by the team, along with the rationale for their selection. (See table 5-1.)

Care Connection: CHF Program Strategies

Once the proposed strategies were finalized, the team reviewed the existing process of CHF patient management to identify where these strategies could best be introduced into the continuum of care. They were integrated into the existing process and a new flowchart (figure 5-6) showing the improved process was designed.

To successfully implement a nontraditional program such as Care Connection: CHF, a wide variety of tools and resources needed to be assembled. Some of hospital-based care components could be merged with the disease management initiative, while in other instances, new resources needed to be developed. Care Connection: CHF program tools and resources and the roles they play in the disease management initiative are listed below.

TABLE 5-1 Improvement Strategies Chosen and Rationale for Choices

Issue	Strategy	Rationale
Physician support	Select physician champion	Physician-to-physician interactions are most effective.
		Cardiologist on staff had participated in the development of and supported nontraditional programs in the past.
Interaction with patients	Heart failure clinic	Advanced practice nurse would see patient with frequency determined by clinical status.
	Cardiac rehabilitation	Provides opportunity to: • Assess weight, medication and diet adherence • Interact with other CHF patients for support
	Community health nurse visits	Allows homebound patients to participate in program and facilitates assessment of status between clinic visits as needed
	Telemanagement	Provides 24-hour-a-day capability for interaction with patients and their families
Program oversight and coordination	Physician advisor	Provides clinical oversight of patient management as well as consultation for difficult cases
	Care coordinator	Coordinates program components, facilitates referrals to other disciplines
		Cardiology case manager on site with the expertise to function in expanded role
Multidisciplinary team participation	Care Connection: CHF team	Include medical center staff having expertise in management of this patient population to facilitate quality, effective disease management
Communication tools	Hot line	Provides contact with team on a 24-hour-a-day basis
	Forms	Standardized forms for assessment, management available to caregivers to promote continuity of care by all disciplines
	On-line intervention summary	Provides immediate access to most recent patient data for all team members
	Program identifier	Identifies patient as a Care Connection participant in all medical center interactions
Patient and family empowerment	Hot line	Provides security and backup for patients and their families throughout program
	Patient pathway	Identifies expectations of patients, their families, and caregivers
	Patient and family education	Provides education regarding medication, visits
		Increases participation and adherence to program participation
Patient management resources	Scales	Key to evaluation of weight gain, medication and diet compliance
	Medication	Frequently, patients unable to access meds due to financial or transportation constraints
	Food	Right types and amounts essential to maintain weight, sodium or caloric intake
	Telephone	Necessary to participate in telemanagement
	Transportation	Patients unable to attend clinic, rehab

FIGURE 5-6 Defined Process of Care

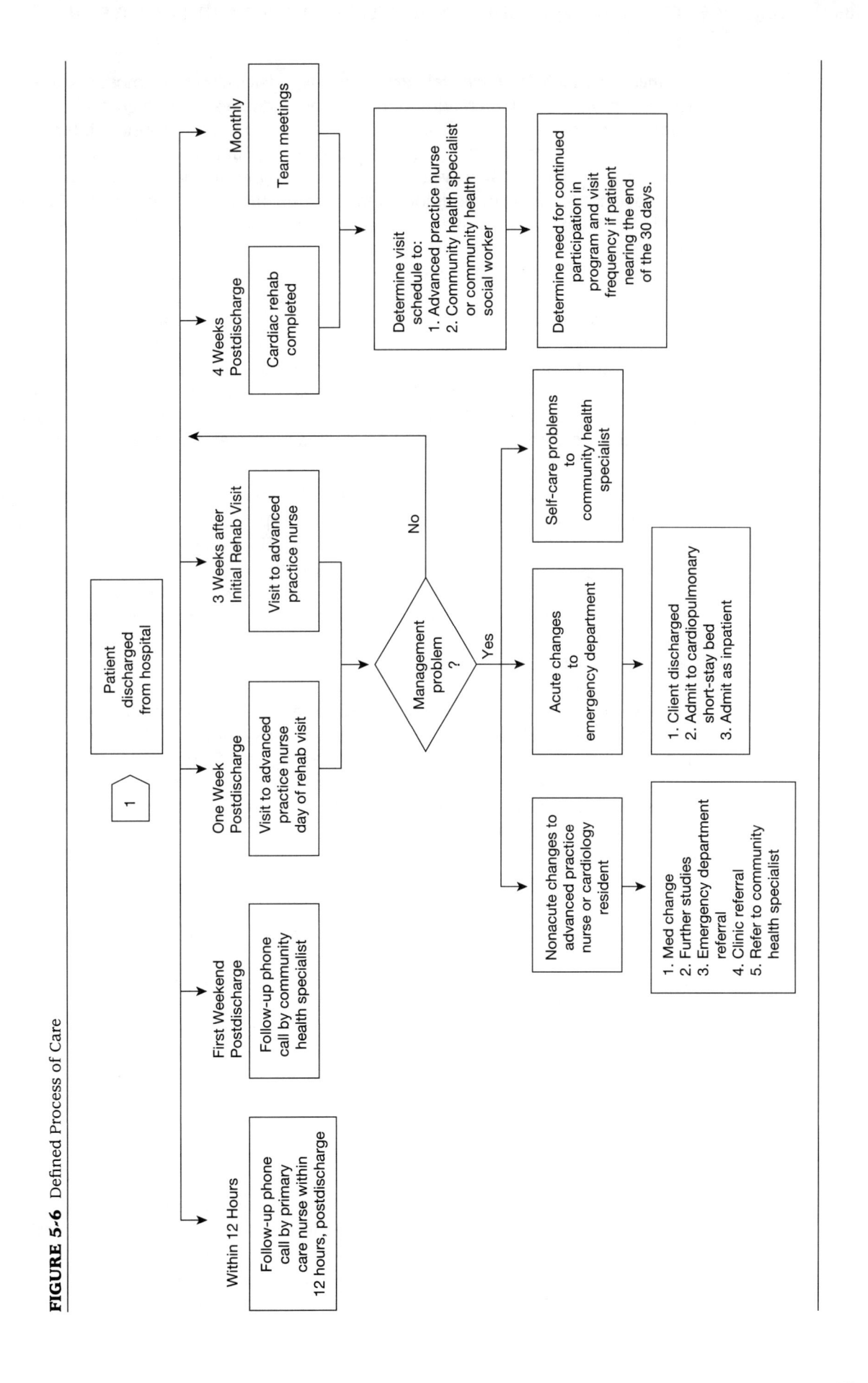

Prospective Plans for Care Delivery An important element of most disease management programs is the creation of treatment guidelines.[10] These guidelines provide a framework for caregiver decision making to ensure that appropriate interventions are used to manage diseases. Treatment guidelines cannot address the therapeutic needs of *every* patient; however, they can be designed for the majority of patients with specific diseases. In addition, treatment guidelines can be developed by the health care team to resolve treatment decisions in which there may be clinically equivalent treatment choices or controversies.[11]

The treatment guidelines developed for the Care Connection: CHF program were displayed in many different formats: clinical pathways, clinical algorithms, and protocols. The format varied according to the intended user of the guideline and the purpose of the tool. For example, pathways provide caregivers with a clinical management tool that organizes, sequences, and times the major interventions of nursing staff, physicians, and other disciplines,[12] whereas clinical algorithms illustrate a complex series of assessment, diagnostic, or treatment decisions.[13] Protocols are descriptions of the recommended course of action in a particular clinical situation.

Clinical pathways: To assure that CHF patients are managed appropriately across the continuum, clinical pathways needed to be developed for the acute care, short-stay, and home care phases. The medical center had CHF pathways in place for patients admitted to general med/surg units, telemetry units, and complicated/uncomplicated critical care units. These hospital pathways were reviewed by the Care Connection: CHF team and revised to include the assessment criteria for determining patients' entry into and discharge from the Care Connection: CHF program and the emergency care components. (See figure 5-7.)

In addition, a subgroup was formed to develop a CHF short-stay pathway. This group was composed of physicians, nurses, social workers, community health specialists, cardiac rehabilitation specialists, and clinicians from the laboratory, radiology, and respiratory therapy. The short-stay pathway (figure 5-8) included the development of criteria that caregivers could use to determine a patient's potential for short stay versus the need for inpatient admission. This pathway defines the hour-to-hour management of the patient, beginning in the emergency department. Admission appropriateness criteria and other key decision points are integrated with the care management recommendations.

Clinical algorithms: Where appropriate, clinical algorithms are used to encourage the critical thinking processes necessary to minimize variation and improve patient outcomes. The algorithms provide clinicians with alternative care options based on the outcome of the patient's physical, psychological, and social assessments. The effectiveness and accuracy of critical thinking principles are integral to selecting the appropriate treatment for achieving optimal patient outcomes.[14] The algorithm developed by the Agency for Health Care Policy and Research for the management of patients with CHF (figure 5-9) forms the basis for disease management in the Care Connection program.[15]

Protocols: Protocols describing appropriate management of CHF-related clinical situations were developed for use in the heart failure clinic and for telemanagement purposes. These protocols were developed jointly by the physicians, the medical residents, and an advanced practice nurse. The protocols closely parallel the algorithm (figure 5-9); however, they provide more comprehensive details about the interventions to be incorporated into the management of the patient.

FIGURE 5-7 Admission, Exclusion, and Discharge Criteria

Admission   Clinical
1. High potential for hospital readmission
2. Frequent CHF exacerbations
3. Referral
4. Physician collaboration with care team

Socioeconomic
1. Patient and family agreement to participate in program
2. Absence of active psychosocial problems that would inhibit attainment of program goals
3. Patient is competent to provide consent to care

Exclusion   Clinical
1. High probability that patient may not benefit from program due to advanced disease state
2. Physician unwillingness to collaborate with care team

Socioeconomic
1. Patient's level-of-care needs cannot be managed safely in the home
2. Lack of support system in the home

Discharge   Clinical
1. Patient no longer requires intensive monitoring
2. Patient demonstrates ability to independently identify signs of disease exacerbation and seek appropriate level of treatment
3. End-stage disease or admission to hospice
4. Patient or family noncompliant with program protocol

Socioeconomic
1. Change in level of care while in community setting
2. Patient no longer willing to participate in program

Specialty Clinics and Services   It was clear that a number of resources were required in order to effectively manage the chronic CHF population. As a result, a variety of services were developed or modified to meet the specific needs of this population and this project. For example, the methodology of the cardiac clinic was modified to provide a clinic specific to heart failure, and a totally new telemanagement process was developed.

Heart failure clinic: The team proposed and implemented a heart failure clinic directed by an advanced practice nurse (APN) along with a collaborating physician. The APN sees patients at intervals determined by each patient's condition, monitors each patient's progress, and modifies the plan of care based on clinical response to interventions. The clinical protocol is used by the APN to manage the average patient's care, with the collaborating physician serving as a resource in complex or complicated cases. For convenience, the clinic is located in an area of the medical center adjacent to cardiac services such as inpatient units, cardiac diagnostics, and cardiac rehabilitation.

Cardiac rehabilitation: Care Connection patients who are physically capable also participate in cardiac rehabilitation. Typically, patients are seen two to three times each week in the rehab program, where their activity, hemodynamic response, exercise tolerance, weight, lung sounds, peripheral edema, and medication adherence are assessed. The primary purpose of this component of the Care Connection: CHF program

FIGURE 5-8 Congestive Heart Failure Short-Stay Pathway

St. Francis Medical Center, Trenton, New Jersey	CONGESTIVE HEART FAILURE SHORT STAY

Admission Date: __/__/__ Discharge Date: __/__/__
Final DRG: _____
Estimated Length of Stay: _____
PMH: _____

This pathway is a "Tool" to facilitate multidisciplinary patient care. Patient care will be tailored to the individual patient and may differ from the pathway. The care pathway does not replace clinical judgement of the professional health care team, including the physician's order.

Shaded boxes represent the goal hour

	Key Indicators are Bolded and Asterisked	UNIT HRS	ED 1 2 3	Cardio–Pulmonary Short Stay 1 2 3 4 5 6 7 8 12 16 20 24
ASSESSMENT/ UTILIZATION	Admission to Cardio–Pulmonary short stay if potential for rapid diuresis and early discharge*			
	Discharge if: Lungs clear, edema < or = 2+*			
	Continue hospitalization if: D/C criteria not met within 24 hours*			
DISCHARGE PLANNING	Nursing assessment for discharge planning			
	Discharge planning assessment (in–home nursing assessment/lab testing)			
TESTS/ PROCEDURES	Admission Chem Screen (0018)			
	CBC with auto diff (5031)			
	Cardiac Profile Q 8 hrs. X 3			
	PT/APTT			
	Pulse Oximetry			
	EKG (2)			
	CXR (1020)*			
	Chem 6 if significant weight loss			
ACTIVITY/ REHAB	Bedrest			
	Progressive Activity			
	Ambulate*			
NUTRITION	4 gm. Cardiac diet			
TREATMENT/ ASSESSMENT/ ELIMINATION	IV Fluids (KVO)			
	Saline Lock			
	Cardiac Monitor			
	Weight*			
	Cardio–pulmonary assessment to include lung sounds, neck vein distention and edema*			
	Assess preadmission diet and fluid intake*			
	VS			
	I&O*			
MEDICATION/ PAIN MNGT	Oxygen PRN			
	IV diuretic*			
	Review Pre–admission meds*			
PATIENT/ FAMILY EDUCATION	Hospitalization			
	Disease specific			
	CHF teaching packet			
NURSING	7:00 AM to 3:30 PM / 3:00 PM to 11:30 PM / 11:00 PM to 7:00 AM	Place Initials in the appropriate box		

Place Initials in the box alongside the standard when completed (Team Coordinator)
Provide a variance explanation code if completed on a day other than the standard (Team Coordinator or ICC)

42

Source: Reprinted, with permission, from St. Francis Medical Center.

is to provide patients with an opportunity to interact with the health care team and to monitor patients' progress. In addition, patients' educational needs regarding diet, activity, and medications are continually reinforced, and patients have the opportunity to interact with others who have similar conditions.

Telemanagement: Telemanagement is a term applied to a number of telephone activities occurring between the team and patients or their families. These activities are

FIGURE 5-9 Clinical Algorithm for Evaluation and Care of Patients with Heart Failure

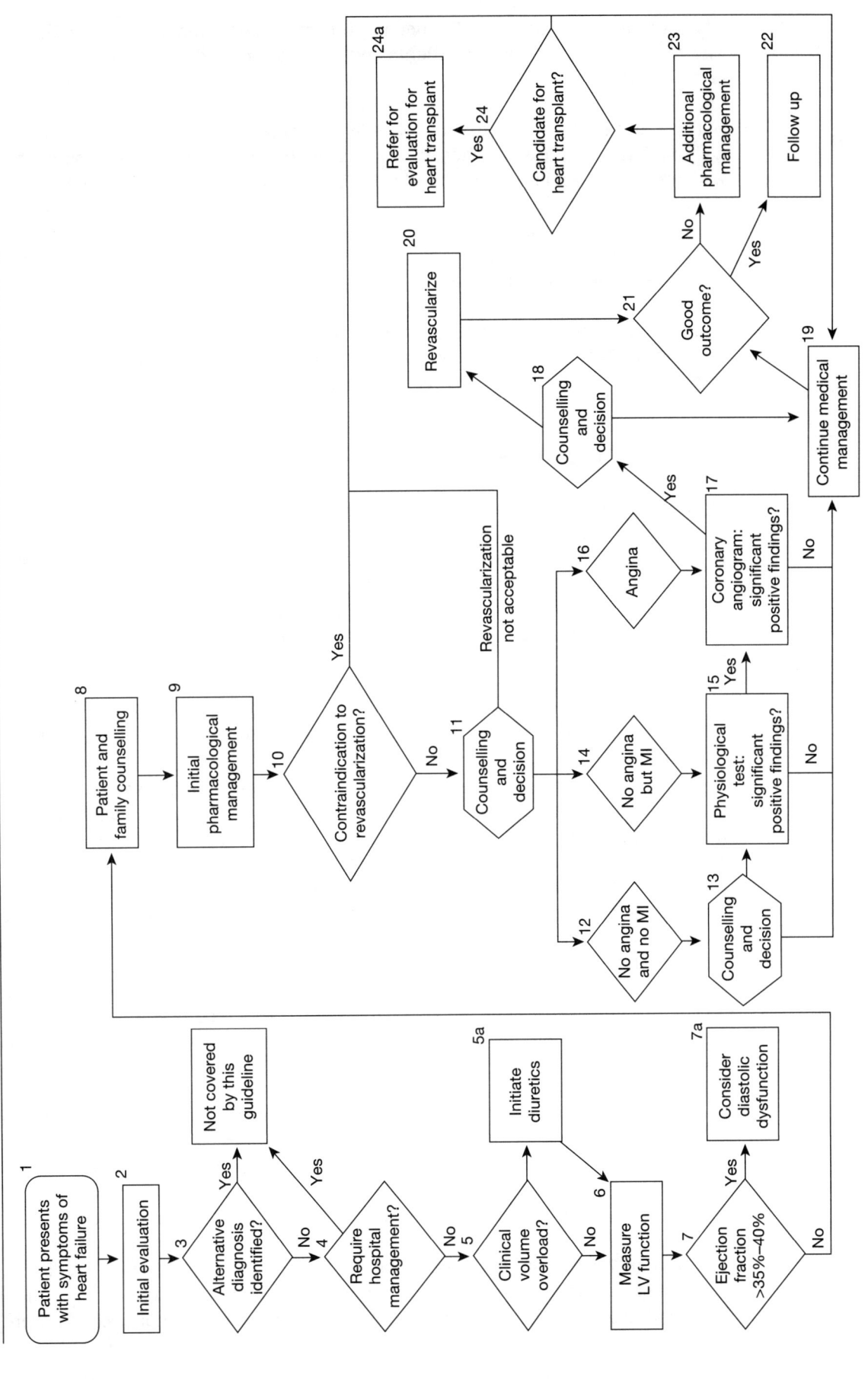

Source: Konstam, M., Dracup, K., Baker, D., and others. *Heart Failure: Evaluation and Care of Patients with Left-Ventricular Systolic Dysfunction, Clinical Practice Guideline No. 11* (publication no. 94-0612). Rockville, MD: Agency for Health Care Policy and Research, Public Health Service, U.S. Department of Health and Human Services, June 1994.

key components of the Care Connection program, since they provide for 24-hour-a-day communication between patients and their care providers. Patients are taught to contact a team member at any time of the day or night when their clinical status changes or other concerns arise. Available communication options include a toll-free hot line and beeper numbers for the APN and care management coordinator. Typically, patients call the APN when the clinic is open. Outside of normal business hours, patients call the hot line number and reach the medical center operator, who connects them with the APN or a medical resident. Depending on the concerns expressed by the patient, the responder may initiate protocol-based interventions, request that a community health specialist visit the patient at home, provide support and counseling, or refer the patient to the emergency department.

Patients and their families are educated about the early signals of change in their clinical status and are encouraged to notify the team immediately when these symptoms occur. Rapid response to patients' concerns and early intervention have proved to be the key to effective CHF disease management and quality-of-life improvements for patients.

Documentation Tools Early in the Care Connection: CHF program developmental phase, it was clear that documentation played an important role. Therefore, a variety of tools were developed to ensure complete and comprehensive record keeping. The first project to be completed was an integrated assessment form designed with multidisciplinary input. The assessment form, while comprehensive, presents some difficulties in its current format and is currently undergoing revision.

Documentation of the patient's clinic visits as well as home visits by the community health specialists are included in the community-based record, a component of the outpatient chart. This file includes patient demographic and historical clinical data, clinical flow sheet, problem list, and medication profile. Other forms are available to document the plan of care as well as the patient's progress throughout the program. All documentation is standardized to conform to the medical center's approved format for outpatient records.

An on-line intervention summary was developed and made available to users of the medical center computerized information system. This module includes fields for documenting basic patient data in the Care Connection program as well as a record of their most recent interactions with the care team. The information is accessible to team members when they wish to review or update a patient's record. Medical residents use the data in the intervention summary to determine a patient's current medications, most recent visit or call, and continuing plan of care.

The intervention summary is also useful for telemanagement activities. Typically this patient population telephones during the night when symptoms develop or when they are frightened or alone. Since patients' outpatient records may not be immediately accessible to telemanagers, the computerized summary allows them to make timely, appropriate recommendations. To date, this has been one of the most valuable tools utilized by Care team members.

A program identifier, contained in the information system and unique to patients in the Care Connection: CHF program, allows admission registrars and medical center staff to recognize program participants wherever they access care. This alert reminds the staff that the patient is a Care Connection participant and encourages them to review the patient's intervention summary prior to making treatment decisions.

The Human Touch Studies have shown that information alone—without direct human contact—does not affect change in practices.[16,17] The Care Connection: CHF program had to be more than pathways, protocols, and documentation tools if it were to succeed. A Gantt project management chart was developed to guide the progress of the disease management initiative and focus the care team's efforts. During the development of the project management chart, the team identified the human resources necessary to operationalize the Care Connection program. Although their roles and responsibilities were modified during program implementation, defining the key players early in the project helped clarify the personnel resources necessary for meeting the goals of the disease management initiative. Descriptions of the roles and responsibilities of the key team members are listed below.

Physician sponsor: The physician sponsor is the project champion, providing advice regarding appropriate medical management of the CHF patient across the continuum. A cardiologist, this sponsor had actively participated in developing the medical center's successful community outreach program for the homebound elderly. The physician sponsor provides direction for the disease management process, answers the care team's questions about program policy, and is available for consultation on complex patient problems. Initially, the physician sponsor also functioned as the collaborating physician for the APN and assisted in the development of the protocols used in the heart failure clinic. The physician sponsor continues to assist with the coordination of care for CHF patients and is currently involved in evaluating program efficacy.

Care management coordinator: The Care Management Coordinator is the cement that holds the program together and assures the provision of care across the continuum. As former care manager for the cardiology service line, the coordinator had developed a rapport with physicians, staff, and patients and was knowledgeable about the problems involved in managing CHF patients. She was actively involved in developing the inpatient CHF clinical pathways and was highly aware of the critical elements of CHF care in the prehospital, acute care, and postdischarge phases of the continuum.

In the Care Connection: CHF program, the care management coordinator ensures that all viable candidates are evaluated prior to entry into the program and refers those who meet admission criteria to the appropriate services. Once patients are admitted to the program, the coordinator oversees their management, identifying elements of care necessary to meet patients' needs and referring patients to appropriate care team members. She initiates problem-solving activities for unique or complex clinical or social situations. Other responsibilities include directing the meetings of the clinical care team and providing coordination and follow-up when patient problems arise outside of normal working hours.

In addition, the care management coordinator gathers and maintains the data necessary for continuous quality improvement activities and program effectiveness evaluations. This data collection and analysis process is very important to the success of the disease management program, particularly because much patient care occurs outside of acute care, such as at home, subacute or rehabilitation facilities, and nursing homes.

Advanced practice nurse: The APN directs the heart failure clinic and coordinates the provision of ongoing care and follow-up. An important member of the care team, she evaluates patients for entry into the program and reexamines each patient's condition on a regular basis (frequency defined by protocol or team recommendation). When necessary she refers patients to other disciplines and collaborates with all provider sites to ensure appropriateness of care.

The APN plays an important role in identifying nonacute changes in the patient's condition and frequently recommends medication adjustments, diagnostic studies, and community health or clinic visits to avoid further deterioration of the patient's condition. Along with other members of the care team, she empowers patients and families by providing them with education. This education promotes patient and family participation in care and increases their perception of control over the disease process.

Primary care nurse: In each care setting the patient has a primary care nurse. This nurse works with the other members of the health care team to coordinate patient care throughout the continuum. Whether in an acute care setting, nursing home, emergency department, or the community, the primary care nurse assists in identifying program candidates and makes program referrals. This care team member coordinates appropriate patient care using the relevant CHF pathway as a guide. She initiates and reinforces patient and family CHF education, reviews discharge and medication instructions, and establishes follow-up plans for patients transferred to another setting. This nurse also provides backup for other team members, participates in team meetings, and provides problem-solving input.

Cardiac rehabilitation nurse: The cardiac rehabilitation nurse collaborates with other care team members to provide ongoing assessment of the patient's condition, coordinates the appropriate rehabilitation component, and makes referrals to other team members. She provides initial rehabilitation consultation, assesses the patient's activity levels, and arranges transportation for postdischarge visits if indicated. Unlike the traditional cardiac rehabilitation program, whose primary purpose is to increase patients' functional capacity, the CHF rehabilitation program provides for ongoing evaluation of the patient's status and offers an opportunity for the patient to interact with and be supported by staff and other patients. The cardiac rehabilitation nurse also participates in team meetings and provides input into patient management issues and problem solving.

Community health specialists: This outpatient component of the program involves a miniteam that includes a community health nurse, social worker, dietician, and, in select cases, other disciplines, such as physical or occupational therapy. The community health nurse provides initial consultation and referral and performs ongoing assessment of the patient's physical condition, socioeconomic status, and environment. Frequently, the nurse visits the patient in the hospital prior to discharge. The nurse confers with the patient's primary care nurse and other acute care providers, completes the initial community readiness assessment, and validates the ongoing plan of care. Other responsibilities include coordinating postdischarge referrals to other members of the miniteam as well as relevant community agencies, such as Meals on Wheels. In addition, community health specialists arrange for necessary in-home support items such as:

- A scale for the patient to use for monitoring weight
- A telephone, if none is present in the home
- Medications, if the patient does not have ready access to a pharmacy
- Appropriate food, if not readily available

Community health specialists also provide and reinforce ongoing education of patients and their families and participate in team meetings and problem solving.

Mission and ministry department and psychological services: Early in the Care Connection: CHF program implementation, team members noted that some of the most dramatic changes in patients' conditions occurred when psychological support was offered to patients and their families. As a result, approximately 9 months into the project, the team was expanded to include members of the mission and ministry department and psychological services. Currently, patients entering the program have a psychological assessment and are given the option of regular visits by one or more of these team members. Preliminary findings suggest that this intervention has been successful in reducing patients' fear and loss of control.

Other disciplines: A number of other disciplines are involved in managing patients in the Care Connection: CHF program. These individuals have other patient care responsibilities in addition to periodically interacting with CHF patients:

- *Primary care physicians:* The physicians make referrals to the program, manage noncardiac medical problems, and consult with CHF team members for complex or unusual problems.
- *Medical residents:* At St. Francis, the resident staff provides backup for the APN in telemanagement (particularly after hours) and in the heart failure clinic.
- *Emergency department:* Physicians and nurses in the emergency department provide initial treatment of patients with acute symptoms and suggest appropriate disposition options. Many times patients are returned home with the support of the community health nurse or admitted as short-stay (less than 24 hours) patients for aggressive management and rapid discharge.

Patient Education Resources   Patient and family empowerment is an important factor in the success of the Care Connection: CHF program. Empowerment comes from providing patients and their families with the proper health education materials and decision support tools and continually reinforcing their role in managing their disease.[18] Several educational tools were developed specifically for involving patients and families in the care management process.

For example, a patient version of a clinical pathway was designed. (See figure 5-10.) The booklet describes the program and outlines expectations for patients and providers in each component or phase of care. The patient is introduced to the pathway by the care coordinator, who gives the booklet at the time of admission into the program. Patients have responded remarkably well to the pathway. It provides them with a road map for disease management, sets expectations of the patient and the care team, stimulates questions regarding care, and provides a resource for medication schedules, appointments, and so on.

In addition, a protocol outlining the symptoms indicative of early CHF onset and CHF complications was developed. (See figure 5-11.) This instruction sheet clarifies appropriate responses based on symptoms and identifies who to call for assistance. The care coordinator or the APN discusses the instruction sheet with the patient upon program entry, and the information is continually reinforced by all caregivers.

Patient education resources are critical to the program's success. Materials are organized in packets so they can be easily shared with patients and their families. The packets contain all needed information about CHF disease pathology, diagnostic studies, treatment, medications, diet, activity, and other relevant topics. By standardizing the educational information used by all health care team members, continuity of care is enhanced.

In addition to education materials designed for patients, a variety of other resources are necessary to support the Care Connection: CHF patient. Program participants are required to have scales and telephones. If patients or their families are unable to obtain these items, they are supplied by the medical center. Transportation is provided when necessary to ensure that patients are able to get to heart failure clinic appointments and cardiac rehabilitation visits.

FIGURE 5-10 Excerpt from Congestive Heart Failure Patient Pathway

◆
Before You Go Home

DIET

Before you leave, your diet will be advanced to a low salt, low cholesterol diet. The dietitian will provide you with diet information.

AVAILABLE INFORMATION

Your nurse will provide you with teaching sheets and booklets about CHF and your medications. There are teaching videos available for you and your family to view. Your nurse and care coordinator are available to answer any questions or concerns you may have.

You may also view the patient education channel (14 and 16) on your hospital television, free of charge, from 8:00 a.m. to 9:30 p.m.

MEDICATIONS

All medications will be reviewed with you and your family before discharge.

DISCHARGE PLANS

A social worker or discharge planner may meet with you and your family to discuss the best discharge plan for you. Options may be:

- Returning to home with or without home health care nurses, physical therapy
- Short term or long term rehabilitation at a skilled nursing facility

Written discharge instructions will be reviewed with you before you go home.

◆
After You Go Home

Here are some key things you will need to do to stay well:

1. Weigh yourself every morning.
2. Take your medications exactly as your doctor prescribed.
3. Follow a healthy, low salt diet.
4. Plan frequent rest periods.
5. Avoid smoking.
6. Call your doctor for:
   - Increased shortness of breath
   - Unexplained weight gain of 2 to 3 pounds within 24 hours
   - New wheezing, chest pain, cough, or fast heartbeat
   - Respiratory infection
   - Increased swelling in legs, feet, ankles, or abdomen

Source: Reprinted, with permission, from St. Francis Medical Center.

PROVIDING EDUCATION AND CONTINUED SUPPORT

Prior to program implementation, the physician sponsor provided Care Connection: CHF education to physicians, residents, and community health specialists (nurses, dieticians, and social workers). This education helped clarify the purpose of the program, the roles of care team members, and the Care Connection referral process.

Physicians

To ensure that physicians were familiar with the program, educational sessions were provided to members of the department of medicine, particularly the emergency department and the cardiology, internal medicine, and family practice sections. These presentations covered the purpose of Care Connection, clinical protocols, typical patient flow, and the physician's role in the process. Each of these groups was initially addressed by the Care Connection: CHF physician sponsor. Subsequently, more detailed information was provided by other members of the CHF care team.

FIGURE 5-11 Patient Instruction Sheet

CARE CONNECTION INSTRUCTION SHEET
CONGESTIVE HEART FAILURE

TELEPHONE: (609) 599-6400

WHO TO CALL:	▶ CARE CONNECTION (599-6400)	EMERGENCY 911
WHEN TO CALL:	▶ *If you notice one or more of the following:* 1. Increased shortness of breath 2. Unexplained weight gain of 2–3 pounds within 24 hours 3. New wheezing, chest pain, cough, or fast heart beat 4. Respiratory infection 5. Increased swelling in legs, feet, ankles, or abdomen ▶ *Your call will be answered:* "St. Francis Medical Center; Care Connection, How may I help you?" ▶ *You will be asked your name and telephone number* ▶ *Within 10–15 minutes, a Care Connection team member will return your call and instructions will be given at that time* • *If your call is not answered within 15 minutes you must re-call the Care Connection number*	▶ *If you notice sudden severe symptoms of:* 1. Chest pain 2. Severe shortness of breath ▶ **Report to the emergency room at St. Francis Medical Center for evaluation** ▶ **Inform the St. Francis staff that you are a Care Connection patient**

General information:
1. The Care Connection hot line number is available 24 hours a day, seven days a week.
2. For calls not related to your heart, please contact your primary care physician or the clinic at St. Francis Medical Center (599-5050).

Residents

Similar education programs were conducted for third-year residents who would be participating in the heart failure clinic and telemanagement activities and providing emergency and inpatient care for CHF patients. Additional training provided to residents included information about their specific roles in the project, use of the protocols, use of the on-line intervention summary, mechanisms for activating community health specialist visits after hours, and additional resources available for patient management.

Community Health Specialists

In the past, strained relationships had existed between physicians and some community health specialists. The physician sponsor and the CHF care team felt that effective communication between physicians and community health specialists was critical to the success of the project. Therefore, the physician sponsor provided an in-depth educational session that included an overview of the Care Connection: CHF program, a review of CHF pathophysiology, medical management, dietary considerations, and clinical parameters requiring consultation with the APN or physician. The participants found this session particularly valuable, and it was videotaped to ensure that all members of the community health team were able to benefit from the session.

Other Departments

Prior to the implementation of the pilot program, educational sessions were conducted on the nursing units. Particular attention was directed to the staff members mostly likely to interact with CHF patients (emergency department, cardiac care unit, cardiac step-down unit). In addition to receiving an overview of the Care Connection: CHF program, these nurses were taught the role of the primary nurse in identifying potential program candidates, methods of referring patients into the program, the short-stay option, the significance of the patient program identifier, and the importance of patient and family education.

The medical center's telephone operators were also instructed in their program role, methods of contacting care team members, the use of a decision tree for determining backup if identified team members are unable to respond within 5 minutes, and principles of communicating with patients and their families. The emergency department and admission registrars and medical record department staff were provided with basic program education and instructed in the use of the patient's program identifier.

Continuing education is provided as the need indicates. For example, in July of each year new residents are oriented to the Care Connection: CHF program and their role in the process.

MEASURING OUTCOMES AND PROVIDING FEEDBACK

The initial objectives for the Care Connection: CHF program were to:

- Improve the perceived quality of life of the patient with chronic CHF
- Decrease emergency department visits
- Decrease inpatient admissions
- Decrease length of stay for admitted patients

Since inception of the program in 1995, data have been gathered to evaluate achievement of these objectives.

Quality-of-Life Measures

Since a major objective of the Care Connection: CHF program was to improve the perceived quality of life for program participants, the team initially considered developing a survey instrument to measure this parameter. However, this was felt to be an extremely time-consuming and difficult project. Therefore, a tool already designed and validated was chosen: the Living with Heart Failure Questionnaire developed by the University of Minnesota.[19] The tool consists of 21 questions designed to measure the patient's perception of physical function, role function, general health, vitality, social function, and mental health. Patients respond to the questions by rating the degree to which their condition has affected their lives over the past month on a scale of 0–5 (0 being not at all and 5 being very much). This survey takes approximately 30 minutes to complete and is administered to patients by the care coordinator prior to program entry and every 3 months thereafter. Changes in patients' perceptions are based on comparisons of their scores at various points in the program.

Measurement results demonstrate the percentage difference in patients' perceptions of quality of life by comparing their initial survey results with their latest completed survey. Sixteen patients in one study demonstrated a significant overall improvement in perceived quality of life of approximately 46 percent.

Utilization Measures

Several outcome measures associated with the utilization-related program objectives are routinely collected by the care management coordinator. The results of utilization studies have thus far shown dramatic improvements far exceeding preprogram projections. (See figure 5-12.) The data reported include 17 patients who had been in the Care Connection: CHF program for 3 or more months. The number of hospital admissions for this population preprogram was 67, with only 15 admissions postprogram. The number of hospital days was 315 preprogram and 87 postprogram. The range of days between hospital admissions was 125 preprogram and 505 postprogram. The number of emergency department visits was 83 preprogram and 21 postprogram.

Distribution of Measurement Data

In addition to the medical center administration, the following groups are informed about measures of Care Connection program success:

- The quality council, the group responsible for overseeing the medical center's continuous quality improvement process and for initiating the Care Connection: CHF program, receives regular feedback of program performance measures.
- The medical center's quality improvement committee receives data that it uses to demonstrate positive outcomes arising from changes in the patient care processes.
- The cardiology section, the group primarily responsible for development and implementation of cardiac care standards, closely monitors the effect of pathway and protocol use for CHF patients.
- The department of medicine, the body overseeing the care provided by the sections of cardiology, internal medicine, and family practice, receives summary reports of the Care Connection: CHF program performance measures.
- The Care Connection: CHF team receives detailed performance measurement reports that it uses to monitor the progress of the project, identify positive outcomes, analyze the care process, and make recommendations for change.

FURTHER PROGRAM ENHANCEMENTS

A number of secondary initiatives have been defined for the continuation and expansion of the Care Connection: CHF program. Some of these initiatives were discussed at program inception but postponed until the foundation components were in place. In other cases the team realized the need for supplemental activities after reviewing the outcome data. Described below are several of the planned program improvements.

Expansion of the Pathway into Home Care

Currently, the CHF clinical pathways address acute care, emergency department, and short-stay management. The next step is to design a home care pathway that includes patient outcomes, key indicators, and home care interventions. The pathway will also

FIGURE 5-12 Program Statistics, Initial Year of Operation

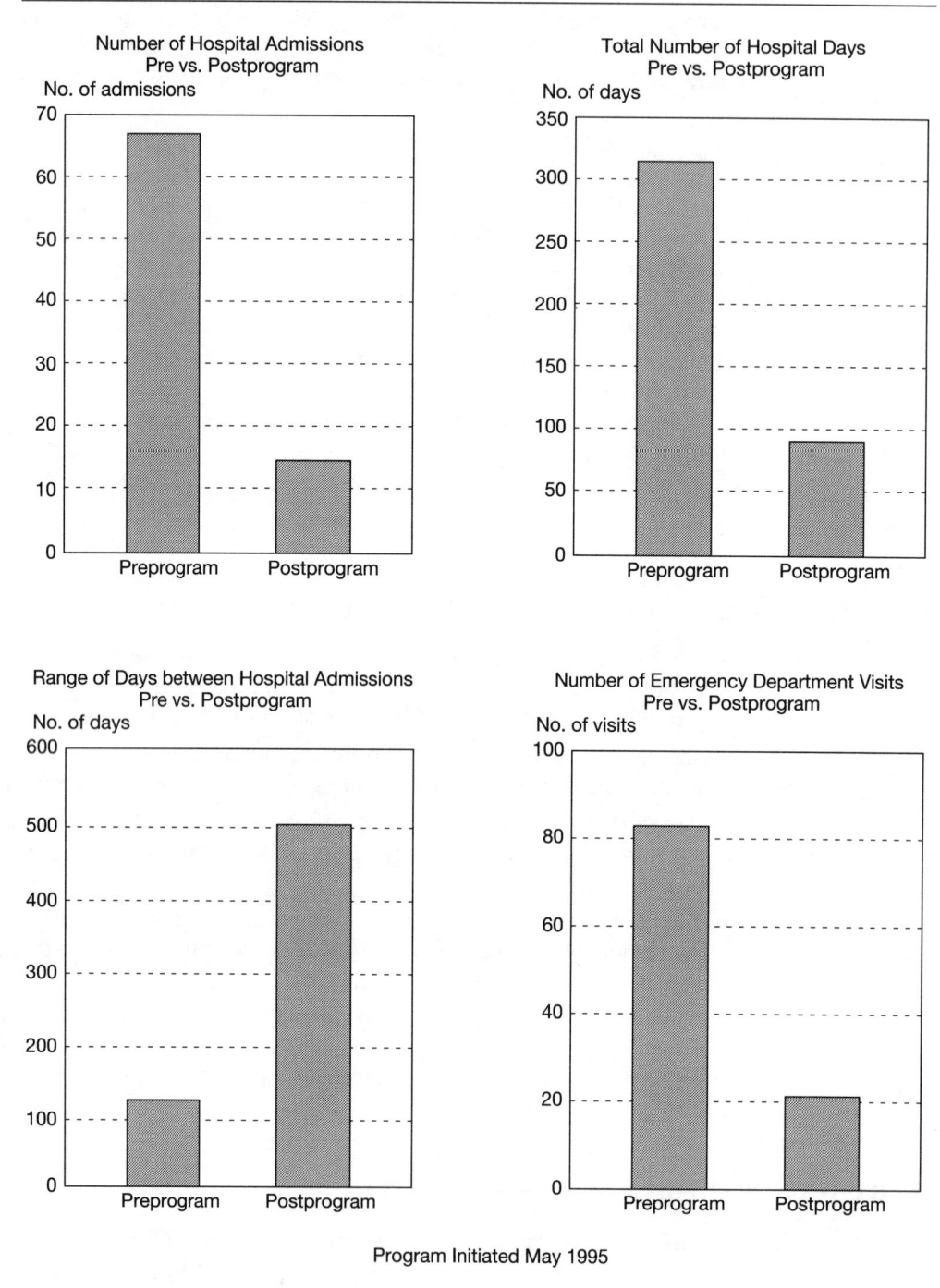

Number of Hospital Admissions Pre vs. Postprogram — Preprogram ~67, Postprogram ~14

Total Number of Hospital Days Pre vs. Postprogram — Preprogram ~315, Postprogram ~88

Range of Days between Hospital Admissions Pre vs. Postprogram — Preprogram ~125, Postprogram ~500

Number of Emergency Department Visits Pre vs. Postprogram — Preprogram ~83, Postprogram ~21

Program Initiated May 1995

help home care providers identify and manage patients' comorbid conditions. A corresponding patient version of the home care pathway is also planned for development.

Implementation in Primary Care Settings

The Care Connection: CHF program has been successfully implemented with a relatively small patient population. However, there is potential for expansion to multiple primary care settings. The first step in this undertaking is educating the primary care physicians on the purpose, components, and outcomes associated with the program. Subsequently, it is our hope to develop similar programs in physician offices, clinics, nursing homes, outreach centers, and senior residence facilities associated with the medical center.

Expansion of Treatment Modalities

Because the CHF patient population is closely monitored by the health care team and has had dramatically positive results using conservative protocols, the team plans to expand the care regimens to include additional therapies such as at-home administration of intravenous Dobutamine therapy.

Placement of Advanced Practice Nurse in Home and Community Settings

At this time program admission criteria require the participants to be able to come to the medical center for heart failure clinic services. This requirement hindered access to the program for some patients. As a next step the team is considering adding a community-based APN to the program team. This individual will see program participants in their homes or in alternative settings, markedly increasing program enrollment as well as improving outcomes for a larger patient population.

Expansion of the Program to Other Chronic Diseases

Given the success of this disease management program, the medical center plans to expand it to other chronic diseases. Diseases that are ideal for continuum-of-care interventions meet one or more of the following criteria:[20]

- They are common in the general population.
- They are associated with potentially wide variation in treatment and approach.
- They have high economic impact.
- They involve high-cost medication usage.
- They are in areas where lifestyle changes or prevention could have a major clinical impact.

St. Francis Medical Center is particularly interested in developing Care Connection programs for patients with asthma, chronic pulmonary diseases, and diabetes. The Care Connection framework, because it is already established and refined, will be used by other teams to develop similar programs for these populations.

SUMMARY

St. Francis Medical Center, like other health care institutions, originally designed nursing-oriented inpatient pathways. Once the pathway initiative became interdisciplinary and caregivers learned to collaborate with one another to achieve predefined inpatient outcomes, the process was ready to be operationalized in the continuum of care.

The Care Connection: CHF program has demonstrated how interdisciplinary teamwork can improve the quality of life for CHF patients and decrease acute care admissions, emergency department visits, and hospital lengths of stay (when inpatient care is required). While the medical center's interdisciplinary pathway initiative had helped to prepare the health care team for this continuum-of-care project, it soon became apparent that pathways could not be the only tool used in guiding patient management decisions. Successful disease management must include the following components:

- A prospective plan for care delivery (can include practice guidelines, protocols, pathways, patient education brochures, and so on)
- Proactive patient intervention techniques and medical treatments designed to achieve desirable outcomes
- Outcome measurement
- Feedback to clinicians

The positive results from the Care Connection: CHF program have allowed caregivers at St. Francis Medical Center to assure delivery of efficient, high-quality care to CHF patients. This model will soon be applied to other patient populations to achieve the medical center's vision of improving the health of its community.

References

1. Zander, K. Managed care and nursing case management. In: G. Mayer, M. Maddin, and E. Lawrenz, editors. *Patient Care Delivery Models.* Rockville, MD: Aspen, 1990.
2. CibaGeneva. *CibaGeneva Pharmacy Benefit Report: 1996 Trends and Forecasts.* Summit, NJ: Ciba-Geneva Pharmaceuticals, April 1996.
3. Terry, K. Disease management: continuous health-care improvement. *Business and Health* 13(4):65–72, 1995.
4. Dearing, G. Standardized disease management improves processes of care. *Outcomes Measurement and Management* 6(5):1–2, 1995.
5. U.S. Department of Health and Human Services. *Aging America: Trends and Projections, 1991 Edition.* Washington, DC: USDHHS, 1991.
6. Health Care Investment Analysts, Inc. *The DRG Handbook.* Baltimore: HCIA, 1993.
7. Ho, K. K., Anderson, K. M., Kannel, W. B., and others. Survival after the onset of congestive heart failure in Framington Heart Study subjects. *Circulation* 88(1):107–15, July 1993.
8. Cardiology Preeminence Roundtable. *Beyond Four Walls: Research Summary for Clinicians and Administrators on CHF Management.* Washington, DC: The Advisory Board, 1994.
9. Brassard, M. *The Memory Jogger II.* Methuen, MA: GOAL/QPC, 1994.
10. Strickland, D. The future of guidelines: health care reform, managed care, and computers will drive the use of guidelines in the years ahead. Special Report on Guidelines. *Business and Health* 12:27–30, 1994.
11. Dearing.
12. Zander, K. Critical pathways. In: M. M. Melum and M. K. Sinioris, editors. *Total Quality Management: The Health Care Pioneers.* Chicago: American Hospital Publishing, 1992, pp. 305–14.
13. Veterans Health Administration Quality Management Institute and Education Center's Clinical Practice Guideline Panel. Clinical Decision Making Aids: Clinical Practice *Guidelines/Clinical Pathways/Clinical Algorithms Position Statement, Version 1.* Durham, NC: Department of Veterans Affairs, Veterans Health Administration. Unpublished report, Aug. 1995.
14. Kleeb, T. Pathways and algorithms. In: R. G. Gift and C. F. Kinney, editors. *Today's Management Methods: A Guide for the Health Care Executive.* Chicago: American Hospital Publishing, 1996, pp. 187–207.
15. Heart Failure Guideline Panel. *Heart Failure: Evaluation and Care of Patients with Left Ventricular Systolic Dysfunction* (publication no. 94-0612). Washington, DC: U.S. Department of Health and Human Services, Agency for Health Care Policy and Research, June 1994.
16. Lee, T. H., and others. Failure of information as an intervention to modify clinical management: a time-series trial in patients with acute chest pain. *Annals of Internal Medicine* 122(6):434–37, 1995.

17. Lewis, L. M., Lasater, L. C., and Ruoff, B. E. Failure of a chest pain clinical policy to modify physician evaluation and management. *Annals of Emergency Medicine* 25(1):9–14, Jan. 1995.
18. Douma, A. The art and science of demand management. *Journal of the Association for Worksite Health Promotion* 2(3):10, summer 1995.
19. Shively, M., and others. Health-related quality of life as an outcome for patients with heart failure. *Journal of Cardiovascular Nursing* 2:89–96, 1996.
20. Donovan, M. R., and Matson, T. A., editors. *Outpatient Case Management: Strategies for a New Reality.* Chicago: American Hospital Publishing, 1994.

CHAPTER 6

Integrating Geriatric Evaluation and Management with a Multidisciplinary Care Planning Process

Jacquelyn Paynter, Katherine Ambrose, and Katherine Dolan

St. Joseph's Hospital is a 200-bed, acute care facility of the Catholic Medical Center of Brooklyn & Queens, Inc., a 1,400-bed multihospital system. Located in Flushing, NY, St. Joseph's offers a full range of acute care and ambulatory services to an inpatient population with an average age of 75 years. The framework from which the Catholic Medical Center's current multidisciplinary care-planning process evolved was a 2-year demonstration project sponsored by the New York State Department of Health using traditional clinical pathways in the case management of patients with diabetes and asthma. As in many organizations, the health care team found it difficult to integrate multidisciplinary care planning and record documentation with the traditional clinical path model.[1-3] Caregivers found paths to be useful for guiding disease-specific care, but the duplication of effort resulting from using two parallel care management systems, coupled with failure to integrate the clinical pathway into the patient's permanent medical record, created significant barriers to achieving buy-in from physicians, nurses, and other disciplines.

When discipline-specific patient assessments cannot be integrated successfully into a single patient management model, the care provided by each discipline continues to be compartmentalized. In the same manner, when clinical pathways cannot be merged with record documentation systems, the path can become burdensome for caregivers, actually interfering with patient care instead of enhancing it. Even when path documentation is used to replace common record entries, difficulties arise when there is a large volume of patients on different clinical pathways, when patients have multiple diagnoses, or when a patient's diagnosis changes during hospitalization.

In 1993 organizational leaders recognized that team cooperation would be enhanced by the development of a patient care management system that could replace duplicative care planning and documentation by integrating the processes of nurses, physicians, rehabilitation staff, social workers, and dietitians into a single collaborative system. Therefore, an organization-wide transition to an enhanced pathway model driven by a collaborative case management team process and a concurrent outcomes and variance management system was executed by a steering committee. The committee was composed of organizational leaders representing physicians, nursing staff, ancillary clinicians, administration, and quality management professionals. On-site educational workshops on case management, variance monitoring, critical pathways, and improving organizational performance and clinical outcomes featured industry experts such as Karen Zander, RN (Center for Case Management, South Natick, MA), and Brent James, MD (Intermountain Health Systems, Salt Lake City, UT). The resulting patient care management system, the *multidisciplinary care plan* (MCP), integrates a generic clinical path with a multidisciplinary documentation system for patient assessment, care planning, intervention, and evaluation. The MCP tool and its development process are described in this chapter.

THE MULTIDISCIPLINARY CARE PLAN DEVELOPMENT PROCESS

The steering committee coordinated the development of the generic MCP tool as a framework for an enhanced clinical pathway approach to care management. After this tool was developed, St. Joseph's began to design MCPs for high-volume, high-risk, or high-cost patient groups, including patients admitted for pneumonia, hip fracture, and laparoscopic cholecystectomy. However, as the feasibility of implementing these diagnostic-specific MCPs was being evaluated it became clear that geriatric patients, regardless of their reason for hospitalization, represented a unique set of challenges. Due to the chronic comorbid nature of their disease-health status and accompanying functional deficits, frail elderly patients are more likely to have longer hospital stays, with higher costs and serious medical complications.[4,5] Patient assessment and care management tools such as the MCP that target the functional outcomes of the elderly are important for two reasons: the growth in the older segment of the population and the trend toward managed care and health promotion and maintenance.[6] Therefore, leaders at St. Joseph's Hospital agreed to design a program specifically targeted to the frail elderly patient. The resulting patient care management model, *geriatric evaluation and management* (GEM), encompasses a collaborative team approach for the case management of functional outcomes that is supported by an integrated, outcomes-driven MCP. The model, described later in this chapter, has proved effective in improving the complex clinical and functional outcomes of the high-risk frail elderly patient.

ORGANIZATIONAL STRUCTURE AND SUPPORT PROCESSES OF THE MULTIDISCIPLINARY CARE PLAN

Effective implementation of a patient care management program requires dedicated leadership and organizational support. In 1993 the MCP model was made an organization-wide priority by top administration, nursing, and physician leadership. At that

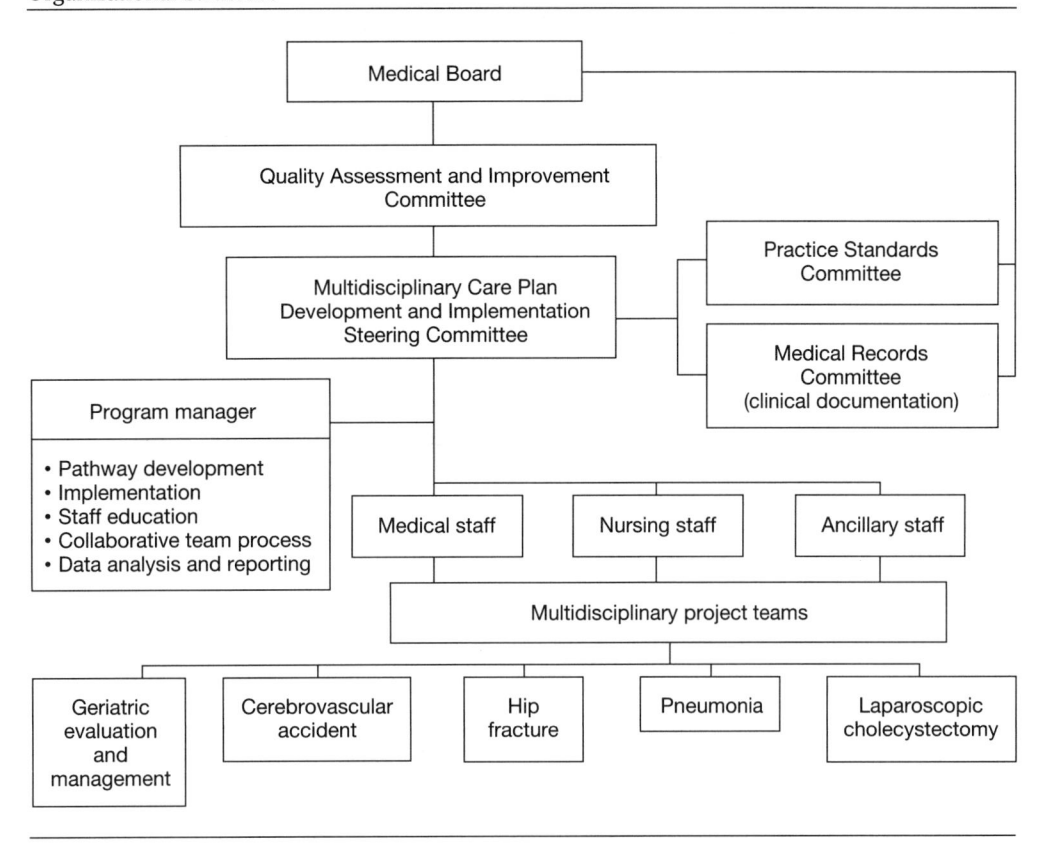

FIGURE 6-1 Integration of Multidisciplinary Care Management Program into Organizational Structure

time a formal organizational structure was designed. (See figure 6-1.) The program was organized under the quality assessment and improvement committee, with relevant groups and committees interacting with care plan development. This organizational structure helped emphasize the importance of the MCP program and eliminated duplicative quality improvement activities. The key committees and support staff are described below.

Development and Implementation Steering Committee

The steering committee comprises organizational leaders representing various disciplines and services. Included on the committee are members from the medical staff, nursing, quality improvement, administration, and key ancillary departments. The steering committee is responsible for setting clinical outcome improvement priorities by comparing the medical center's utilization and patient outcomes with internal and external benchmarks, evaluating different program models, and reviewing the literature. The following factors are taken into account when choosing projects:

- High volume, high costs, or high risks
- Evidence of significant improvement opportunities based on performance measurement or variance data results
- Relevance to the mission of the organization
- Potential for success
- Impact on patient satisfaction

Also, the steering committee establishes and supports project teams. It coordinates the MCP approval process with relevant groups, such as discipline-specific or departmental leaders, the practice standards committee, the medical records committee, and the medical board. In addition to monitoring the progress of each clinical outcome improvement project, the committee reviews data evaluating project effectiveness and makes recommendations for further improvement.

Multidisciplinary Project Teams

Project teams include physicians, nurses, physical therapists, respiratory therapists, dietitians, social workers, pharmacists, and other relevant health care professionals. Team members are selected for their professional experience and knowledge of the clinical process chosen for improvement. The teams are responsible for identifying standards of care for the patient population, comparing actual practice against industry standards, developing the clinical pathway, and implementing appropriate interventions to promote expected patient outcomes and resolve variances.

Program Manager

The program manager coordinates the MCP program. This individual is responsible for providing staff education, supporting MCP development and implementation, coordinating staff education, analyzing MCP variance data, and reporting progress to the steering committee. The project manager also oversees program operations, project time lines, and case management activities.

Case Managers

Nurses having clinical, utilization management, and discharge planning expertise serve as unit-based case managers. It is their responsibility to collaborate with physicians and other health care team members to establish and monitor patient care throughout the acute care stay on that unit. Each case manager is also responsible for an ongoing comprehensive assessment of the patient's condition to assure that optimal clinical outcomes are achieved. Health care utilization management is coordinated for approximately 30 to 35 patients. However, case managers are not direct caregivers. Their specific responsibilities include the following:

- Facilitate ongoing communication with health team members to meet identified patient outcomes.
- Identify patient-, system-, and practitioner-related pathway variances and collaborate with multidisciplinary team members to resolve them.
- Monitor the patient's clinical progress throughout the hospital stay and coordinate postdischarge planning assessments.
- Coordinate collaborative multidisciplinary team rounds.
- Facilitate effective use of the MCP by the health care team.
- Solicit feedback from members of the multidisciplinary team to facilitate MCP program revisions as needed.
- Identify additional patient populations for case management and participate in the development of MCPs.
- Analyze aggregated MCP variance data to identify trends and opportunities to improve systems, practice, and patient outcomes.

Administrative, Clerical, and Informational Support

Case managers, along with direct caregivers, identify and document variance information. The quality improvement department staff is responsible for trending variance data, physician and staff education, and dissemination of variance reports.

THE NATURE OF THE MULTIDISCIPLINARY CARE PLAN

The MCP is a care management system used by the health care team to manage and document the patient care delivery process and achieve targeted outcome goals. It is maintained as a permanent part of the patient's record and includes the following components:

- Clinical pathway timeline
- Assessment and care-planning tools
  - Admission database
  - Nutritional screen
  - Discharge-planning assessment
  - Physical therapy screen
  - Patient education assessment
- MCP variance management system
- Variance action response (VAR) record
- Quality assurance (QA) variance monitor

These components, except the QA variance monitor, are bound together in a booklet (the MCP). The MCP is a permanent part of the medical record. As patients are admitted, the booklets are used by caregivers for clinical assessment, care planning, and medical record documentation. The QA variance monitor is a scannable form that is not part of the patient's medical record. The specific use of each of the MCP components is described below.

Clinical Pathway

Following the format of traditional clinical paths, the clinical pathway section of the MCP details expected tests, treatments, outcomes, infusion therapy, consults, pastoral care, nutritional services, respiratory services, physical therapy, speech therapy, social services, and discharge preparations. A generic (or blank) multiple-page pathway form is available for caregivers to document expected interventions and outcomes. Predefined interventions and expected outcomes may be incorporated into the generic MCP for specific diseases or procedures (for example, diabetes, pneumonia, or laparoscopic cholecystectomy) and for special populations such as frail elderly patients.

To develop an individualized plan of care, each discipline caring for the patient documents planned interventions and expected outcome goals based on clinical assessments and their professional standards. Physician orders are written on the physician order sheet and transcribed onto the MCP by the unit clerk or the staff nurse. An organizational initiative is planned to automate the entire clinical record. Once this is complete the order entry process, diagnostic test results, and physician documentation will be integrated with the MCP.

Assessment Tools

Each MCP includes standard assessment tools used for all patients. These assessment tools include the following.

Admission Database The admission database is completed by the staff nurse. It includes patient demographics, admission source, admitting diagnosis, a preliminary (working) diagnosis-related group (DRG) and target length of stay, medical history, medication history, allergies, advance directives, substance use, mobility, sensory status, nutrition and eating patterns, elimination and toileting, discharge planning needs, patient's pressure ulcer potential, and falls risk while hospitalized.

Nutritional Screen As part of the admission database, the nutritional screen (figure 6-2) is initiated by the staff nurse during the admission assessment. The dietitian completes part B of the screen and is responsible for documenting the patient's nutritional risk and need for interventions on the MCP's nutrition section for all patients within 24 hours of admission. This individual also conducts a complete nutritional assessment for high-risk patients and develops a plan of care with the patient's physician to meet the patient's nutritional needs.

Discharge Planning Assessment The discharge-planning assessment (figure 6-3) is completed by the social worker. This form is completed within 24 hours of the patient's admission and is used to document the patient's posthospital needs and the tentative discharge plan.

Physical Therapy Screen The physical therapy screen (figure 6-4) is completed by the physical therapist for all patients referred for assessment. This form is used to document the patient's ability to follow commands, bed mobility, transfers, ambulation status, interventions required, rehabilitation potential, recommendations, and requests for medical assessment (if necessary).

Patient Education Assessment The patient education assessment (figure 6-5) is an interdisciplinary tool that includes an evaluation of the patient's learning needs, readiness, and barriers; identification of methods used; and an evaluation of teaching effectiveness. Included on the form are patient education parameters recommended by the Joint Commission on Accreditation of Healthcare Organizations (JCAHO): diagnosis, symptoms to report, medications, diet, equipment, and community resources.[7]

Reassessment of Patients Each discipline is responsible for reevaluating and documenting the patient's status as follows:

- Nurses assess body systems every 8 hours and as needed to identify clinical variation in the patient's condition as well as outcomes and interventions.
- The social worker, case manager, and nurse collaboratively evaluate the patient's discharge plan and progress along the pathway. They also identify system-related variances and patient-related variances that could affect the discharge plan.
- Physical therapists assess the patient's progress toward achieving functional outcome or rehabilitation goals.
- Dietitians assess the patient's progress toward achieving nutritional outcome goals.
- Physicians evaluate the patient's progress toward achieving disease-specific treatment goals and functional outcomes. They are also responsible for overall care management.

FIGURE 6-2 Nutritional Screening and Assessment

Part A: Completed by nurse on admission

Nutrition/Eating	No	Yes	Description
Special diet needs	__	__	_____
Dentures Partial plates	__	__	Upper __ _____
Full	__	__	Lower __ _____
Weight change over past 3 Mo:	__	__	_____
Loss __ Gain __ #Lbs. ____			
Problems:			
Nausea/vomiting	__	__	_____
Edema/swelling	__	__	_____
Diarrhea/constipation	__	__	_____
Nothing by mouth (NPO)	__	__	_____
Swallowing/chewing	__	__	_____
Fever/infection	__	__	_____
Trauma/fractures	__	__	_____

Part B: Completed by dietitian

Nutritional Services	Nutritional Screen	Nutritional Assessment
	• Low nutritional risk Basic care services: daily menu selection, preferences, tolerances • Moderate nutritional risk Nutritional intervention to be documented on MCP form • High nutritional risk Nutritional assessment to be completed by dietitian	Date: _____ Patient at nutritional risk O_2 _____ IBW _____ %IBW _____ UBW _____ ABW _____ ____ %Wt Chg. ____ week(s) ____ month(s) ____ Potential drug/nutrient interactions: ____ Pertinent lab data: _____ Estimated needs: Kcal: _____ Protein: _____ Other: _____ Present nutrition intake estimated @ _____ and compared to needs is: __ Meeting needs __ Not meeting needs Nutritional education is: __ Indicated __ Not indicated Nutritional plan of care: _____ D/C Plan:

Source: Catholic Medical Center of Brooklyn & Queens, Inc., Multidisciplinary Care Plan, Jan. 1995.

This multidisciplinary care-planning model meets JCAHO's requirements for patient assessment, patient education, and team collaboration.[8] During a recent JCAHO survey, the MCP process was cited as an "avant garde approach to collaborative patient care."

The Multidisciplinary Care Plan Variance Management System

Upon admission, patients are assessed, and an individualized plan of care based on this assessment is written by health care team members. The plan of care includes

FIGURE 6-3 Discharge-Planning Assessment

DISCHARGE REFERRAL

☐ HOME ☐ SOCIAL WORK ☐ OTHER _____

_____
_____

RN Signature _____ Date _____

| DATE | DAY _____ | DAY _____ | DAY _____ |

Patient Interviewed: ☐   Next of Kin Contacted: ☐

Mental Status/Adjustment to Illness: _____

Prior Living Arrangements: _____
_____

Prior Services: _____

Insurance: _____

Ambulation/Activities of Daily Living: Prior _____ Current _____

Support Systems Available (Name, Phone, Relationship)

1) _____

2) _____

Referrals:
_____
_____

Assessment:

Initial Discharge Plan:

Signature _____ Title/Dept: _____ Date: _____

Source: Catholic Medical Center of Brooklyn & Queens, Inc., Multidisciplinary Care Plan, Jan. 1995.

specific, time-limited goals established with input from the patient or family. These goals are translated into expected outcomes. As the patient progresses through the hospitalization, the multidisciplinary team continuously assesses the patient's progress toward goal attainment. If the patient does not proceed as expected, a variance, any discrepancy between actual and expected outcomes, is identified.[9] All members

THE NATURE OF THE MULTIDISCIPLINARY CARE PLAN   111

FIGURE 6-4 Physical Therapy Screen

	Admission Day Date _____

PT/OT	**Screen**
	
	Mental status:
	    follows 0 1 2 3 step commands
	
	Bed mobility:
	Rolling dependent max mod min assist
	Sidelying to sit dependent max mod min assist
	
	Transfers:
	Sit to stand dependent max mod min assist
	Commode to stand dependent max mod min assist
	
	Ambulation: dependent max mod min assist
	Weight-bearing restrictions _____
	Walker Quad cane Straight cane Crutches Wheelchair
	Other _____
	
	Interventions:
	___ No physical therapy required
	___ Out-of-bed team
	___ Daily physical therapy (assessment and goals)
	___ Maintenance physical therapy (3×/wk)
	
	Rehabilitation Potential:
	Poor ___ Fair ___ Good ___ Excellent ___
	
	Discharge Recommendation:
	___ Acute rehab ___ Home with PT
	___ Subacute rehab ___ Skilled nursing
	___ Outpatient rehab ___ No further PT needed
	
	Medical Assessment for Physical Therapy Referral:
	___ Physical therapy recommended to attending physician
	___ Patient is not a candidate for physical therapy
	
	                                                                  _____ M.D.

Source: Catholic Medical Center of Brooklyn & Queens, Inc., Multidisciplinary Care Plan, Jan. 1995.

of the multidisciplinary team are responsible for identifying and resolving variances 24 hours a day.

A variance may be either positive or negative. For example, if the expected length of stay is 5 days and the patient progresses faster than expected and is discharged in 4 days, a positive variance would be reflected in aggregated quality improvement reports. Conversely, if an individual patient develops a nosocomial infection or if there is a system delay in obtaining the results of a diagnostic test, a negative variance is identified. The multidisciplinary team is charged with promptly identifying potential or actual negative variances to expedite appropriate health care delivery, thereby promoting optimum outcomes.

There are three major categories of variances: patient related, practitioner related, and system related. Patient-related variances are identified when a condition, decision, or refusal occurs. The variance may be due to patient choice or an involuntary condition or occurrence. Practitioner-related variances are identified when a situation occurs involving response time, availability, or a decision made by a practitioner involved in the patient's care. System-related variances are the most commonly

FIGURE 6-5 Patient Education Assessment

Patient Education Assessment: (check all that apply)
- ___ Cultural/religious practices
- ___ Emotional barriers
- ___ Desire and motivation
- ___ Physical or cognitive limitation
- ___ Language barriers
- ___ Present understanding of illness
- ___ Discharge status (home, community, family)
- ___ Legal representative or agent involved

Language spoken _____   Interpreter _____
Person(s) involved in teaching _____

Key:

Teaching Methods	Evaluation of Learning
E - Explanation	1 - Identifies key points
D - Demonstration	2 - Verbalizes understanding
R - Role play	3 - Returns demonstration
A/V - Audiovisual	4 - Performs skill independently
H - Handout	5 - Applies knowledge
G - Group discussion	6 - No evidence of learning

Education Plan

Learning Outcomes: The patient or family, legal representative or agent demonstrates or verbalizes knowledge of:	Teaching Methods (use key)	Date and Initial	Evaluation (use key)	Date and Initial	Resources Used
1. Illness/health maintenance					
2. Signs/symptoms to report					
3. Anticipated length of stay					
4. Medications/food-drug interactions					
5. Treatments/equipment/procedures					
6. IV therapy					
7. Changes in daily living (work, exercise, activity, safety)					
8. Diet					
9. Available community resources					
10. Other					

Source: Catholic Medical Center of Brooklyn & Queens, Inc., Multidisciplinary Care Plan, Jan. 1995.

identified, especially when a new MCP is introduced into the patient care process. Some examples of common system-related variances are:

- Delays due to high service demand or scheduling problems
- Certain departments may be closed after hours and on weekends
- Tests not performed due to broken or malfunctioning equipment

FIGURE 6-6 Variance Action Response Record

DOCUMENTATION CODES (C):					
V - VARIANCE A - ACTION/INTERVENTION R - RESPONSE					
C	DAY ____ DATE ____	C	DAY ____ DATE ____	C	DAY ____ DATE ____

Source: Catholic Medical Center of Brooklyn & Queens, Multidisciplinary Care Plan, Jan. 1995.

- Communication deficit (for example, request for a consult never delivered to intended party)
- Delays in obtaining patient consents

Documenting Variances

Using a charting-by-exception methodology, clinicians document that interventions are completed and outcomes met by entering their signatures. Interventions or outcomes that are *not* met are circled, and the responsible caregiver documents the variance and its cause, the action taken to address the variance, and the patient's response in the VAR section of the MCP. (See figure 6-6.) Only clinical variances are documented on the VAR record. For system variances a separate QA variance monitor form is used. This scannable form is not part of the patient's permanent medical record.

The quality improvement department staff is responsible for gathering variance data contained in records of discharged patients. It also is responsible for entering information contained on the QA variance monitor form into the department database. Information in this database is used by the department to prepare variance reports for the organization's quality improvement committees.

Daily Bed Rounds Concurrent MCP variance monitoring is the principal mechanism used to identify and resolve variances as they occur. In addition, each unit has a unit-based multidisciplinary team composed of the case manager, staff nurses, social worker, dietitian, pharmacist, physical therapist, and medical house officer. This team meets each weekday to discuss each patient on the unit. Bed rounds have been shown to be a successful strategy for managing the day-to-day patient care process to efficiently move patients through their hospitalizations.[10] At St. Joseph's Hospital, daily bed rounds for the 30 to 35 patients on each unit take approximately 30 minutes.

During daily bed rounds the multidisciplinary team primarily discusses variance resolution, not variance identification. Caregivers are expected to resolve variances as soon as possible. If the variance is unresolved by the time rounds occur, the team collaborates on variance resolution plans and an appropriate team member assumes responsibility for initiating the team-recommended action. The next day this person reports on the progress of variance resolution, and this is documented as an action/intervention on the VAR record. (See figure 6-6.)

During the team meeting the patient's current status is compared to the patient-specific outcome goals. The members of the team discuss and document the patient assessment, care plan, interventions, and expected outcomes. Since the bed rounds are conducted outside the patient's room, the team has the opportunity to see the patient firsthand. The patient and family (if present) may be involved in the team's discussions and thus in the care-planning and evaluation process. Using the patient's MCP as a guide, the staff nurse caring for the patient briefs the team on the patient's progress and discusses any variances and discharge-planning needs. If a physician's order is required, the order is written by the physician member of the bed rounds team, or the attending physician is contacted by a designated team member.

GERIATRIC EVALUATION AND MANAGEMENT

GEM is a collaborative team approach to case management that focuses on improving functional outcomes for the at-risk frail elderly patient. A substantial portion of hospitalized elderly patients are debilitated with poor mobility, decreased cognitive function, multisystem failure, and multiple comorbidities.[11,12] These functional problems affect the patients' overall quality of life. Quality-of-life evaluations encompass health status factors such as presence, absence, or risk of disease; socioeconomic factors such as the ability to handle finances and socialize in the community; and environmental factors such as housing and safety. Health status evaluations encompass physical, mental, and social factors, including actual symptoms of illness as well as levels of functioning. Using functional status measures, caregivers can accomplish five tasks:[13]

1. Detect patient's disease or dysfunction.
2. Assess the extent of patients' disease and dysfunction.
3. Select treatments and other interventions.
4. Assess patients' need for community resources.
5. Evaluate the effects of these interventions.

The geriatric MCP is a 28-page document that is integrated into the generic MCP format and includes a geriatric-specific clinical pathway. The geriatric pathway portion of the MCP is used by the multidisciplinary team to apply appropriate geriatric management strategies aimed at reaching predetermined goals along a defined time line. The assessment tools are used throughout the patient's hospitalization to determine baseline and functional improvements. These measurement tools were selectively derived from widely recognized functional status evaluation instruments. (See table 6-1.)

The MCP is designed to address conditions that commonly affect the functional status of the elderly, including:

- Impaired senses
- Impaired cognition

TABLE 6-1 Assessing Functional Status in Clinical Settings

Functional Status Indicator	Definition	Measurement Tools
Activities of daily living	Degree to which the person has limitations in self-care, basic mobility, and incontinence	Katz Basic ADL Assessment
Cognitive function	Degree to which a person is alert, oriented, able to concentrate, and able to perform tasks such as concentrating	Folstein Mini-Mental Exam
Affective function	Degree to which a person feels depressed, anxious, or generally happy	Brink/Yesavage Depression/Anxiety Scale
Social-role function	Degree to which a person is limited in visiting friends or in participating in community activities	Targeted Health History
Physical health	General appearance, speech patterns and content, mood, handgrips, muscle strength and mobility, gait, use of assistive devices, incontinence, health habits, nutrition, and medication usage	Targeted Health History and Physical Exam

- Impaired mobility
- Poor nutrition and hydration
- Impaired skin integrity
- Stress and depression
- Incontinence
- Polypharmacy

THE GERIATRIC EVALUATION AND MANAGEMENT PROGRAM DEVELOPMENT PROCESS

In 1993 the MCP development and implementation committee at St. Joseph's Hospital selected frail elderly patients as a high-priority population for clinical outcome improvements. This group of patients was chosen because published studies had shown that a functional status approach, combined with multidisciplinary team assessments, is an effective patient management strategy for these patients.[14-16] Research suggested that comprehensive GEM programs are useful models for providing care.[17] Methods to detect disability, assess disease severity, measure patient progress over time, and plan for long-term care are all important components of an effective GEM program. Therefore, it was the committee's assertion that a GEM program, supported by the already existing MCP model, would provide an effective vehicle for improving the complex clinical and functional outcomes of high-risk frail elderly patients at St. Joseph's Hospital.

Create a Team

A GEM project team composed of a geriatrician, geriatric clinical nurse specialist, dietitian, physical therapist, pharmacist, respiratory therapist, social worker, case manager, home care coordinator, and quality management professional was formed to provide GEM services. The GEM team conducts biweekly clinical rounds to assess the functional status of selected high-risk frail elderly patients, develop a plan of care, and evaluate patient progress and intervention effectiveness. The expertise and leadership provided by the geriatrician and the geriatric nurse are essential for the ongoing success of the GEM program.

FIGURE 6-7 Pressure Ulcer Potential Scoring System

Parameter	0	1	2	3	Score
Physical condition	Good	Fair	Poor	Very bad	
Mental state	Alert	Lethargic	Semicomatose	Comatose	
Nutritional status	Good	Fair	Poor	Very bad	

Count the Conditions below as Double

Activity	Ambulatory	Walks with help	Chair bound	Bed bound	
Mobility	Full	Slightly limited	Very limited	Immobile	
Incontinence	None	Occasional	Usually incontinent	Totally incontinent	

Key: Total score of 10 or more = at risk. **Total Score** [ ]

Source: Catholic Medical Center of Brooklyn & Queens, Inc., Multidisciplinary Care Plan, Jan. 1995.

Define the Target Population and Exclusions

The first step in designing the GEM program was to identify the target population that would benefit the most from focused team interventions. Because GEM is not disease specific, the target population needed to be defined based on risk factors, not diagnoses. To aid in identifying the appropriate patient population, the GEM project team considered the literature definition of frail elderly persons. Burke and Walsh define *frail elderly persons* as those people who are, usually, over the age of 75 and have accumulated continuing chronic health problems that make them particularly vulnerable to physical, mental, and financial losses as well as to the loss of social resources, social roles, and housing independence.[18] This definition was modified slightly to identify those patients who would be considered candidates for the GEM program at St. Joseph's Hospital, where program candidates are those persons who meet the following criteria:

- Aged 70 years or older *and*
- At high risk for development of a pressure ulcer *or*
- Meet the polypharmacy criteria of more than five prescribed medications

The patient's pressure ulcer potential (PUP) is based on factors known to influence development of pressure ulcers: nutritional status, mobility, activity level, mental status, incontinence, and overall physical condition. Each of these factors is assessed by the staff nurse using the PUP scoring system shown in figure 6-7. An overall PUP score of 10 or more indicates the patient is at risk for pressure ulcer development. Frail geriatric patients are identified during the admission assessment process. Any patient meeting one or more of the criteria is placed on the geriatric MCP and assessed for referral to the GEM team.

Define Program Goals

The GEM project committee established clear, measurable goals to give the program direction and for use when evaluating its effectiveness. The goals focused on the GEM committee's key objectives for pursuing the project and were as follows:

- Improve functional outcomes of the frail elderly through collaborative outcomes-driven case management.

- Reduce fragmentation of the health care delivery system through increased coordination of services across the continuum of care.
- Ensure customer satisfaction (patients and families, nursing homes, physicians, staff) by providing coordinated outcomes-driven care.
- Reduce costs by:
  — Decreasing hospital lengths of stay
  — Preventing complications
  — Decreasing inappropriate service utilization
  — Standardizing practice and product use

Define Program Benchmarks

An important step in the project development phase was to clarify current practices and system and patient outcomes and determine how they differ from optimal expectations. To establish improvement goals and strategies the GEM project committee evaluated past geriatric care performance data such as length of stay, timeliness and appropriateness of clinical interventions, and outcome measurement parameters. Project team members reviewed the literature and comparative data.[19-21] The information they gathered helped them develop more effective systems for managing geriatric patients and identify appropriate GEM program targets based on internal or external "best practice" benchmarks.

The project team considered a number of factors in developing its performance measures or "benchmark indicators," including the following:

- Appropriateness of interventions—for example, selection and use of drugs, diagnostic tests, procedures, supplies, and ancillary services such as rehabilitation, respiratory, and nutritional services as well as the appropriate interpretation of test results and use of treatments
- Timeliness of services—for example, scheduling, performing, and reporting results of diagnostic tests and procedures, ancillary service interventions, and consultations
- Efficiency and effectiveness of care—for example, optimal timing, interventions, and equipment and supply use for procedures and drug therapy as well as the appropriate length of stay

The benchmarks identified to evaluate the impact of the GEM program on patient outcomes as well as the performance of health care delivery systems are shown in table 6-2.

Define Interventions Necessary to Achieve Program Goals

Research indicates that patients' functional status is the most important factor in recovery from illness and health maintenance among elderly populations.[22] Therefore, the GEM program treatment plan was designed around appropriate assessment and interventions addressing the frail elderly patient's functional status. The care functions believed to have a significant impact on the hospital's ability to coordinate safe, timely discharge for frail elderly patients are described below.

Behavioral and Psychosocial Functions The patient's level of consciousness, orientation and cognitive status, and the impact of lethargy, disorientation, and dementia are considered when establishing the patient's activities of daily living. Program

TABLE 6-2 Geriatric Evaluation and Management Program Benchmarks

Benchmark Indicator	Benchmark Source
National pressure ulcer incidence = 7%	National Pressure Ulcer Advisory Council, 1994
Nutritional screening within 24 hours of admission	Nutritional Screening Initiative (NSI), *Nutrition Intervention Manual for Professionals Caring for Older Americans*, 1993
Nutritional intake within 75% of protein/calorie requirements	USDHHS, Public Health Department, AHCPR, *Pressure Ulcer Treatment Clinical Guideline*, 1994
Serum albumin ≥ 3.5	USDHHS, Public Health Department, AHCPR, *Pressure Ulcer Treatment Clinical Guideline*, 1994
Foley catheter < 72 hours	Internal benchmark
Bed rest < 24 hours	Internal benchmark
Nosocomial MRSA infection rate; monthly trended comparisons	Internal benchmark
Advance directives/self-determination = 100%	New York State Health Care Proxy Law
Polypharmacy ≥ 5 drugs	National Council on Patient Information, *Priorities and Approaches to Improving Prescription Drug Use by Older Americans*, 1987

interventions, such as recreational activities, are designed to improve patients' mental status outcomes and to foster the maximum level of independence, self-determination, and patient satisfaction.

Self-Determination Advance directives and involvement of the patient in decision making are important factors to incorporate into any care management program. The patient's desires or the existence of a health care proxy is determined upon admission and reassessed throughout the hospital stay.

Grooming and Hygiene Personal cleanliness affects skin integrity as well as the patient's overall feeling of well-being. This functional outcome is also an important basic activity of daily living for which the maximum level of independence should be maintained.

Activity and Mobility The importance of optimizing physical mobility and activity level is well documented.[23] This functional element greatly affects patient wellness and recovery from illness as well as the prevention of complications such as pressure ulcers, pneumonia, deep vein thrombosis, poor appetite, loss of strength, and poor bowel motility. A patient who can walk or transfer himself or herself from bed to chair to toilet is infinitely more capable of expeditiously returning to the community. It is estimated that each day in bed translates into one week more of convalescence.[24]

Skin Integrity The maintenance of skin integrity is a high priority for the hospitalized frail elderly patient because of a high incidence of risk factors such as poor nutritional status, incontinence, immobility, sensory impairment, and overall poor physical condition secondary to the aging process, disease, or injury. The incidence of nosocomial skin breakdown can be markedly reduced with proper care and attention to the skin. By determining the patient's PUP score (figure 6-7), the staff can develop an individualized patient care plan to prevent skin breakdown or heal existing pressure ulcers.

Nutrition and Hydration Nutrition and hydration coupled with mobility and hygiene are the most significant factors in the healing of pressure ulcers as well as in the patient's overall recovery from illness. It is often difficult to ensure that older pa-

FIGURE 6-8 Falls Risk Scoring System

Risk Factor	Indicators	Value	Score
History	History of previous falls	2	
Physical status	Fatigability/weakness	2	
	Dizziness/balance problems	1	
	Impaired mobility	1	
	Sensory impairment	1	
	Seizure disorder	1	
	Alteration in elimination	1	
Mental status	Confused	2	
	Impaired memory/judgment	2	
	Disoriented to person/place/time	2	
	Lack of familiarity with immediate surroundings	1	
	Inability to understand/follow instructions	1	
Medication	Drugs that have diuretic effect	1	
	Drugs that suppress thought process and/or create hypotensive effect (narcotics, sedatives, psychotrophics, hypnotics, tranquilizers, antihypertensives)	1	
	Drugs that increase GI motility (laxatives, enemas, cathartics)	1	
		Total Score	_____

Source: Catholic Medical Center of Brooklyn & Queens, Inc., Multidisciplinary Care Plan, Jan. 1995.

tients receive enough food and water. Many patients have long-standing disease processes, and in the days, and sometimes weeks, prior to their hospital admissions they may not have achieved proper nutritional intake. When they arrive at the hospital they may have severe nutritional compromise and high risk for the development of pressure ulcers. An appropriate care plan that includes feeding mechanisms (hand feeding, nasogastric and gastrostomy tubes, and routine evaluation of total protein and caloric and fluid intake) is essential to maintain the nutritional health of the frail elderly patient.[25] Failure to assess patients' nutritional status and take appropriate action can result in significantly higher morbidity and mortality and marked increases in hospital lengths of stay.

Safety The falls risk evaluation (figure 6-8) is used by caregivers to evaluate patients' risk of falling while in the hospital. The assessment is based on the patient's history of previous falls, physical condition (weakness, dizziness, balance problems, impaired mobility, sensory impairment), mental status (confusion, impaired memory or judgment, disorientation, lack of familiarity with surroundings, inability to understand instructions), and current medications (drugs that have a diuretic effect, suppress the thought process, or increase gastric motility).

The results of this risk assessment are considered by caregivers as they design treatment strategies for reducing patient accidents and injuries during the hospital stay.[26] The goal is to minimize the use of patient restraints by increasing observation, maintaining the bed in the low position, keeping the side rails up as appropriate, assisting patients with bathroom privileges, and providing nonskid slippers.

Bowel and Bladder Elimination or Incontinence Maintenance of effective bowel and bladder elimination patterns through routine assessment and care-planning interventions is a key factor in promoting the patient's overall well-being. Since incontinence affects skin integrity and the patient's self-esteem,[27] an effective program for toileting (where appropriate) and personal hygiene must be instituted to ensure that the patient's elimination is sufficient and dignity is maintained.

Medication Management Polypharmacy is defined as the concurrent use of five or more drugs.[28] By assessing the patient's medication regimen, caregivers can design treatment plans that minimize drug interactions as well as manage the common side effects that might otherwise go unnoticed or unreported.[29]

Define Pathway Boundary

The project team chose to start with a hospital-based pathway that would be initiated for all patients meeting the age, polypharmacy, and PUP score criteria. While the GEM MCP focuses on improving or maintaining the functional status of frail elderly patients, the tool also provides the framework for disease-specific care management. Although not yet fully developed, the GEM MCP model will eventually be extended to the posthospital or community health environment including ambulatory and home care services to prevent deterioration of patients' functional status and reduce hospital readmissions.

Define Caregiver Involvement

The project team agreed that an interdisciplinary collaborative model was the most important success factor for the GEM program. Therefore, all members of the health care team involved in caring for frail elderly patients participate in the multidisciplinary assessment and care-planning process as follows:

- *Geriatrician:* Acts as medical champion and expert in gerontological health; provides leadership for the GEM project team as well as specialty consultations on frail elderly patients at risk for or experiencing actual declines in their functional status
- *Geriatric clinical nurse specialist:* Provides specialty consultation and evaluation of nursing interventions and makes recommendations on the use of treatments and interventions, such as special products and equipment; also assists staff nurses and the multidisciplinary team with specialized assessments
- *Attending physicians and house officers:* Evaluates patient status, establishes the diagnosis, prescribes appropriate therapeutic interventions, and oversees overall patient care activities
- *Nurse manager:* Oversees day-to-day nursing care and has 24-hour responsibility for a patient care unit
- *Primary nurse:* Assesses patient status, plans needed care, provides nursing interventions, and evaluates actual patient outcomes against expected outcomes
- *Dietitian:* Assesses nutritional status, recommends appropriate interventions, and monitors patient response and progress
- *Pharmacist:* Assesses medication usage relative to appropriateness, interactions, side effects, and polypharmacy
- *Physical therapist:* Assesses functional status (activity, mobility) and delivers therapeutic interventions prescribed by the attending physician
- *Social worker:* Assesses psychosocial status, intervenes with patient and family, coordinates overall discharge plan, and assists with placement, durable medical equipment arrangements, and home care planning
- *Case manager:* Serves as team leader for daily multidisciplinary team rounds, monitors pathway variances, and provides discharge planning assessments; also evaluates the appropriateness, timeliness, and effectiveness of resource utilization to ensure the patient progresses along the pathway as expected

THE GERIATRIC EVALUATION AND MANAGEMENT PROGRAM TOOLS

The geriatric MCP expands the scope of the standard MCP. It encompasses the routine tests and treatments and the functions important to the care of the geriatric patient:

- Behavioral and psychosocial factors
- Grooming and hygiene
- Mobility and activity
- Skin integrity
- Nutrition and hydration
- Safety
- Medication management
- Bowel and bladder elimination and incontinence

These functional care elements serve as the clinical pathway framework for the geriatric MCP's interventions and outcomes section (figure 6-9), the core of the geriatric MCP. The entire GEM MCP tool incorporates all of the components of the generic MCP described in earlier sections of this chapter and also provides the functional status interventions and outcomes of the geriatric-specific clinical pathway shown in figure 6-9. Within the first 24 hours of admission to the GEM program, the patient's GEM MCP is implemented by the nurse and individualized to the patient's needs based on the findings of interdisciplinary assessments, diagnoses, and physician orders.

COLLABORATIVE MULTIDISCIPLINARY TEAM ROUNDS

The geriatric MCP is the blueprint used by the multidisciplinary team to guide care for frail elderly patients. Once or twice a week at regularly scheduled times, the GEM team meets to discuss GEM program patients. This team includes the following members:

- Geriatrician
- Geriatric clinical nurse specialist
- Staff nurse
- Case manager
- Dietitian
- Nursing unit director or clinical nurse manager
- Medical residents
- Pharmacist
- Social worker
- Physical therapist

The GEM team provides specialty consultation by assessing the status of frail elderly patients at high risk for pressure ulcers or decline in functional status. Functional elements evaluated by the GEM team include each patient's mobility, skin integrity, incontinence, nutritional status, and drug utilization patterns.

Prior to GEM rounds, the staff nurse assembles pertinent patient information, including:

- Patient's name and age
- Patient's current prescribed diet and average daily intake

FIGURE 6-9 Geriatric Multidisciplinary Care Plan Interventions and Outcomes

	Day 1 Date _____	Day 2 Date _____	Day 3 Date _____	Day 4 . . .[a] Date _____	Day 8 Date _____
Behavior			Maintain/improve patient's usual behavioral pattern		
Grooming/Hygiene			Maintain/improve patient's ability to groom self		
Skin integrity	Maintain/improve patient's skin integrity PUP Score _____ Implement skin and tissue protocol				Reassess PUP _____ Pressure ulcer will evidence improvement in stage/size
Nutrition/Hydration	Total intake • 75% prot/cal requirement • 1800 cc/day + unless contraindicated				No unplanned weight loss/gain (3–5 lbs.) Follow-up nutritional assessment Patient weight: _____
Mobility		Out of bed/chair or ambulate Progress activity as appropriate to patient's condition			
Safety	Falls risk score Prevent injuries • Bed in low position • Call light in reach • Frequent observation as required or q2h • Maintain safe environment Implement fall prevention protocol				Reassess falls risk score
Medication administration	No adverse drug reactions Reduce polypharmacy			Review culture results and sensitivity pattern Antibiotics reviewed	
Elimination	No Foley except for strict I&O for incontinent patients Implement elimination protocol	Maintain/improve usual bowel/bladder pattern			

Source: Catholic Medical Center of Brooklyn & Queens, Inc., Geriatric Multidisciplinary Care Plan, Jan. 1995.
[a] For brevity, days 5 through 7 were omitted.

- Status of pressure ulcers (community or hospital acquired, stage, size, and treatment, and whether the ulcer[s] are improving, worsening, or remaining the same)
- Laboratory test results (culture reports, blood chemistry)
- Status of antibiotic usage and signs or symptoms of immunosuppression
- Elimination status
- Mobility status
- Mental status

Unlike the daily bed rounds, the GEM rounds are conducted for the purpose of recommending interventions specifically related to geriatric MCP functional outcomes. The geriatric clinical specialist and the geriatrician speak with the patient and examine the status of any pressure ulcers. They report to their findings at the GEM rounds, where the team develops a specialized plan of care for the GEM program patient.

The GEM rounds last approximately 30 minutes. The discussions focus entirely on the small group of elderly patients who are at risk for pressure ulcer development, malnutrition, or other undesired functional outcomes. From 5 to 10 minutes are spent reviewing each patient's status and developing patient-specific care plans. During GEM rounds, functional outcomes for each patient are assessed and documented. This information is used to evaluate the progress of individual patients and assess the overall effectiveness of the GEM program. The GEM team monitors each patient's progress, focusing on the functional status indicators that affect the frail elderly population's risk for pressure ulcer development and malnutrition. Because of their chronic frail condition, GEM patients remain on the GEM program until discharge.

GERIATRIC EVALUATION AND MANAGEMENT PROGRAM EVALUATION

MCP patient outcome and systems performance data, including those gathered from the geriatric MCP, are reported quarterly to hospital and departmental quality assurance committees, the medical board, and specialty committees (nutritional, skin care, pharmacy, therapeutics, and so on). The data are used by these groups to improve the effectiveness of the care planning process. The MCP steering committee receives monthly reports of variance data to identify patterns of avoidable system-, patient-, or practitioner-related variances. A sample GEM program functional outcomes report (demonstration data only) useful for identifying clinical intervention and institutional system improvements is illustrated in figure 6-10.

When the geriatric MCP was first developed by the GEM project team, considerable effort went into defining objective outcome measures that could be evaluated by the multidisciplinary team. (See table 6-2.) Variances from these outcomes are used in planning the care for individual patients and to evaluate GEM program effectiveness. GEM outcome measures are not meant to be all inclusive. Rather, they focus on the reasonably obtainable elements of care considered to be most important to achieving desirable patient outcomes.

CONCLUSION

The GEM program has proved effective in improving geriatric outcomes by increasing process efficiency, administering appropriate and effective interventions, and

FIGURE 6-10 Sample Geriatric Evaluation and Management Program Functional Outcome Indicator Report

Functional Category	Performance Measure	Preprogram Intervention	Postprogram Intervention
Nutritional status	Body weight +/− 5 lbs. of target weight	36%	60%
	Protein/calorie intake maintained for 75% of patient's nutritional need	35%	51%
Mobility	Bed rest for more than 24 hours after admission	93%	96%
	• Out of bed at least once a day	17%	39%
	• Turn patient every 2 hours while in bed and every hour while in a chair	84%	99%
Skin integrity	Nosocomial pressure ulcer incidence	11%	6%
	• Implemented skin care protocol	92%	100%
Medication usage	Polypharmacy (defined as >5 prescribed medications)	92%	62%
	• Average number of prescribed medications per patient	10	5.5
Elimination	Foley catheter > 72 hrs	51%	41%
Mental status	Disorientation	75%	68%
	Lethargy	38%	36%
Resource utilization	Reduce length of stay	15.1 days	9.63 days
	Average age	82 years	86 years

Note: This data simulation illustrates how performance improvements and opportunities can be reported to clinicians and organizational leaders and used to achieve programmatic goals. In this example, the bed rest, dietary intake, mental status, and Foley catheter use data show some gains, but programmatic interventions are needed to determine how to improve this functional outcome measure further.

decreasing length of stay. In the 2.5-year period following program implementation, the following improvements have been achieved:

- *Improved efficiency and decreased length of stay:* The GEM program's clinical process improvement activities have resulted in significant cost savings as evidenced by reductions in patients' lengths of stay and complications (for example, infections and pressure ulcers) and improvements in the timeliness of ancillary interventions.
- *Improved functional and clinical outcomes:* GEM patient outcome data have revealed substantial reductions in nosocomial pressure ulcers, reductions in nosocomial methicillin-resistant *staphylococcus aureus* infections, reductions in antibiotic costs per day, increases in nutritional screening of all patients within 24 hours of admission with an increased number of patients achieving their target weights, and a remarkable reduction in the average number of prescribed medications per patient.

Similar geriatric management approaches have been successfully implemented by a number of institutions, with reported reduction in inpatient resource utilization, improved patient satisfaction, and positive functional status outcomes.[30] The key elements to the effectiveness of the GEM program at St. Joseph's Hospital are the geriatric MCP and the concurrent multidisciplinary collaborative team case management process augmented by specialty consultations from experts in gerontology.

Lessons Learned

Other organizations wishing to launch similar multidisciplinary care management models should consider the lessons learned by St. Joseph's Hospital:

1. Promote medical staff support through participation in the early stages of the project and selection of physician champions to spearhead clinical pathway development.

2. Establish a formal leadership structure (for example, steering committee) that includes medical, nursing, ancillary, and administrative leaders.
3. Define a systematic process for program development, approval, implementation, and evaluation.
4. Establish a mechanism for two-way communication with internal and external customers.
5. Implement an effective and ongoing physician and staff education program that includes information about program philosophies, goals and objectives, methods, tools, and results.

Future Directions

The MCP and GEM programs at St. Joseph's Hospital continue to evolve. Future goals include:

- Automation of patient lifetime records, focusing on health maintenance and prevention
- Expansion of the case management process to include geriatric outreach in primary care and postacute care settings in collaboration with home care and skilled nursing facility providers and through the development of subacute care capabilities. Frail elderly patients could be managed across the entire continuum of care.
- Development and expansion of wellness tools and health-related quality-of-life measures
- Continued progress in developing organizational expertise in caring for the geriatric patient, focusing on ongoing team building and coordination
- Expansion of the patient education resource center to include hospital pharmacist involvement in food-drug and drug-drug interactions and polypharmacy education

Summary

The St. Joseph's Hospital MCP has proved to be an effective care management system. The duplicative care planning and documentation systems of hospital caregivers have been replaced by a single collaborative system. In addition, the MCP has also provided a mechanism for measuring actual patient care against a predetermined process and outcome time line. Team bed rounds have fostered unity among staff and physicians, with members of the team reporting greater satisfaction with the patient care process. The MCP format illustrates the benefits of creating clinical pathways that can be used as a framework for multidisciplinary documentation. The St. Joseph's experience substantiates the importance of administrative and clinical management support. Such backing helped to ensure adequate resource investment, program visibility, and overall integration of the various program elements across disciplines and into the organization's existing operational and quality improvement structures.

Data show that a collaborative case management approach supported by an integrated outcomes-driven MCP pathway model effectively manages and improves care for patients with specific diagnoses or procedures and also for high-risk frail elderly patients. The GEM program, which evolved from the MCP model, included many of the features of the MCP process as well as some unique additions:

- Support from experts on a geriatric evaluation team
- Intense, focused patient assessment and reassessment

Over the 3-year period in which the MCP program evolved and the GEM program was implemented, quality and utilization performance measures showed continued improvements. Today the program is viewed as a highly integrated, patient-centered system yielding significant improvements in patients' functional status, decreases in infection rates, and reductions in lengths of stay.

The GEM results suggest that a fully integrated system focusing on maintaining and improving the functional status of hospitalized geriatric patients can produce meaningful improvements in patient outcomes. A significant increase in hospital admissions occurred after the benefits of the MCP process and the GEM program were shared with referring physicians and nursing homes in the St. Joseph Hospital market area.

References

1. Spath, P. L., editor. *Clinical Paths: Tools for Outcomes Management.* Chicago: American Hospital Publishing, 1994.
2. Hofmann, P. A. Critical path method: an important tool for coordinating clinical care. *Joint Commission Journal of Quality Improvement* 19(7):235–46, July 1993.
3. Lumsdon, K. Rule 1 on critical paths: proceed with caution. *Hospital and Health Networks* 67(22):56, Nov. 20, 1993.
4. Rubenstein, L. V., and others. Effectiveness of a geriatric evaluation unit: a randomized clinical trial. *New England Journal of Medicine* 331:1664–70, 1984.
5. Hendrickson, C., and others. Consequences of assessment and intervention among elderly people: a three year randomized controlled trial. *British Medical Journal* 289:1522–24, 1984.
6. Wasson, J. Decision making for improved outcomes in elder care. *Group Practice Journal,* pp. 67–69, July-Aug. 1994.
7. Joint Commission on Accreditation of Healthcare Organizations. *Comprehensive Accreditation Manual for Hospitals.* Oakbrook Terrace, IL: JCAHO, 1996, pp. 211–21.
8. JCAHO.
9. Zander, K. Quantifying, managing and improving quality using variance concurrently. *The New Definition* 7(4), fall 1992.
10. Zander, K. Health care team meetings: sharing responsibility for cost and quality of care. *The New Definition* 4(2), spring 1989.
11. Rubenstein and others.
12. Hendrickson and others.
13. Wasson.
14. Williams, T. F., and others. Appropriate placement of the chronically ill and aged: a successful approach by evaluation. *JAMA* 226:1332–35, 1973.
15. Rubenstein and others.
16. Hendrickson and others.
17. Rubin, C. D., and others. A randomized clinical trial of outpatient geriatric evaluation and management in a large public hospital. *Journal of the American Gerontological Society* 36:342–47, 1988.
18. Burke, M., and Walsh, M. Care of the frail elderly. In: *Gerontological Nursing.* St. Louis: Mosby, 1992, pp. 1–42.
19. Hendrickson and others.
20. Rubin and others.
21. Topp, R. Development of an exercise program for older adults: pre-exercise testing, exercise prescription and program maintenance. *Nurse Practitioner* 16(10), Oct. 1991.
22. Williams and others.
23. Topp.

24. Eliopoulos, C. Activity and exercise. In: *Manual of Gerontological Nursing*. St. Louis: Mosby, 1995, pp. 337–47.
25. Fishman, P. Detecting malnutrition's warning signs with simple screening tools. *Geriatrics* 49(10):39–43, 1994.
26. Hill, B., and others. Reducing the incidence of falls in high risk patients. *Journal of Nursing Administration* 18(7,8):24–27, July–Aug. 1988.
27. Newman, D. K. The treatment of urinary incontinence in adults. *Nurse Practitioner* 14(6):21–32, June 1989.
28. Ferentz, K. The primary care setting: managing medical comorbidity in the elderly depressed patient. *Geriatrics* 50(suppl. 1), S-25–S-27, 1995.
29. Kurfees, J. F., and Dotson, R. L. Drug interactions in the elderly. *Journal of Family Practice* 25(5):477–88, 1987.
30. Rubenstein and others.

CHAPTER 7

Mapping Home Care Services

Sheila Hawley and Bonnie Davis

In the early 1990s many acute care facilities were designing and implementing clinical paths. Very few caregivers outside of hospitals were acquainted with the benefits of paths or how to integrate them into patient care processes. The resulting decline in hospital lengths of stay had a significant impact on out-of-hospital providers. Patients were leaving the hospital at higher acuity levels, which translated into the need for more intense postdischarge services. The principal caregiver for these discharged patients was home health care services, causing home care to be the most rapidly growing health care provider.

As health care services shifted from institutional services to the home, payers and consumers expressed concern about cost and quality. These groups began to demand that home health agencies become more accountable for quality patient care and cost containment.[1] Such demands forced home health agencies to consider the same strategies that hospitals implemented when they had faced similar challenges in the 1980s. Like hospitals, home health agencies had to assure that patient care processes were stabilized, appropriate, efficient, and cost-effective. Home care services had to improve patient outcomes while minimizing overall resource use.

Following the lead of hospitals, many home health agencies began to explore the use of patient management tools such as the clinical path, which identifies interventions in a predicted sequence based on a time line for a particular diagnosis or procedure, thereby achieving targeted patient outcomes within a specified time period.[2] However, whereas inpatient clinical paths include the tasks required of physicians, nurses, and other disciplines, the home care path is more nursing oriented, with assessment and education the primary interventions. Inpatient paths include short-term clinical outcomes associated with the hospital period of care, whereas the outcomes on home care paths are usually related to patient and caregiver independence in the care and maintenance of the disease process. Ideally, the two types of paths can be integrated, with the inpatient path including a home care referral intervention as well as activities related to information transfer at the time of hospital discharge.

CLINTON'S EARLY PATH INITIATIVE

In early 1993 Clinton Memorial Hospital Home Health Agency leaders began to investigate how clinical pathways and other coordinated care initiatives might help the agency meet the anticipated demands of managed care. Although the eastern part of the United States had yet to feel the full impact of managed care, the agency's leaders wanted to get a head start in the coming transition. They believed that many of the needed changes they anticipated would take several years to accomplish: decrease visit frequency per patient, cut costs, increase productivity, and increase the quality of care. To accommodate these changes the agency first had to change its philosophy from a Medicare model to a managed care model. This shift meant retraining staff from the nurses to the aides to educate them on the goal of patient care: to maximize patient independence rather than foster dependence on home care services. This attitudinal change process took approximately 18 months and resulted in shorter lengths of stay and decreased costs.

Of all the initiatives that might have been chosen, the agency leaders selected clinical pathways as their first project. This patient management tool seemed to be ideal for defining the entire home care process efficiently while promoting quality patient care and effective resource use. As an added benefit, clinical paths could help streamline patient care documentation. It was apparent, however, that home care pathways would need to look different than those designed for hospitalized patients. Essentially, home care paths would have to "go beyond" the traditional hospital path and cover a wider array of services from many different disciplines. Because no material existed on home care paths in 1993, the caregivers at Clinton Home Health Agency decided to develop their own unique pathway model. The result, Clinton HomeCare-Paths, took approximately 1 year to develop and was achieved in three stages.

Forming a Development Committee

The path development committee included the home care manager, the home care coordinator, and a clinical nurse specialist who was also the agency's continuous quality improvement representative. This committee established the goals for the clinical path program, which included the following:

- Decrease overall time required for patient education
- Improve patient teaching methods
- Enhance patient care continuity
- Improve consistency among caregivers
- Decrease paperwork for the nursing staff (other disciplines would be added at a later date)

Developing Clinical Paths for Selected Patient Groups

The committee members, with input from other home care staff, were primarily responsible for designing the first four Clinton HomeCare-Paths. The first step was to identify patient populations that represented high-volume, high-risk, high-cost, or high-interest categories. The patient groups chosen for the first paths were congestive heart failure (CHF), chronic obstructive pulmonary disease (COPD), insulin-dependent diabetes mellitus (IDDM), and acute or chronic wound care.

Developing Path Format and Goals

Developing the format for the HomeCare-Paths was a more difficult process than selecting the patient populations. The primary goals were to:

- Design a user-friendly format
- Make it comprehensive enough to cover all routine patient care parameters
- Incorporate the nursing visit documentation and the care path into one form
- Require very little narrative documentation for the nursing staff

With input from the nurses, a standardized format for documenting *each* home visit was designed. (See figure 7-1.) Unlike traditional clinical paths, which typically illustrate the patient's progression as steps in a continuum on one page, the Clinton home care nurses chose to design paths that illustrate one visit per page in a multiple-page path document. Each page on the home care path is comparable to one column (or day) on a hospital path. A "one page per visit" format would provide sufficient space for the home care nurse to record all relevant patient assessment, intervention, and outcome information.

The routine assessments performed on all patients were included at the top of the standard form. Space was provided at the bottom of the form for documenting diagnosis-specific interventions and outcomes.

Once the final format was chosen, the path development committee filled in the diagnosis-specific content based on its review of current literature references, nursing practice standards, and the agency's historical experience. In the initial development phase, the Clinton HomeCare-Paths were designed with Medicare reimbursement regulations in mind. For example, a 9-week visit period was allowed before the patient's clinical needs were reassessed. Even working within these parameters, Clinton Home Health Agency found that most of its paths specified fewer nursing visits than had previously been provided to patients having the same diagnosis. This situation was also true when comparing Clinton's HomeCare-Paths with those designed by other home health agencies. Many of Clinton's paths suggested a lower number of nursing visits for each diagnosis while still achieving optimal patient outcomes.

To improve program effectiveness, the committee agreed to keep it simple. The Clinton HomeCare-Path system was designed as a two-step process:

1. The first nurse responsible for seeing a patient initiates the HomeCare-Path packet specific to the patient's diagnosis or procedure. The path packet contains everything needed for delivery of care for that patient, including all the educational materials.
2. At each visit the nurse records information on the forms contained in the packet. No additional chart forms are necessary unless the patient develops a new condition.

HOMECARE-PATH NURSING DOCUMENTATION TOOLS

In January 1994 Clinton Home Health Agency implemented its first four clinical paths. One of the greatest efficiency advantages of these patient management tools has proved to be the reduction in paperwork. Before the introduction of clinical paths, nurses dictated each of their home visit notes to a medical transcriptionist. Because the dictated-to-transcribed turnaround time averaged approximately 2 weeks, this process caused a considerable delay in completion of nursing notes. In addition, the transcription services cost the agency more than $16,000 annually. Even though the paths greatly streamlined documentation, during path implementation the nurses

FIGURE 7-1 Standardized Home Visit Form

Clinton Memorial Hospital
HOME HEALTH AGENCY
610 West Main Street ❖ Wilmington, Ohio 45177
(513) 382-9380

HOMECARE-PATH — VISIT

Patient Name _____ MR# _____

Nursing Assessment of Signs & Symptoms: Problem (+) No Problem (-)   WM - Written Material   NA - Not Applicable

☐ NEUROLOGICAL	☐ RESPIRATORY	☐ G.I.	☐ G.U.	☐ MUSCULO/SKELETAL

☐ Alert
☐ Anxious
☐ Confused
☐ Disoriented
☐ Lethargic
☐ Vertigo
☐ Sensory
	☐ Clear A & P
	☐ Crackles
	☐ Rhonchi
	☐ Cough/SOB
	☐ Wheezes
	☐ O₂
	☐ Describe lung sounds
		☐ Nausea/Vomiting
		☐ Anorexia
		☐ Diarrhea
		☐ Constipation
		☐ Bowel sounds
		☐ Last BM _____
			☐ Burning/pain
			☐ Frequency/urgency
			☐ Hesitancy
			☐ Distention/retention
			☐ Incontinent
			☐ Catheter
			   Size _____
				☐ Weakness
				☐ Bed/chair bound
				☐ Balance/gait unsteady
				☐ Functional status
				   ☐ Independent
				   ☐ Assist
				   ☐ Dependent
				☐ Assistive Device
				   ☐ Cane
				   ☐ Walker
				   ☐ Wheelchair
				☐ Other:

☐ VITAL SIGNS
☐ Temp. _____
☐ Pulse _____
☐ Resp. _____
☐ B/P _____
	☐ CARDIOVASCULAR
	☐ Arrhythmia
	☐ Chest pain
	☐ Peripheral Pulses
	☐ Edema:
	   RUE ___ LUE ___
	   RLE ___ LLE ___
		☐ DIET/HYDRATION
		☐ Regular
		☐ ADA _____
		☐ Blood sugar _____
		☐ Appetite
		☐ Weight _____
			Urine _____
			Color _____
			Odor _____
			Clear _____
			Cloudy _____
				☐ PAIN
				☐ Location
				☐ Intensity
				   0-10 _____
				☐ Pain Med. Effectiveness

☐ HOME SAFETY	☐ PSYCHOSOCIAL
	Strengths:
	☐ Family Support
	   ☐ Willing
	   ☐ Available
	   ☐ Able
		☐ SKIN
		☐ Color
		☐ Turgor
		☐ Dry
		☐ Wound
		☐ Other:
			☐ MED COMPLIANCE
			☐ New
			☐ Changes
			☐ Other:
				HHA SERVICE Y N
				Patient satisfaction ☐ ☐
				HHA to continue ☐ ☐
				HHA POC revised ☐ ☐
				HHA following
				assignment ☐ ☐

☐ OTHER	☐ LAST MD APPT.			

A carepath is meant to serve as a general framework for handling the care of a patient with a particular health problem. It should be recognized that pathways are not meant to establish legal standards of care. Seriously ill patients may not be appropriate to manage with a pathway.

NURSING INTERVENTION/EDUCATION	COMPLETED	NOT COMPLETED	COMMENTS

PATIENT OUTCOME	MET	NOT MET	EXPLAIN VARIANCE

PLAN

TIME IN	TIME OUT	DATE	RN SIGNATURE	PATIENT INITIAL

© 1994 Clinton Memorial Hospital   GENLFORM.PM5

Source: Reprinted, with permission, from Clinton Memorial Hospital, copyright 1994.

found it difficult to make the transition from long, narrative, dictated chart notes to the checklist format. After 2 to 3 months the staff began to feel more comfortable using this new charting-by-exception methodology. After a full year of using the first four clinical paths, the staff nurses were eager for more to be developed. The documentation tools that proved to be so successful are described in this section.

Care Plan

The first form in the path is the care plan. (See figure 7-2.) The plan includes details of the patient assessments that are to be completed at each visit, all relevant nursing diagnoses, and long-term and short-term patient goals. The plan is individualized for a particular patient by entering the dates when the patient goals are expected to be met. Listed below the goals is the recommended frequency of nursing care visits. Although based on the Medicare reimbursement model, the number of visits can be revised according to patient need.

Assessment Visit Checklist

The next form in the path is the assessment visit checklist (figure 7-3), which is completed only at the assessment visit. Nurses use this form to indicate that all the routine tasks required on the first visit have been completed and the patient has achieved the predetermined outcomes. Routine tasks include completing the Bill of Rights, advance directives, consent forms, safety plan, and discharge plan and fulfilling accreditation requirements. The checklist has been especially helpful for improving consistency among different caregivers as well as continuity of patient care. The form also helps to ensure that all required documentation is completed for each intervention and outcome on the first visit.

Patient involvement in the care is also documented on the assessment visit form. The nurse goes over the interventions and expected outcomes with the patient or the patient's family, and the plan can be modified based on patient or family input. Once this discussion is completed, the patient initials the form to indicate that the information was provided and that he or she participated in and understood the care plan.

Visit Notes

The next HomeCare-Path form is for documenting the actual nursing visit notes. (See figure 7-4.) The note is a one-page form, with the top half containing a comprehensive checklist of all systems assessments that must be completed along with required information: date of last physician appointment, aides' supervisory visits, patient's safety, and psychosocial needs. The bottom half of the form contains the nursing interventions expected for the visit based on the patient's medical diagnosis and the nursing diagnoses listed on the care plan. Patient outcomes are documented below the interventions and coincide with the interventions. Variance documentation will be discussed later in this chapter.

The "WM" at the end of some of the nursing interventions stands for "written material." This material is standardized and included in the HomeCare-Path packet that the nurse takes along to the patient's home.

The visit note form is printed on two-part carbonless NCR paper. The nurse completes the original, leaves the copy with the patient, and returns the original to the agency office. When the patient is visited by the next nurse (frequently a different staff person), the copy is available for review, thereby promoting continuity of patient care. The only documentation left for the nurse to complete after each home visit is the charge slip.

FIGURE 7-2 Care Plan for Congestive Heart Failure Patients

Clinton Memorial Hospital
Home Health Agency
Wilmington, Ohio 45177

CHF — CARE PLAN
HOME CARE PATH

Patient Name _____ Date _____

MR# _____

ASSESS/MONITOR EACH VISIT:

Complete Cardiopulmonary Assessment with vital signs, B/P, respiratory status (cough, color, mental status, lung sounds) pedal pulses, edema, weight, medication compliance, functional status, diet/hydration, O_2 compliance, emotional status, need for referrals.

NURSING DIAGNOSIS:

1. Alteration in cardiac output: decreased, r/t decreased contractility.
2. Alteration in fluid volume: excess, r/t decreased cardiac output.
3. Alteration in nutritional intake less than body requirements r/t impaired absorption of nutrients secondary to low cardiac output.
4. Potential ineffective coping r/t disease process.
5. Potential alteration in skin integrity r/t edema.
6. Decreased activity tolerance r/t decreased cardiac output.
7. Knowledge deficit r/t disease process and signs and symptoms of early failure.
8. Knowledge deficit r/t medication schedule, actions and side effects.

SHORT/LONG TERM GOALS:

1. Patient/caregiver will be able to access HHA appropriately by _____.
2. Patient/caregiver will be knowledgeable in home safety, medications, home O_2 (if applicable) by _____.
3. Patient/caregiver will understand the pathophysiology of CHF disease process by _____.
4. Patient/caregiver will understand early signs and symptoms of CHF by _____.
5. Patient/caregiver will understand appropriate diet to obtain sufficient nutrients to maintain body function by _____.
6. Patient/caregiver will demonstrate good symptom management by _____.
7. Patient/caregiver will understand good skin care to maintain intact skin integrity by _____.
8. Patient's condition will improve or be maintained at current level.

RECOMMENDED FREQUENCY:

1-3xwkx5, qowx4, prn x4 for cardiopulmonary complications, prn x2 for venipuncture, and prn x2 for constipation.

© 1994 Clinton Memorial Hospital   CHFINFO.PM5

A carepath is meant to serve as a general framework for handling the care of a patient with a particular health problem. It should be recognized that pathways are not meant to establish legal standards of care. Seriously ill patients may not be appropriate to manage with a pathway.

Source: Reprinted, with permission, from Clinton Memorial Hospital, copyright 1994.

FIGURE 7-3 Assessment Visit Checklist

Clinton Memorial Hospital
HOME HEALTH AGENCY
610 West Main Street ❖ Wilmington, Ohio 45177
(513) 382-9380

HOMECARE-PATH ASSESSMENT VISIT

Patient Name _____ MR# _____

Date _____ Time In _____ Time Out _____   WM - Written Material   NA - Not Applicable

NURSING INTERVENTIONS	COMPLETED	NOT COMPLETED	COMMENTS
1. Assess patient for appropriateness for Home Care and level of learning.			
2. Complete admission packet (process) - Bill of Rights, Advance Directives, Consent Form - obtain appropriate signatures.			
3. Assess environmental and psychosocial needs.			
4. Do physical/outcome assessment.			
5. Instruction: a. Call system - WM.			
b. Emergency numbers - WM.			
c. Home safety/disaster plan - WM.			
d. Medication safety/schedule - WM.			

6. Evaluate need for referrals:
   MOW _____   PT _____
   LSW _____   ST _____
   HHA _____   OT _____
   Other _____			

7. Discuss general plan of care and tentative plan of discharge.			
8. Other			

PATIENT OUTCOME	MET	NOT MET	EXPLAIN VARIANCE
1. Verbalizes Home Health call system.			
2. States two measures to promote home/medication safety. a.			
b.			
3. Other			

SIGNATURE	PATIENT INITIAL

© 1994 Clinton Memorial Hospital   PASSVST.PM5

Source: Reprinted, with permission, from Clinton Memorial Hospital, copyright 1994.

FIGURE 7-4 Nursing Visit Note Form for Congestive Heart Failure Patients

Clinton Memorial Hospital
HOME HEALTH AGENCY
610 W. Main Street ❖ Wilmington, Ohio 45177
(513) 382-9380

CHF — HOMECARE-PATH — VISIT #1

Patient Name _____ MR# _____

Nursing Assessment of Signs & Symptoms: Problem (+)   No Problem (-)   WM - Written Material   NA - Not Applicable

☐ **NEUROLOGICAL**
☐ Alert
☐ Anxious
☐ Confused
☐ Disoriented
☐ Lethargic
☐ Vertigo
☐ Sensory

☐ **VITAL SIGNS**
☐ Temp. _____
☐ Pulse _____
☐ Resp. _____
☐ B/P _____

☐ **HOME SAFETY**

☐ **OTHER**

☐ **RESPIRATORY**
☐ Clear A & P
☐ Crackles
☐ Rhonchi
☐ Cough/SOB
☐ Wheezes
☐ O_2 _____

☐ **CARDIOVASCULAR**
☐ Arrhythmia
☐ Chest pain
☐ Peripheral Pulses
☐ Edema:
   RUE _____ LUE _____
   RLE _____ LLE _____

☐ **PSYCHOSOCIAL**
Strengths:
☐ Family Support
   ☐ Willing
   ☐ Available
   ☐ Able

☐ **LAST MD APPT.**

☐ **G.I.**
☐ Nausea/Vomiting
☐ Anorexia
☐ Diarrhea
☐ Constipation
☐ Bowel sounds
☐ Last BM _____

☐ **DIET/HYDRATION**
☐ Regular
☐ ADA
☐ Blood sugar _____
☐ Appetite
☐ Weight _____

☐ **SKIN**
☐ Color
☐ Turgor
☐ Dry
☐ Wound
☐ Other: _____

☐ **G.U.**
☐ Burning/pain
☐ Frequency/urgency
☐ Hesitancy
☐ Distention/retention
☐ Incontinent
☐ Catheter
   Size _____
Urine _____
Color _____
Odor _____
Clear _____
Cloudy _____

☐ **MED COMPLIANCE**
☐ New
☐ Changes
☐ Other:

☐ **MUSCULO/SKELETAL**
☐ Weakness
☐ Bed/chair bound
☐ Balance/gait unsteady
☐ Functional status
   ☐ Independent
   ☐ Assist
   ☐ Dependent
☐ Assistive Device
   ☐ Cane
   ☐ Walker
   ☐ Wheelchair
☐ Other:

☐ **PAIN**
☐ Location
☐ Intensity
   0-10 _____
☐ Pain Med. Effectiveness

HHA SERVICE   Y   N
Patient satisfaction ☐ ☐
HHA to continue   ☐ ☐
HHA POC revised   ☐ ☐
HHA following   ☐ ☐
assignment

NURSING INTERVENTION/EDUCATION	COMPLETED	NOT COMPLETED	COMMENTS
1. Instruct patient/caregiver on medication #1-3 - WM.			
2. Instruct patient/caregiver on Home O_2 if applicable - WM			
3. Begin instruction to patient/caregiver on pathophysiology/disease process CHF - WM.			
4. Instruct patient/caregiver on low/no salt diet - WM.			
5. Instruct patient/caregiver on importance of weighing every day or as ordered by M.D., and record - WM.			
6. Other			

PATIENT OUTCOME	MET	NOT MET	EXPLAIN VARIANCE
1. Verbally returns medication administration and major side effects for each medication taught today.			
2. States 3 - O_2 safety measures, if applicable.			
3. Verbally defines CHF.			
4. States 3 foods high in sodium to avoid.			
5. Verbally understands when to weigh and record.			
6. Other			

PLAN

TIME IN	TIME OUT	DATE	RN SIGNATURE	PATIENT INITIAL

© 1994 Clinton Memorial Hospital   CHF1-12.PM5

Source: Reprinted, with permission, from Clinton Memorial Hospital, copyright 1994.

One visit form is available for each expected visit, based on the patient's diagnosis. The number of visits in a care path can range from 3 to 12. For example, a patient requiring home care for intravenous therapy is expected to need 3 visits, whereas the care path for a patient with a condition such as chronic CHF includes 12.

A generic version of the visit form (figure 7-1) was developed to document visits for patients who are not on a care path or who have been on a path and need visits beyond the established number. The interventions and outcomes section of this form is blank. The nurse fills in the interventions and outcomes at the time of the visit as well as whether they were completed.

Copaths

A copath is used for patients who have significant comorbidities or secondary diagnoses. It is a comprehensive, flexible tool that allows the nurse to document patient assessments and education related to the secondary disease process. It is a separate tool from the care path but can be used simultaneously with it or independently. For example, patients with a primary diagnosis of CHF would be on the CHF care path; if they also had IDDM as a secondary diagnosis, they would be on an IDDM copath. (See figure 7-5.)

A copath is used as a documentation tool to record assessment and education of the secondary diagnosis. The primary nurse determines when a copath is needed based on the patient's or caregiver's knowledge level and management of the secondary diagnosis.

CARE PATHS AND PERFORMANCE IMPROVEMENT

The Clinton HomeCare-Path system promotes and enhances the performance improvement activities of the home health agency. Performance measurement data are readily available from the nursing notes and the variance reporting process. The variance report form (figure 7-6) is completed when there is any change in the patient's plan of care. Variances can be negative (patient progresses slower than anticipated) or positive (patient progresses faster than anticipated).

An example of a negative variance: The patient is ill on the second home visit and unable to complete the scheduled interventions. The variance is documented on the report form, and the interventions are rescheduled for the third visit.

An example of a positive variance: At the first home visit the patient is able to complete all the education requirements for the first visit and those expected to be completed on the second. This variance is noted on the report form, and the patient advances to the third-visit level for his or her education-related interventions.

Performance Improvement

Nursing notes and variance data are used in improvement activities. For example, during performance improvement activities, care providers discovered that patient weights were not being documented at each home visit. The staff was notified about this deficiency and urged to improve its performance. However, further analysis showed little change and after discussion with the staff it became apparent that the problem was related to the path format, not just the care providers. Shading was added to the path for those interventions most important to the process of care. (See figure 7-4.) By shading *lung sound assessment, weight,* and *edema assessment,* for example, the staff is reminded of the importance of each of these evaluations for each CHF-related home care visit.

138 CHAPTER 7 MAPPING HOME CARE SERVICES

FIGURE 7-5 Copath for Insulin-Dependent Diabetes Mellitus Patients

Clinton Memorial Hospital
Home Health Agency
Wilmington, Ohio 45177

INSULIN DEPENDENT DIABETES MELLITUS CO-PATH

Patient Name_____ MR#_____

Start of Care _____ This Diagnosis is: ____ New ____ Exacerbation ____ Chronic Condition

M = Met   **NM = Not Met**   **N/A = Not Applicable**

GOALS: Patient/caregiver will demonstrate understanding of disease process and self-care management.

DATES:

PATIENT OUTCOMES:

1. I. Instruct on definition/causes of IDDM.
   O. States definition/causes of IDDM.
2. I. Instruct on proper blood sugar monitoring.
   O. Demonstrates proper blood sugar monitoring.
3. I. Instruct on insulin injection.
   O. Demonstrates proper insulin injection (including site rotation).
4. I. Instruct on proper needle disposal.
   O. Demonstrates proper needle disposal.
5. I. Instruct on s/s of Hypoglycemia and Tx.
   O. States 2 s/s of Hypoglycemia and Tx.
6. I. Instruct on s/s of Hyperglycemia and Tx.
   O. States 2 s/s of Hyperglycemia and Tx.
7. I. Instruct on ADA diet/daily calorie allowance.
   O. States ADA diet, including daily calorie allowance.
8. I. Instruct on causes of Hypo/Hyperglycemia.
   O. States 2 causes each of Hypo/Hyperglycemia.
9. I. Instruct on diabetic ketoacidosis
   O. States definition of diabetic ketoacidosis and emergency number to call.
10. I. Instruct on action and side effects of insulin.
    O. States action and side effects of insulin.
11. I. Instruct on measures to prevent long-term effects of insulin/consequences of noncompliance.
    O. States 3 measures to prevent long-term effects/consequences of noncompliance.
12. I. Instruct on skin care.
    O. States s/s of skin problems to report.
13. I. Instruct on good skin/foot care.
    O. Demonstrates good skin/foot care.

NURSE SIGNATURE

© 1994 Clinton Memorial Hospital Rev. 4/96   IDDMCOPT.PM5

Source: Reprinted, with permission, from Clinton Memorial Hospital, copyright 1994.

FIGURE 7-6 Variance Report Form

**Clinton Memorial Hospital
Home Health Agency**
Wilmington, OH 45177

HOMECARE - PATH VARIANCE REPORT

Care-Path Diagnosis _____
Care-Path Start Date _____
Care-Path Stop Date _____
Pt. D/C Date _____

Nurse: _____

Please give a brief explanation of variance under the appropriate category.

VISIT	DATE	INTERV./ OUTCOME	PATIENT TOO SICK	PATIENT OR NURSES' DECISION	PATIENT'S CAREGIVER DECISION	COGNITIVE STATUS	LACK OF CAREGIVER	SECONDARY LACK OF EQUIPMENT	DIAGNOSIS INTERFERENCE	OTHER
VISIT 1										
VISIT 2										
VISIT 3										
VISIT 4										
VISIT 5										
VISIT 6										
VISIT 7										
VISIT 8										
VISIT 9										
VISIT 10										
VISIT 11										
VISIT 12										
VISIT 13										
NURSE SIGNATURE										

© 1994 Clinton Memorial Hospital Rev. 9/95

PTHVARPT.PM5

Source: Reprinted, with permission, from Clinton Memorial Hospital, copyright 1994.

TABLE 7-1 Comparison of Prepath and Postpath Outcome Measures

Measure	Prepath Data	Postpath Data
Cost per patient	$3,300	$1,400
Median cost	$1,300	$700
Total cost	$84,600	$36,800
Average visits per patient	23	10
Mean length of stay	106 days	70 days
Mean number of hospital readmissions	1.16	0.68
Documentation of diet teaching	44%	100%
Documentation of medication teaching	80%	100%
Patient disposition		
Self-care	12%	16%
Home with assist	32%	40%
Extended care facility	20%	4%
Hospital admit	28%	24%
Expired	8%	4%
Hospice	0%	12%

Outcome Measurement

Outcome measures are documented at the end of each patient visit when the nurse notes the patient's response to the interventions. The number of visits provided to each patient is easily tracked along with the length of stay in the program, hospital readmissions, and program readmissions. By using these outcome data the home health agency can, for example, evaluate all patients on a particular path, pinpoint problem areas, and target improvement needs. For example, if variances are repeatedly occurring because of unavailable supplies, appropriate steps can be taken to procure the necessary supplies.

Cost-Effectiveness Research

A retrospective research study of Clinton Home Health Agency patients conducted by Mancuso, a graduate student at the University of Michigan, examined CHF patients before and after implementation of the care paths.[3] Results of the study, which covered the period from 1990 to 1996, are shown in table 7-1. Fifty cases were studied: 25 preimplementation and 25 postimplementation. The average age of patients in the study was 77 years.

This study showed that the cost per patient to provide home care prior to paths was $3,300, dropping to $1,400 after paths were implemented. Total cost savings for the 25 patients was $47,800, which can mean the difference between an agency's failure and its survival in the managed care and capitated environment. Average visits per patient decreased by 13. Table 7-1 shows other outcomes measured by this study. For example, documentation of patient dietary teaching was improved by the care paths, from 44 percent to 100 percent. In addition, patients' average length of stay in home care decreased significantly after care paths were implemented, from 106 days to 70 days.

Data like these have been shared with local managed care companies to illustrate the benefit of contracting with Clinton Home Health Agency. Having access to such data enables home health agencies to demonstrate their cost-effectiveness to managed care companies.

Benchmark Project

In the future, Clinton Home Health Agency hopes to begin a benchmark project with other agencies that are using the same HomeCare-Paths. This will allow more valid comparisons between agencies when the same data collection tools are used for similar patient populations. Such a comparative project will allow all involved agencies to identify problem areas affecting quality of care, cost of care, and agency efficiency.

INTERDISCIPLINARY PATHS

A long-term goal for Clinton HomeCare-Paths is to incorporate other disciplines into the path system. In mid-1995 Clinton Home Health Agency began expanding its nurse-oriented clinical path model into an interdisciplinary tool, a change that is currently under way. The Clinton HomeCare-Path system had been implemented for approximately 2 years before the path concept was discussed with physical therapists, speech therapists, social workers, and occupational therapists. This interdisciplinary expansion phase has been much more difficult than expected; staff resistance has been significant.

The goals for incorporating other disciplines into the HomeCare-Path system were the same as for the nursing staff: pathways would be developed for each discipline's high-volume, high-risk, high-cost, and/or high-interest patient populations. The only requirement is that the path format used by other disciplines be similar to the nursing care paths.

Some of the other disciplines were initially resistant to the concept of paths in general. As with the nurses, their traditional care-planning processes did not involve the use of checklists and predefined interventions, and they, too, were accustomed to narrative charting. Speech therapists and occupational therapists were the most open to the idea of care paths. To date, occupational and physical therapy have developed a care path for patients with problems in their lower extremities (figure 7-7), and physical, occupational, and speech therapy have developed a care path for patients with nervous system disorders (figure 7-8).

At first the physical therapists felt that, because their patients are at varying levels of ability at the start of therapy, it would be very difficult to develop a "standard" care path for patients having a particular diagnosis. To overcome this problem, physical therapy, like occupational therapy, decided to group its care paths into body system categories rather than diagnoses. Currently, a physical therapy HomeCare-Path has been created for patients with lower extremity and nervous system problems, and other paths are expected to be developed. Physical, occupational, and speech therapy plan to work more closely together on future care path development because of their similar patient populations and outcome goals.

The social worker had traditionally documented lengthy narrative visit notes and found the concept of charting by exception hard to accept. However, after completing a care path for community information resources related to the patients' diagnosis and needs, the social worker is becoming accustomed to using checklists and preprinted interventions. Plans are under way to develop other social-service-related HomeCare-Paths.

FIGURE 7-7 Occupational Therapy Visit Note Form

Clinton Memorial Hospital Home Health Agency
Wilmington, Ohio 45177

OCCUPATIONAL THERAPIST LOWER EXTREMITY ORTHOPEDIC — HOMECARE-PATH — VISIT #1

Patient Name _____ MR# _____

DME = Durable Medical Equipment   WM - Written Material

☐ ADL	☐ UE STRENGTH	☐ COGNITION	☐ SAFETY	☐ FUNCTIONAL TRANSFERS
☐ Dependent	☐ Normal	☐ Alert	☐ Good	☐ Dependent
☐ Max @	☐ Good	☐ Confused	☐ Fair	☐ Max @
☐ Mod @	☐ Fair	☐ Lethargic	☐ Poor	☐ Mod @
☐ Min @	☐ Poor	☐ Uncooperative		☐ Mid @
☐ Supervision				☐ Supervision
☐ Independent				☐ Independent

OCCUPATIONAL THERAPY INTERVENTION	COMPLETED	NOT COMPLETED	COMMENTS
1. Instruct patient/caregiver on precautions - WM.			
2. Instruct administrator ADL equipment - WM.			
3. Instruct/recommend DME - WM.			
4. Instruct on UE strengthening ex. - WM.			
5. Instruct on proper transfer technique.			
6. Other			

PATIENT OUTCOME	MET	NOT MET	EXPLAIN VARIANCE
1. Verbalizes precautions and contraindications if precautions are not followed.			
2. Verbally understands use of ADL equipment.			
3. Verbally understands use of DME.			
4. Demonstrates UE strengthening program if applicable with written handout.			
5. Verbally understands transfer technique.			
6. Other			

Assessment: _____

PLAN

TIME IN	TIME OUT	DATE	OT SIGNATURE	PATIENT INITIAL

© 1996 Clinton Memorial Hospital   OTHRP1-4.PM5

Source: Reprinted, with permission, from Clinton Memorial Hospital, copyright 1996.

FIGURE 7-8 Occupational, Physical, and Speech Therapy Care Path for Patients with Nervous Disorders

Clinton Memorial Hospital
Home Health Agency
Wilmington, Ohio 45177

OCCUPATIONAL, PHYSICAL & SPEECH THERAPY FOR NEUROLOGY—HOMECARE-PATH

Patient Name _____ Date _____

MR# _____

CLINICAL DIAGNOSIS:

_____
_____
_____

OCCUPATIONAL, PHYSICAL AND SPEECH THERAPIST DIAGNOSIS: (CHECK ALL THAT APPLY)

____ 1. Impaired mobility: bed transitions, gait, wheelchair, toilet, tub.
____ 2. Limitation of motion interfering with function of limb.
____ 3. Potential for injury: joint dislocation, strain, sprain, nonunion, skin breakdown.
____ 4. Pain.
____ 5. Cognitive deficit.
____ 6. Knowledge deficit; client/caregiver.
____ 7. Safety concerns.
____ 8. Joint effusion/lower extremity edema.
____ 9. Nonfunctional strength.
____ 10. Nonfunctional endurance.
____ 11. Need for adaptive equipment.
____ 12. Balance deficits.
____ 13. Multiple medical problems interfering with progress.
____ 14. Impaired ADL.
____ 15. Impaired homemaking.
____ 16. Impaired coordination.
____ 17. Impaired auditory/reading comprehension.
____ 18. Impaired verbal/written expression.
____ 19. Motor speech impairments.
____ 20. Swallowing difficulties.
____ 21. Impaired perception.
____ 22. Impaired sensation.

SHORT/LONG TERM GOALS:

____ 1. Bed mobility independence.
____ 2. Transitions independence.
____ 3. Safety in all mobility/transitions.
____ 4. Independent gait with or without assistive device.
____ 5. Caregiver or client independent with assistive devices/adaptive equipment.
____ 6. Functional strength is > 3+/5 of involved extremity.
____ 7. Functional endurance is > 2/3.
____ 8. CG/client is independent with home exercise program.
____ 9. CG/client is independent with precautions.
____ 10. Resumption of prior activities in home.
____ 11. ADL independence.
____ 12. Improve auditory/reading comprehension to functional status.
____ 13. Improve verbal/written expression to functional status.
____ 14. Improve intelligibility of speech to be understood.
____ 15. Improve safety and efficiency of swallowing to meet nutritional needs without risk of aspiration.
____ 16. Demonstrates knowledge regarding specific communication/cognitive/swallowing deficits.
____ 17. Demonstrates knowledge regarding safety precautions.
____ 18. Improve cognitive skills so that pt. may function safely at home.
____ 19. Improve coordination for ADL independence.

RECOMMENDED VISIT FREQUENCY:

2-5xwk/4-6wks. for treatment and teaching client/caregiver
1-3xwk/2-4wks. for treatment and teaching client/caregiver
1-2xwk/2wks. to advance activities, monitor needs and continue teaching client/caregiver.

© 1997 Clinton Memorial Hospital

POSTNFO.PM5

A carepath is meant to serve as a general framework for handling the care of a patient with a particular health problem. Seriously ill patients may not be appropriate to manage with a pathway. It should be recognized that pathways are not meant to establish legal standards of care.

Source: Reprinted, with permission, from Clinton Memorial Hospital, copyright 1997.

CONCLUSION

Home care clinical paths have proved to be a useful tool for guiding the delivery of home care services, ensuring that patients achieve the most desirable outcomes within a reasonable time period. When Clinton Memorial Hospital Home Health Agency began to investigate clinical paths in 1992, very few home health agencies had begun to develop these tools. Therefore, Clinton's leaders designed their own model to accommodate the needs of their rural patient population and their agency's internal staffing and structure. Many positive benefits came out of this initiative. However, home health agencies, like all health care organizations, must realize that path development is costly. Clinton Home Health Agency estimated its path-related costs to be approximately $7,500 to develop the first four pathways. These costs include research, designing and formatting, and printing. After the initial start-up expense of the first four pathways, the costs are now approximately $325 to develop and produce each new pathway.

The agency has estimated a total annual savings of $73,699 based on the utilization of the 20 paths it has implemented. These savings are primarily related to documentation efficiency. Other home health agencies may wish to minimize their pathway start-up costs by investing in one of the many home care path systems now available on the market.

The most important lessons learned by the caregivers involved in the Clinton HomeCare-Path system were that process changes must be simple, user friendly, and cost-effective to assure staff buy-in and implementation success. As the environment becomes dominated by managed care organizations and risk contracting, home care agencies that have not implemented paths or similar patient care management tools will fail to exist.

References

1. Mancuso, L. The effects of clinical pathways on costs and patient outcomes in home care. Master's thesis, University of Michigan, 1996.
2. Zander, K., and Etheredge, M. L. *Collaborative Care: Nursing Case Management*. Chicago: American Hospital Publishing, 1989.
3. Mancuso.

CHAPTER 8

Incorporating Case Management into Home Care

DeAnne Mosher

In 1992 Clinton Memorial Hospital Home Health Agency, Wilmington, OH, embarked on a clinical path initiative. The agency's path development process and the resulting HomeCare-Path system is described by Sheila Hawley and Bonnie Davis in chapter 7 of this book. The agency has realized many benefits from these care paths, including increased patient participation in care, more consistent care planning and documentation, enhanced new-employee orientation, and the elimination of home care service disruptions caused by the use of agency nurses. However, leaders at Clinton Home Health Agency soon realized that care paths were not enough to satisfy the demands of the managed care environment. Several improvement goals existed that could not be addressed by the care path tool alone:

- Increase overall agency efficiency
- Decrease agency costs
- Improve patient satisfaction
- Improve patient self-care skills
- Strengthen the nurses' organizational skills

Reminiscent of their 1992 literature search for examples of home health clinical paths, leaders at Clinton Home Health Agency did not find much information about home health initiatives that might help address these issues. What they did find was a good deal being written about hospital-initiated case management. In this system hospital case managers assume responsibility for intrahospital coordination of patient care services and effective use of resources. The case management process seemed to complement hospitals' clinical path efforts and at the same time offer solutions to problems that paths alone could not address. The concept of case management in home care is not new, though in 1995 many home health agencies had not formally adopted the case management prototype.

The case management delivery model seemed to be an ideal improvement step for Clinton Home Health Agency. In 1995 every staff nurse in the agency was considered to be a primary care nurse, whether full-time or part-time staff. As primary care nurses, each had his or her own patient caseload. A clinical coordinator was responsible for obtaining all patients' insurance verifications, negotiating for visits, managing the referral process, and making patient assignments to the nurses and other disciplines. Because this model of home services delivery is prevalent in the industry, it was difficult for leaders and staff to think beyond their existing circumstances. However, changes were necessary if the agency were to increase efficiency and decrease costs. Therefore, the leaders needed to examine the current processes objectively. What they found was that the primary care nursing model used at Clinton Home Health Agency had its flaws. For instance:

- The part-time nurses were unable to fulfill their role as primary care nurses because other staff had to take over patient visits when the part-time nurses were unavailable.
- Nurses with specialty training in obstetrical care, enterostomal therapy, chemotherapy administration, and so on, were expected to assume primary care nursing roles. However, they were unable to meet their specialty service obligations in addition to seeing routine patients.

Case management was chosen as the agency's next managed care strategy because it seemed to offer many advantages that would benefit the staff and the patients. For example:

- It can reduce hospital readmissions. Home care case managers can teach patients to make better use of health care resources and participate actively in healing and self-care. Patients' immediate responses to therapy can be optimized, which in turn will improve their long-term outcomes.
- It can increase cooperation among home health care team members. Through better communication and clearly defined roles, a case management model fosters partnership and improves working relationships among health care team members.
- It can lower per-patient home care costs. By improving coordination among the home caregivers, costly duplication of services and administrative delays can be reduced or eliminated.
- It can improve patient satisfaction. The home care case manager can help patients and their families deal with the often frustrating system of health care, bringing greater satisfaction to the entire experience.
- It ultimately promotes staff empowerment and professionalism. By increasing caregivers' autonomy and accountability, case management has the potential to empower nurses and increase job satisfaction, thereby reducing staff turnover.

This chapter describes the process by which Clinton Home Health Agency transformed its primary care nursing model into a case management delivery system. Although the experiences depicted are those of a small rural home health agency, the insights gained from them apply to all home health agencies.

DEVELOPMENT OF THE CASE MANAGEMENT MODEL

The first challange that faced agency leaders was to define case management, formulate a goal statement, and specify the new roles for the home health nurses. In the search for a definition that was meaningful for home care providers, the origins of case management were traced back to the turn of the century. At that time patients received much of their health care at home, and public health nurses served as care coordinators. Today this model of care coordination, known as *case management*, is being performed by many different disciplines working for many different employers: managed care health plans, HMOs, large employer groups, hospitals, public health departments, home care agencies, and so on.[1] Each case management program offers a slightly different range of care coordination activities. For example, acute care hospitals and home health care agencies usually view case management as a strategy for coordinating services while the patient remains within the facility or continues receiving care from the agency.[2,3] A few acute care hospitals have developed community-based programs, so their case management services follow patients outside the hospital.[4] Payer-initiated case management and long-term case management offered by public health departments tend to cover the entire continuum of care regardless of the location in which service is provided. All case management programs, however broad or limited in scope, include the activities of assessment, planning, implementation, and evaluation.

In selecting the definition of case management for Clinton Home Health Agency, leadership had to consider the scope of services to be offered and the probable role of the home caregivers in tomorrow's managed care environment. After carefully evaluating these issues and reviewing the case management definitions used by other groups, Clinton Home Health Agency adopted the following definition:

> At Clinton Memorial Hospital Home Health Agency, case management is the process of coordinating an individual client's total health care services to achieve optimal quality care delivered in a cost-effective manner. The process integrates assessment, planning, implementation, and evaluation components.

Next, the purpose of case management at the agency had to be established. Borrowing from the language of the Case Management Society of America, the following purpose statements were formulated:[5]

- Interject objectivity and information where it is lacking.
- Maximize efficiency in utilization of available resources.
- Allow multidisciplinarians in various settings to work collaboratively during different phases of a patient's illness, thereby maximizing the resources available in the public or private health system according to individual needs.
- Promote the optimal allocation of health dollars.

The Role of the Nurse Case Managers

The full-time nurses at Clinton Home Health Agency were transformed into case managers having primary care responsibilities for a defined caseload of patients. They assumed roles as planners, coordinators, educators, negotiators, and communicators, taking over many of the responsibilities previously delegated to the clinical coordinator. These new case management roles were defined as described below.

Planner The case manager is responsible for defining and implementing a patient care treatment plan without compromising outcomes or inappropriately increasing costs:

- The planning process includes the patient as the primary decision maker and considers the patient's goals as an integral part of the plan.
- For each step in the process, contingencies are incorporated into the overall plan to anticipate treatment and service complications.

- Plan modifications, based on the results of monitoring and reevaluation, are initiated to accommodate changes in treatment or patient progress.

Coordinator The case manager is responsible for coordinating all health care services required for the patient, including but not limited to:

- Physician office visits
- Transportation
- Home medical equipment
- Nurse and home health aide visits
- Home safety evaluations
- Medical supplies
- Infusion therapy needs
- Home and outpatient needs
    Physical therapy
    —Occupational therapy
    —Speech therapy
    —Social worker visits

Educator The case manager is responsible for providing patients and providers with information regarding:

- Health plan subscriber benefits and eligibility
- Treatment plan and alternative choices
- Navigation of the health care delivery system

Negotiator The case manager is responsible for negotiating with payers for appropriate patient visit frequency.

Communicator Case managers serve as the central contact between the physician, insurance company, and patient. They are responsible for assuring that communication flows freely among all parties involved in the patient's care. The part-time nurses would serve as "visit" nurses. As such they provide routine care for patients but do not have case management responsibilities. They assist the case managers in carrying out the patient care activities planned by the managers for their patients.

The Case Manager's Job Description

Clinton Home Health Agency's home health director outlined two requirements for the case manager's job description:

1. The job description and the employee performance evaluation had to be included on one form.
2. The performance evaluation had to be criteria based to meet the standards of the Joint Commission on Accreditation of Healthcare Organizations.

The case manager job description from Clinton can be seen in figure 8-1.
  Some home health organizations only employ clinical nurse specialists or master-prepared registered nurses as their case managers. Caregivers having these credentials are not readily available in small rural communities such as Wilmington, OH. Therefore, the nurse case managers at Clinton Home Health Agency are not required

FIGURE 8-1 Nurse Case Manager Job Description and Performance Evaluation

POSITION TITLE: Case Manager: Nursing
REPORTS TO: Clinical Supervisor
JOB SUMMARY The Case Manager, Nursing, is a Registered Professional Nurse who understands the organizational Quality Statement and complies with the organization's quality commitments. And has the responsibility, accountability and authority for providing coordinated, comprehensive nursing care in accordance with the objectives, policies and procedures of Clinton Memorial Hospital and its Home Health Agency for the sick or disabled neonate, pediatric, adolescent, adult and geriatric client, according to the individual RN's abilities and competencies.

QUALIFICATIONS AND REQUIREMENTS:
1. Graduate from an approved program of nursing.
2. Current Ohio nursing license.
3. Minimum of one (1) year medical-surgical hospital nursing.
4. Valid Ohio driver's license and a car.

PERFORMANCE LEVELS
5 - Far Exceeds Standards
4 - Exceeds Standards
3 - Meets Standards
2 - Needs Improvement
1 - Far Below Standards

Responsibilities/Performance Criteria

Behavior/Function	Performance Criteria	A Points	B Relative Weight	C Point Value A × B
A. Professional Responsibilities • Case Management	1. Acts as case manager for primary patients in accordance with role and responsibilities defined by agency		.06	
	2. Coordinates care with: a) Primary RN case manager b) Other disciplines c) Other agencies		.05	
	3. Communicates care with: a) Team members: nursing b) Other disciplines c) Home care coordinator d) Patient and family		.05	
	4. Acts as associate case manager in absence of case manager			
• Clinical Abilities	1. Assessment of health status a) Demonstrates the knowledge and the skills necessary to provide care, based on the psycho/social, educational, safety, and related patient needs appropriate to the age of the patients served b) Physical c) Psychological d) Social/Family		.05	
	2. Able to correlate physical processes of illness, complications and relate to patient		.05	
	3. Plan of care reflects achievable, measurable, expected outcomes		.03	
	4. Technical/Procedure skills a) Current/updated/competent b) Follows agency policies/procedures; standards		.03	
	5. Develops a plan of care for home health aides (HHAs) and supervises/teaches HHA regarding individual patient needs		.04	
	6. Applies teaching/learning principles for patient and family		.03	

149

FIGURE 8-1 *Continued*

Responsibilities/Performance Criteria		PERFORMANCE LEVELS		
		5 - Far Exceeds Standards			
		4 - Exceeds Standards			
		3 - Meets Standards			
		2 - Needs Improvement			
		1 - Far Below Standards			
Behavior/Function	**Performance Criteria**	**A** Points	**B** Relative Weight	**C** Point Value A × B
• Manages Own Practice	1. Organized in approach to time and tasks		.02	
	2. Delegates nonnurse tasks to support personnel (HHA)		.02	
	3. Able to deal with problems in order of priority		.02	
	4. Able to make independent decisions		.05	
	5. Able to analyze a situation and develop a plan		.03	
	6. Adjusts schedule if unexpected problems occur		.04	
B. Responsibility to Agency • Knowledge • Communication • Functions within Clinton Memorial Hospital system • Performance Improvement/Risk Management Program	1. Understands/complies with rules and regulations governing home health care		.05	
	2. Clinically current and competent in nursing with specific emphasis in the area of home health nursing and age specific, as appropriate		.04	
	3. Keeps home care team leader informed of major changes in clients		.04	
	4. Submits orders and medical updates in a timely manner and in accordance with Clinton Memorial Hospital system		.04	
	5. Written documentation complete and reflects skilled care provided		.03	
	6. Shares new concepts and ideas with peers		.02	
	7. Good interpersonal communication skills with: a) "Customer service" oriented b) Patients and family c) Colleagues d) Physicians		.04	
	8. Communicates and behaves in a manner consistent with the organization's quality statement and quality commitments		.04	
	9. Assumes responsibility for agency and patients on weekends and evening on-call as needed.		.03	
	10. Able to be a "marketing person" for agency		.02	
	11. Maintains continuing education units required for Ohio license		.02	
	12. Current CPR (basic life support) certification		.02	
	13. Participates in TQM/CQI program a) Continually evaluates patient care b) Utilizes feedback from quality studies in improving practice		.04	

FIGURE 8-1 *Continued*

OVERALL PERFORMANCE RATING

☐ Outstanding (3.5–4.0)   ☐ Needs Improvement (0.5–1.49)
☐ More than Satisfactory (2.5–3.49)   ☐ Unsatisfactory (0–0.49)
☐ Satisfactory (1.5–2.49)

Evaluator's Response
_____
_____

Employee's Response
_____
_____

Signature of Employee _____ Date: _____

Signature of CHS Group Leader _____ Date: _____

APPROVAL:
  Group Leader _____ Date: _____
  Human Resources Team Leader II _____ Date: _____
  Executive Director _____ Date: _____
  President & CEO _____ Date: _____

Source: Reprinted, with permission, Clinton Memorial Hospital.

to have advanced degrees. They are, however, supervised by a case-management-certified registered nurse.

Guiding Principles for Case Managers and Visit Nurses

The precepts governing Clinton Home Health Agency's home care case managers were defined before the process was implemented. As noted later in the chapter, these responsibilities were refined as opportunities for improvement were identified. The initial responsibilities were defined as follows:

1. Case managers will perform all patient assessments except obstetrical (OB) cases, unless they have special OB training.
2. There will be no ceiling on the number of cases assigned to a case manager. The acuity of the case manager's patient load will be considered in determining the maximum number of cases assigned. For example, a case manager could adequately manage more low-acuity patients than high-acuity patients.
3. Case managers will be expected to complete 90 to 120 total monthly visits, with an assessment visit equaling two visits. This range in expected number of visits allows for flexibility throughout the month to accommodate documentation requirements and unforeseen patient assessment volumes.
4. Case managers will work together to prevent the occurrence of simultaneous vacations.
5. When one case manager is on a planned vacation or is off work as the result of a long-term illness, the remaining case managers, with support from the clinical supervisor, will fulfill the furloughed manager's responsibilities, including patient

assessments, visit assignments, and management of any issues or problems that arise. During a case manager's short-term illness, the clinical supervisor will fulfill the case manager's responsibilities.

Guiding principles were also defined for the visit nurses. These are registered nurses who may be employed part or full time by the agency. Their guidelines are as follows:

1. Visit nurses will be expected to make one patient visit for each hour worked.
2. It is the responsibility of the visit nurses to obtain their own visit schedules from the case managers or home health care coordinator.
3. The visit nurses will return all completed visit paperwork to the office at the end of each day worked.
4. When the agency census is low, visit nurses will be expected to participate in agency-related activities such as quality improvement, chart review, or other activities assigned by the clinical supervisor, manager, or director.
5. Visit nurses will not be expected to attend weekly team meetings. Because patient update information and assignments will be communicated to visit nurses outside of the meetings, they will have time for more patient visits.

Case Management Tools

The case managers delegate patient visits to the visit nurses using the visit nurse schedule board. (See figure 8-2.) Each case manager uses a different color marking pen to fill in the information on the schedule board. This color-coded system allows the visit nurse to know at a glance who the case manager is for a particular patient.

The patient update form (figure 8-3) is reviewed at the weekly team meetings and distributed to the visit nurses. Information on this form is kept up-to-date to ensure

FIGURE 8-2 Visit Nurse Schedule Board

	Monday		Tuesday		Wednesday		Thursday		Friday
Date:	10/28		10/29		10/30		10/31		11/1
Edda	LOC	Sue	LOC	VN	LOC	VN	LOC	VN	LOC
1. J. Smith 2. T. Jones 3. S. Davis 4. E. Toms 5. R. Abel 6. P. Green 7. 8.	Blan Sabina Blan Cuba Wilm Wilm	Mick Rice Long Dye	W.C. W.C. P.W. Wilm						
Pam	LOC	VN	LOC	VN	LOC	VN	LOC	VN	LOC
1. C. Sams 2. W. Baker 3. Y. Abt	Wilm Wilm Sabina								
VN	LOC	VN	LOC	VN	LOC	VN	LOC	VN	LOC
1. 2. 3.									

FIGURE 8-3 Patient Update Form

Patient Name	Admit Date	Discharge Date	Case Manager	Home Health Aide	Social Services	Physical Therapy/ Speech Therapy/ Occupational Therapy	Update
T. Smith	10/28		Sue	✓	✓		
J. Jones		10/29					
B. Rice							Antibiotics discontinued
C. Alt							Started on parenteral fluids
D. Toms	10/27		Pam			PT only	

that the visit nurses have the latest information for their on-call books and for visit coverage purposes. The update form is very simple to use. If a patient is discharged from home care, the patient's name and discharge date are entered. If a patient is admitted to the hospital, the patient's name, admission date, case manager's name, and home services that had been started are entered. New information about a current patient is entered in the column labeled "update."

The last tool developed was the case managers' schedule board. (See figure 8-4.) This board has an erasable surface and is used to identify patients assigned to each of the case managers, the social worker, and the rehabilitation therapists. It is updated at least weekly at the team meetings and more often if necessary.

Selection of Patients for Case Management

Based on the reported experiences of hospital-based and payer-based case management initiatives, not all patients benefit from care coordination. Case management services are usually aimed at those groups of patients who have a progressive disease and the potential for consuming large amounts of health care resources. These patient populations include:[6]

- Cardiac patients
- Patients with chronic pain
- Patients with respiratory problems (chronic and acute)
- Cancer patients
- End-stage renal disease patients
- Patients with cerebral vascular conditions
- Patients with central nervous system injuries
- Patients who have had an amputation

In addition to selected patient populations, case management services may be offered to patients in the following situations:[7]

- Patients requiring long-term care outside the hospital
- Patients having a history of lengthy or costly hospital admissions
- Patients having multiple specialty referrals or services

FIGURE 8-4 Case Manager Schedule Board

Case Manager Nurse (Blue)		Case Manager Nurse (Red)		Social Worker
E. Toms F. Long C. Sams W. Baker	Physical Therapy D. Toms	J. Smith T. Jones B. Dye Y. Abt	Intravenous C. Alt Physical Therapy	T. Smith Occupational Therapy Physical Therapy
		Case Manager Nurse (Green)		D. Toms
		S. Davis B. Abel	Intravenous P. Green Physical Therapy Management and Evaluation R. Mick B. Rice	Speech Therapy

- Patients having a history of multiple emergency department visits
- Patients having multiple prescriptions
- Patients having a known history of chaotic patterns of family care or who come from dysfunctional families

Approximately 80 percent of the patient population served by Clinton Memorial Hospital is discharged without home care services. Of the remaining 20 percent, those who are referred to the home health agency usually represent patients with high-risk diagnoses or situations that would benefit from longer-term case management. Therefore, Clinton Home Health Agency decided to implement case management for all patients referred to it. Some patients would require a greater intensity of case management than others, but all would need case management nonetheless.

Calculation of Staffing Needs

To determine the number of case managers that would be needed to support this new patient care delivery model, a detailed analysis was conducted of current and projected needs for patient visits and staffing. Visit projections for Clinton Home Health Agency were then calculated using the step-by-step process outlined next. Although the values shown in each step reflect the Clinton experience, this model can be used by any home health agency.

Step 1: Calculate Projected Number of Patient Visits Data from 1994 were used to calculate the projected number of patient visits for 1995. The following formulas were used:

(a) Average length of stay (LOS) in the home health agency = Number of total days divided by the number of total patients

2979 ÷ 72 = 41

(b) Percentage of time that patient is on service in the Medicare 62-day certification period = Average LOS divided by the number of days in certification period (62) multiplied by 100

(41 ÷ 62) × 100 = 0.65 × 100 = 65%

(c) Number of visits per LOS per certification period = On-service percentage of certification period times expected number of visits by discipline in certification period

0.65 × 23 = 14.95

(d) Number of visits per certification period = Number of visits per LOS per certification period times the number of referrals per certification period

15 × 72 = 1080

(e) Number of visits possible per year = Number of visits per certification period times the number of certification periods per year (5.7 per year)

1080 × 5.7 = 6156

(f) Number of visits possible per month = Number of visits possible per year divided by 12

6156 ÷ 12 = 513

There was a 28 percent increase in the nurse visits in 1994 as compared with 1993. This same rate of growth was expected in 1995, so the number of possible visits per month was multiplied by 0.28. The monthly nurse visit projections for 1995 were calculated to be 657.

Step 2: Determine Projected Staffing Requirements After determining the anticipated patient visits for 1995, the staffing requirements were projected. The following assumptions were made in these calculations:

- One full-time equivalent (FTE) = One full-time (37.5 to 40 hours per week) position
- To determine an FTE, the average or expected number of hours worked per week is divided by the maximum number possible, without overtime.
  - *Example:* A person works three 8-hour days per week, or 24 hours per week. This equates to 0.6 FTE (24 ÷ 40).
  - *Example:* A person works from 8:00 am to 2:30 pm, 5 days a week. This equates to 0.81 FTE (32.5 ÷ 40).

Based on these assumptions, the number of days per month each FTE works was computed. To arrive at this figure, the following information was used:

A full-time (40 hours per week) staff person works 21.5 days per month.

5 days per week × 4.3 weeks per month = 21.5 days

A 4-day-per-week employee works 17.2 days per month.

4 days per week × 4.3 wks per month = 17.2 days

A 3-day-per-week employee works 12.9 days per month.

3 days per week × 4.3 wks per month = 12.9 days

A 2-day-per-week employee works 8.6 days per month.

2 days per week × 4.3 wks per month = 8.6 days

TABLE 8-1 Number of Possible Nurse Home Health Visits per Month

Staff Category	Total Number in Category	Expected Visit Productivity per Day		No. of Work Days per Month	No. of Possible Visits per Month
Full time	4	20	×	21.5	= 430
Part time (4 days/week)	1	5	×	17.2	= 86.0
Part time (3 days/week)	1	5	×	12.9	= 64.5
Part time (2 days/week)	1	5	×	8.6	= 43.0
		Total possible nurse home visits per month			623.5

The 1995 staffing projections for Clinton Home Health Agency, based on a staff of four FTEs and three part-time nurses, are shown in table 8-1. The monthly visits for 1995 were projected to be 657, and the total possible visits per month, based on existing staffing levels, was calculated to be only 624. Thus it appeared that 33 additional visits each month could *only* be accomplished if more staff were hired. However, agency leaders chose not to expand the staff. This decision was based on their previous experience with care paths, which had resulted in a decreased number of visits per patient. Case management was expected to further decrease the per-patient visit numbers, so it was agreed that the existing staff could handle the projected patient load.

Step 3: Determine the Number of Case Managers and Visit Nurses Needed First the number of visits the part-time (PT) nurses can perform in a month was clarified. Visits were calculated at the rate of one per hour.

PT nurse, 2 days per week × 8 hours per day = 16 hours per week = 16 visits per week
PT nurse, 3 days per week × 8 hours per day = 24 hours per week = 24 visits per week
PT nurse, 4 days per week × 8 hours per day = 32 hours per week = 32 visits per week
Total possible: 72 visits per week
× 4 weeks per month
Total possible visits per month: 288

By subtracting the total number of visits per month that can be performed by visit nurses (288) from the total number of monthly projected visits (624), it is clear that the case managers would have to complete 336 patient visits each month. As shown by the data in table 8-1, the case managers were expected to be able to complete 430 visits per month. Therefore, it appeared they would be able to meet the projected requirements. However, the case managers must perform patient assessments, and these count as two visits.

To determine whether the four case managers would be able complete all the patient assessments plus their other duties, another calculation was necessary. Based on 1994 data, an average of 50 patient assessments are completed each month. Therefore, each of the case managers would likely have 12.5, or 13, assessments per month. This translates into 26 assessment-related visits each month (one assessment equals two routine visits). Assuming each case manager works 21.5 days per month and completes four visits each day, each could be expected to complete 60 nonassessment visits and 26 assessment visits each month (total expected visits = 86).

To ensure that case managers are not overwhelmed with too many assessment visits on any particular day, three scheduling options were defined:

1. Case managers can complete three nonassessment visits and one assessment visit in one day.

2. Case managers can complete two assessment visits in one day.
3. Case managers can complete four to five nonassessment visits in one day.

CASE MANAGEMENT GETS OFF THE GROUND

The first 6 months of the case management program were turbulent ones. This situation was not unexpected, given the significance of the process change. Visits were missed, diagnostic tests were not performed as ordered, and the case managers and visit nurses did not communicate well with one another. No one was working as a team, though it must be said that the nurses had yet to be fully trained in some important case management activities: insurance verification, visit negotiations, and initial intravenous procedure start-ups.

Even in this difficult environment, everyone was trying hard to make case management work. In April 1996 the staff met to identify case-management-related situations needing improvement and developed action plans to remedy the situations. Out of this meeting came several case management system improvements, including those listed below. The case management process greatly improved as a result, and people began to work together as a team.

Communication Difficulties Resolved

Communication difficulties between case managers and visit nurses required development of the new tools. For each of their patients case managers began maintaining a calendar. (See figure 8-5.) At the top of the calendar, the case manager notes the patient's name, visit frequency, other home health agency services being provided for the patient, and the care path, if any, being used. The date of the case manager's assessment visit is noted, along with routine visits and any diagnostic tests or assessments to be completed at these visits. The visit nurse adds pertinent patient findings, such as weight, lung sounds, and blood pressure.

In addition to the patient calendar, it was agreed that visit nurses would have access to the patient's face sheet (figure 8-6) at each visit, as well as a copy of the patient's treatment plan, medication profile, and recent laboratory reports.

Responsibilities Clarified

Responsibilities of case managers and visit nurses required further clarification. The need for each nurse, whether a case manager or a visit nurse, to problem solve at each visit was reinforced. These interventions might include calling the physician from the patient's home to verify medications or answering patient and family questions.

Patient Assignments Modified

Because of the large geographic area covered by Clinton Home Health Agency nurses, the patient assignments required modification. Case managers had been assigned patients who were geographically close together, but this had not been done for visit nurses. Because these nurses had to cover a large geographic area, they had difficulty getting to patients' homes in time to draw blood for fasting lab work or drug-level determinations. Consequently, visit nurses were teamed up with a case manager so they were responsible for the same geographic area. A home health aide eventually was added to the team.

FIGURE 8-5 Patient Calendar Showing Wound Care Path

JUNE

Bear, Teddy June 4 - Aug 4 Wound Care Path
RN 1-3 wk X 4 wks qowk 5, prn 4 wound, prn 2 Resp.
Aide 2-3 X wk X 3 wks, 1-2X wk X 2 wks

SUNDAY	MONDAY	TUESDAY	WEDNESDAY	THURSDAY	FRIDAY	SATURDAY
MAY S M T W T F S 　 　 1 2 3 4 5 6 7 8 9 10 11 12 13 14 15 16 17 18 19 20 21 22 23 24 25 26 27 28 29 30 31	JULY S M T W T F S 　 1 2 3 4 5 6 7 8 9 10 11 12 13 14 15 16 17 18 19 20 21 22 23 24 25 26 27 28 29 30 31					1
2	3	4	5 visit cont teaching Wound Care & Sorbsan	6	7 visit T-101° purulent drainage odor called MD, culture obtained started on Ciprok X needs LSW	8
9	10 visit (cm. fax note to Dr. Jones)	11	12 M.D. Appt. 10:30	13 visit	14	15
16 FATHER'S DAY	17 visit	18	19	20	21 FLAG DAY	22
23	24 begin qowk visit	25	26	27	28	29
30						

Lungs. esp L base
Nutrition
Cough
Temp
Pedal edema
WT
L Chest incision
   Medication Compliance

158

FIGURE 8-6 Face Sheet

CLINTON MEMORIAL HOSPITAL HOME HEALTH AGENCY FACE SHEET	Date Code	Date No Code	Advance Directives ☐ Pt has living will ☐ Pt has durable Health Care POA ☐ None of the above ☐ Copy in chart
Referral Date Acceptance Date			
Client Name (Last, First, MI) [ ] Verified Spelling		Medical Record No.	Age	Sex M F [ ] [ ]
Address (Street, Apt. No., City, State, Zip Code)		County	Telephone
Marital Status S M W D	Date of Birth	Soc. Security No.	Client's Retirement Date: Spouse's Retirement Date:
Primary Care Person (Relationship)	Telephone	Emergency Contact (Relationship)	Telephone
Insurance Company/Policy No./Address/HMO [ ] Verified No. with Card/Medicare HMO		Guarantor	Referral Source
Attending Physician (Address and Phone)		Other Physician(s) (Address and Phone)	
Date Patient Last Saw M.D.:	Institution Providing Prior Care:	Admission:	Discharge:
Principal Diagnosis Related to Admission		Date of Onset	
Other Pertinent Diagnosis		Date of Onset	
Surgery Relevant to Care and Date Performed		Equipment/Supplier	

Directions to Home
 	
Ambulance Preference _____
  Phone No. _____
Pharmacy Preference _____
  Phone No. _____
		Allergies	

		Medications (Current meds, new 30 days, changes 60 days)	
Information taken by			
R.N. Signature/Date			

Referral Date
  HHA _____
  PT _____
  ST _____
  MSW _____
	Diet		

Form No.: 600-H Revised: 09/06/91 Revised: 1/3/92			

Source: Reprinted, with permission, Clinton Memorial Hospital.

PRELIMINARY MEASURES OF CASE MANAGEMENT EFFECTIVENESS

The case management program at Clinton Home Health Agency is still in its infancy. As noted, the process continues to undergo revision. Therefore, many formal measures of case management effectiveness have yet to be instituted. Some preliminary data are available for a few measures, the results of which are described below.

Patient Satisfaction

One of the primary goals of the case management process was to improve patient satisfaction. Thus far, satisfaction scores have dropped below pre–case management levels. Once the communication and scheduling processes are stabilized, these scores should improve.

Patient Care Skills

Measures are also in place to determine whether case management has helped improve patients' self-care skills, decrease hospital readmissions, and decrease costs. To evaluate these issues, 25 charts of patients with congestive heart failure were studied and compared with similar patients treated with care paths alone or without care paths or case management. The results are shown in table 8-2. Although care paths had improved patients' self-care skill levels, case management further improved upon that level. Case management also appeared to decrease total costs and average visits per patient.

Length of Home Care Service Days

One surprise in the data was the inability of case management to decrease the length of home care service days beyond what had already been achieved with the care paths. This finding is probably related to the traditional thinking of home care nurses. Even though patients may be ready for discharge before they reach the end of the Medicare 62-day certification period, they are kept as clients. Clinton Home Health Agency will work to reorient the nurses' thinking to promote discharges when patients

TABLE 8-2 Case Management vs. Paths vs. Prepath Performance for Congestive Heart Failure Patients

	Prepath Data (25 patients) 10/93–4/94	Path-Managed Data (25 patients) 10/95–4/95	Path Plus Case Management Data (25 patients) 10/95–4/96
Cost per patient	$3,300	$1,400	$1,372
Median cost	$1,300	$700	$1,007
Total cost	$84,600	$36,800	$31,548
Average visits per patient	22.04	9.52	9.4
Median visits per patient	8	6	7.2
Average length of home care service days	43.8 days	37.4 days	37.6 days
Patient disposition, %			
Self-care	12	16	61
Home with assist	32	40	4
Extended care facility	20	4	4
Hospital admit	28	24	9
Expired	8	4	17
Hospice	0	12	0

FIGURE 8-7 Use of PRN Nurses

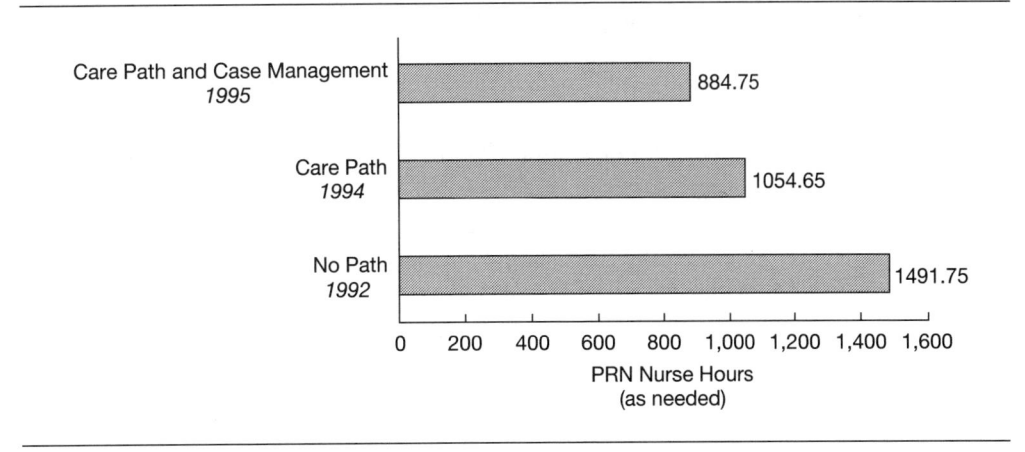

Category	PRN Nurse Hours
Care Path and Case Management 1995	884.75
Care Path 1994	1054.65
No Path 1992	1491.75

no longer require medically necessary services, even if they have not reached the end of the Medicare certification period.

Home Care Nurses' Organizational Skills

Another goal of case management was to improve the organizational skills of the home care nurses. Three observations related to this goal have been noted to date:

1. A great deal of planning was required on the part of the visit nurses, who were expected to perform one visit per hour worked. Coordinating travel distances and meeting the special needs of patients, such as drawing fasting blood levels, was a challenge they were able to overcome.
2. For the case managers, efficient use of their time became critical. They had to complete the necessary paperwork for an increased number of cases, coordinate patient care across all disciplines, assess all new patient referrals, and provide for routine visits.
3. The case managers and the visit nurses learned to work as a team. They came together and resolved many of the obstacles that arose during initiation of case management.

Other improvements that can directly be attributed to the case management delivery model include the following:

- By decreasing the visit nurses' nonproductive team meeting time, Clinton Home Health Agency was able to make them available for more direct patient care activities.
- The case managers handle all physician contacts. By "bundling" the issues that need to be discussed, rather than having several nurses making multiple calls to the same doctor, the physicians' time is better spent.
- Improved patient care coordination has resulted in a decrease in the use of agency nurses (figure 8-7), resulting in cost savings for the agency.

CONCLUSION

Clinton Memorial Hospital Home Health Agency's change from a primary care nursing model to a case management delivery system did not occur without incident. However, caregivers have begun to work together in a cooperative team effort. Case managers are learning to trust the judgment of their peer professionals, an issue that was most difficult to overcome. Open communication between visit nurse and case manager is critical to the success of the patient care process. All nurses must feel secure about their own nursing skills and knowledge as well as those of their team members.

Beyond cooperation, case management has moved the caregivers toward the "one less visit" mind-set. By fostering patient independence, rather than the dependence that was previously created, the agency staff is beginning to learn that more is not necessarily better. Case management has helped the home care nurses to evolve to the next level of success after care paths, while maintaining or improving patient satisfaction, decreasing costs, and increasing efficiency.

References

1. Satinsky, M. A. *An Executive Guide to Case Management Strategies.* Chicago: American Hospital Publishing, 1995.
2. Lulavage, A. RN-LPN teams: toward unit nursing case management. *Nursing Management* 22(3):58–61, Mar. 1991.
3. Sinnen, M. T., and Schifalacqua, M. M. Coordinated care in a community hospital. *Nursing Management* 22(3):38–42, Mar. 1991.
4. Rogers, M., Swindle, D., and Riordan, J. Community-based nursing case management. *Nursing Management* 22(3):30–34, Mar. 1991.
5. Case Management Society of America. *Standards of Practice for Case Management.* Little Rock, AR: Case Management Society of America, 1995.
6. Donovan, M. R., and Matson, T. A., editors. *Outpatient Case Management: Strategies for a New Reality.* Chicago: American Hospital Publishing, 1994.
7. St. Coeur, M., editor. *Case Management Practice Guidelines.* St. Louis: Mosby, 1996.

CHAPTER 9

Reducing Length of Stay and Improving Outcomes

Kevin Turley and Kerry M. Turley

Total quality management (TQM) provides a framework for improving quality by eliminating variation in the production of a product or a service.[1] In the early 1990s health care providers began to apply this model to patient care delivery. A TQM tool known as the *critical pathway method* (CPM) is a technique used to improve uniformity in the delivery of hospital patient care. While variations from the pathway were expected, they were markedly reduced from those in a less controlled setting.[2] Physician-directed diagnostic and therapeutic plans were initially developed for certain inpatient or outpatient populations with specific disease entities such as asthma. The pathways served as tools for standardizing care delivery to patient populations. Pathway variations were analyzed, and the information used to refine the pathway for the individual patient group.[3] The CPM was most applicable to homogeneous populations, where common interventions were easily identified and outcomes definable. This method was used by many organizations to reduce hospital stays and improve quality of care.[4]

A major weakness of the CPM was its reactive nature. The industrial technique of decreasing process variation was applied to patient care in an attempt to reduce negative variation. By reducing negative variation, caregivers hoped to limit hospital lengths of stay. Variations from the path were collected and analyzed *after* a patient's episode of care and used to improve the care provided to future hospital admissions.[5] This approach, in a sense, represented a traditional quality assurance strategy whereby the process is inspected and aggregate data gathered during inspections are analyzed after the fact. This strategy helped caregivers identify pervasive, population-wide variations; however, it lacked the ability to discriminate negative variances at the individual patient level. Even with these limitations, the traditional CPM did assist organizations in recognizing the cause of gross variations so they could make necessary changes in patient care processes.[6,7]

This chapter describes how cardiac surgery caregivers evolved from the traditional CPM tool into a proactive patient care management approach that allows their congenital patients to advance along the path according to their clinical needs. Kevin

164 CHAPTER 9 REDUCING LENGTH OF STAY AND IMPROVING OUTCOMES

Turley, a congenital cardiovascular surgeon practicing at California Pacific Medical Center (CPMC) and Kaiser Northern California in San Francisco, was instrumental in developing a holistic patient care approach that involves patient and family empowerment, dynamic case management, and a pathway that allows patients to "outperform" the system.

THE EVOLUTION OF CARDIAC SURGERY PATHWAYS

In 1991 Turley and colleagues applied the CPM to patients with congenital heart disease. They found this patient population to be very heterogeneous, and for this reason, the *reactive* CPM approach was found to have limited value. Although variation analysis helped cardiovascular caregivers identify some gross infrastructure problems, patient-specific problems could only be detected sporadically.

A second model, an *interactive* pathway methodology, was thus developed and applied to patients with congenital heart disease.[8] Using this model, daily assessments of the patient's progress were performed by a clinical nurse coordinator—case manager (CNC-CM), and variances from the pathway were noted. This coordinator's role was modeled after that of heart transplant coordinators, who follow patients from preoperative assessment, through operative intervention, and into the postoperative experience. The nurse coordinator identified appropriate responses to the pathways and documented patients' reasons for not responding.

Because of the intrinsic nature of the nurse coordinator's approach, the success of this interactive pathway soon became evident. By monitoring patients' progress, the CNC-CM had an opportunity to affect patients' progression during their episodes of care. More important, however, it was realized that patients' and families' interaction may be able to accelerate this progress.[9]

In 1994 the authors reported their initial experience with the interactive pathway model, which involved 172 patients undergoing congenital heart surgery.[10] These patients were compared with 114 similar patients treated by Kevin Turley at his prior hospital who were not managed with a critical pathway. The findings are summarized below.

The interactive CPM resulted in an overall decrease of 44 percent in average length of stay (6.2 days for patients not on a pathway versus 3.7 days for pathway patients).[11] The pathways markedly reduced variation in patient care processes, as evidenced by:

- A change in length-of-stay standard deviation from 2.65 to 1.01
- A change in length-of-stay range from 4–14 to 3–7, $p < 0.0001$

When average length of stay in the intensive care unit (ICU) was examined, comparable results were noted. Overall, critical pathway–managed (CPM) patients demonstrated a decrease in:

- Mean ICU average length of stay (non-CPM = 2.05 days; CPM = 1.25 days)
- Standard deviation (non-CPM = 1.13; CPM = 0.48)
- Range in ICU lengths of stay (non-CPM = 1–7 days; CPM = 1–3 days)

The percentage of change for CPM patients was −39 percent. This was significant at $p < 0.01$.

Outcome data for CPM patients were compared with that for non-CPM patients. Studies showed no significant differences in mortality, readmission rates, unscheduled emergency room or clinic visits, or negative family satisfaction survey results.

Although marked reductions in total hospital and ICU lengths of stay were achieved for this heterogeneous population of congenital heart surgery patients, it soon became apparent that the interactive CPM failed to recognize the possibility of positive variation in a heterogeneous patient population and failed to encourage patients to outperform the plan. Therefore, a third model—the *proactive* approach—was developed. This model was entitled the *cardiovascular radical outcome method* (CV-ROM). To fashion this approach the organization had first to deal with caregivers' bias, a dominant element in health care delivery. Bias exists in every clinician's actions and approaches to patient care and in the health care delivery system itself. For example, when excellent clinical results have been obtained in the past by keeping surgical patients in the hospital for a specific time period, it is difficult to question the wisdom of this practice. Often caregivers' treatment decisions reflect yesterday's attitudes, yet today's health care environment invites questioning of these long-standing preferences. Customary practices may have been effective, but they do not necessarily represent quality patient care. Quality must be defined by the patient's response, not caregiver bias.

Unlike the interactive pathway model, in the proactive approach the delivery system is responsive to the patient's performance, and most important, positive variation is possible. The system participants include the patient's family, the CNC-CM, the surgeon planner, and the physician and nurse implementers. The surgeon planner defines the plan and collaborates with the CNC-CM and physician and nurse implementers to develop the process for the family.

These participants work together to develop the pathway *with* and *for* the patient. Concurrently, the CNC-CM and the surgeon planner identify positive factors, such as family support and athleticism, and comorbidities, such as congenital kidney or liver disease, in the development of the plan. They work with the physician and nurse implementers to move the family and the patient along the pathway.

The CV-ROM approach has been found to be very effective for complex cardiac surgery patients. Recent studies demonstrated its utility in the most heterogeneous and complex of cardiac surgery subgroups: adult patients with chronic congenital heart disease. These are patients in whom secondary changes have occurred and for whom the family-directed CV-ROM approach would appear to be less applicable.[12,13]

THE CARDIOVASCULAR RADICAL OUTCOME METHOD

Having experienced reactive and interactive critical pathway patient management models, the authors evolved to a proactive design. The first two models, based on traditional critical pathway strategies, relied heavily on the identification of negative variances and regular examination of aggregate data to identify improvements that could be applied to future patients. The proactive model relies on real-time feedback to positively influence changes in the patient's progression through the episode of care.

The patient discharge decision is captured in the critical question, What are we doing special for you today in the hospital that cannot be done at home? Each day the patient and his or her family are asked this question, and they and the caregivers understand its meaning. When the answer is "Nothing," they expect the patient to be discharged to home care. Clearly, the centerpiece of the proactive approach is patient and family empowerment. The nursing care model known as *active and accountable family participation* complements the empowerment process.

A second critical element of the CV-ROM process is the cardiovascular CNC-CM. This person oversees the patient's progress throughout the entire episode of care. The CNC-CM is closely involved with the patient and the pathway preoperatively and postoperatively. The postoperative period begins immediately after surgery and is continued for 1 month after discharge from the hospital.

A third important component of the CV-ROM process is the information system. To provide real-time support of the proactive CV-ROM model, a flexible computer-based feedback system was designed.

The Proactive Pathway Model

All members of the health care team are involved in the pathway at various points along the cardiac surgery episode of care. Team members include the pediatric cardiac surgeon, administrative and patient coordinator, CNC-CM, pediatric intensive care staff nurses, pediatric ward primary care nurses, pediatric social worker, pediatric cardiologists, and pediatric intensivist.

The pathway starts when the patient's surgery date is scheduled and continues for 1 month postdischarge. The surgeon planner designs the pathway with the CNC-CM, and each staff member becomes involved at the appropriate time.

Seven critical moments were identified as "hinge points" in the congenital heart surgery pathway:

1. Introduction
2. Empowerment
3. Operation
4. Extubation
5. Ambulation
6. Alimentation
7. The critical question

These hinge points represent specific decision moments where, depending on the patients' response, they can:

- Advance faster than the pathway suggests
- Continue with the standard pathway protocol
- Have their progress decelerated

The standard inpatient cycle is completed by the 3rd hospital day. A traditional pathway format is used to illustrate the x-axis of time and the y-axis of the recommended treatment plan. However, a z-axis has been added. The z-axis illustrates the ROM levels (or progression steps) that are possible. Patients may be on ROM 1 (3-day hospitalization), ROM 2 (4-day hospitalization), ROM 3 (5-day hospitalization), and so on. Figure 9-1 demonstrates the standard ROM grid formed by the x-axis of time, the y-axis of individual pathways, and the z-axis of ROM levels corresponding to hospitalizations of 3, 4, 5, and 6 or more days.

The decisions made at each of the seven critical moments dictate which level the patient will be on. Patients outperforming the planned pathway move to a lower level and to a shorter hospitalization.[14] Likewise, patients may move to a higher ROM level if factors cause a slowdown in their progression. The typical issues taken into consideration at each critical moment are listed below.

Moment 1: Introduction The CNC-CM evaluates the family's expectations and cooperation with the plan of care. At this point comorbidities are identified and blood transfusion arrangements are made.

Moment 2: Empowerment A family interview is conducted by the CNC-CM less than 1 week before surgery. At this point the family dynamics are identified, cooperation is again assessed, and comorbidities are further defined. The interview results are considered by the surgeon planner, and a pathway is constructed.

FIGURE 9-1 Standard Radical Outcome Grid

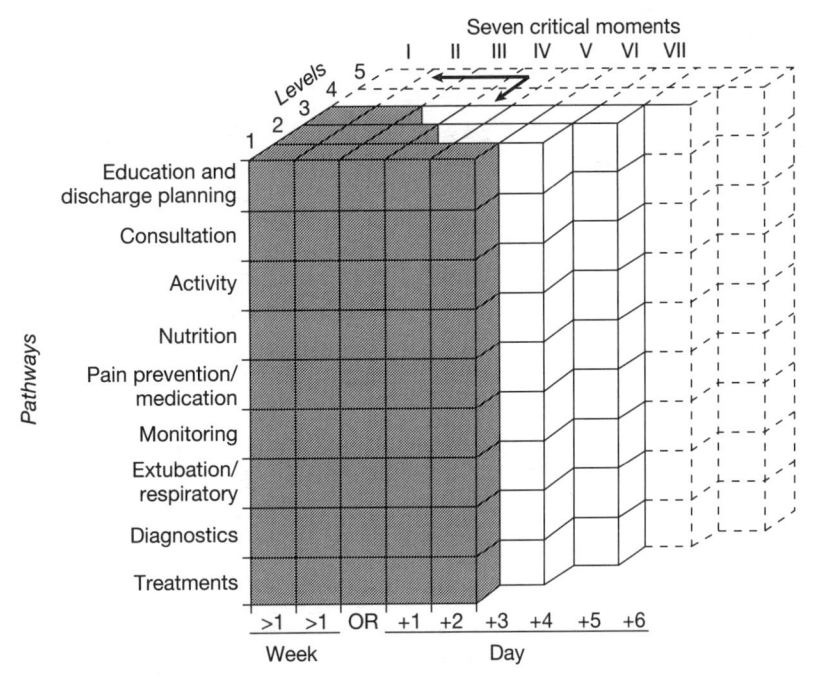

A case of tetralogy of Fallot with a planned 5-day hospitalization, radical outcome method (ROM) 3, in which the patient experiences early extubation and progresses to early ambulation with movement to ROM 2 and, ultimately, ROM 1, which is discharge on the third postoperative day. The critical moments function as hinge points at which movement can occur to a lower level, shorter pathway design, and length of stay.

Source: Reprinted, with permission, from Turley, K., Tyndall, M., Turley, K. M., and others. Radical outcome method: a new approach to critical pathways in congenital heart disease. *Circulation* 92 (suppl. II): II-245–II-249, 1995; published by the American Heart Association.

The surgeon planner provides an in-depth construct based on the standard pathway plans. A simple pathway plan, representing ROM 1, is described in figure 9-2. At the ROM 1 level the patient is expected to stay in the hospital 3 days. The pathway is expanded and contracted by the surgeon based on the patient's experience, preoperative diagnosis, and comorbidities identified in preoperative sessions.

Moment 3: Operation The nature of the operative procedure, complications, and anesthetic management influence the patient's ROM level of pathway progression. The surgeon planner determines whether the patient can outperform the pathway, should continue with the standard protocol, or requires deceleration.

Moment 4: Extubation Early extubation for selected patients results in marked acceleration in pathway progress. The anesthesiologist and intensivist, in concert with the surgeon planner, assess the patient's readiness for this procedure.

Moment 5: Ambulation Following removal of the patient's chest tube and other monitoring devices, the patient's ability to begin ambulation is assessed by the CNC-CM and surgeon planner. At this point in the pathway, patient and family feedback is important to the clinicians. By providing adequate postoperative pain prevention through regularly scheduled analgesics, antipyretics, and nonsteroidal anti-inflammatories, clinicians can give patients the opportunity to outperform the planned pathway. It is the patient and family response that dictates a positive result.

FIGURE 9-2 Simple Pathway (Radical Outcome Method 1)

Pathway	>1 week	<1 week	Day −1	OR	Day 1	Day 2	Day 3
Education and Discharge Planning	Begins at scheduling: Family—length of stay and what to expect w/surgery.	Ambulatory program w/inspiration spirometer and Cough Bear taught. Practice "pulling chest tubes." Wound care. Postop expectations	Family plan reinforced with postop expectations	Family support.	Assessment of family care and support.		Chest tube stitch removed—CNC. Discharge teaching re: wound care, activity level, diet, follow-up appts. w/cardiology and CV surgeon given.
Consultation	Begins at scheduling: Blood needed identified, family blood typing process begun.	Thursday prior to OR: Surgery risk/benefits. CNC explains "family assignments." Final check for DD blood, home study request, child care after discharge arranged.	Intensivist. Cardiac anesthesia.				
Activity	Special problems.		Ad lib.	Bed rest.	OOB in chair for entire day. Ambulate q 1 hr. for 10 min. Patient in street clothes.	OOB in chair and play room. Ambulate q 45 min.–1 hr. for 10 min.	Ad lib. Out of bed all day.
Nutrition	Evaluation.		Regular diet. NPO 2400 hr.	NPO	NPO Peripheral IV D₅'N @ 2/3 maintenance.	0600 hr. liquids given. 0800 hr. Adv. to regular diet. DC IV	Regular diet.
Pain Prevention/ Medication		Allergies reviewed. Prior anesthetic, analgesic history.		Acetaminophen q 4 hr. pr. MS IV prn.	Acetaminophen q 4 hr. pr. MS IV prn.	Acetaminophen q 4 hr. po. Ibuprofen po.	Discharged on Acetaminophen and Ibuprofen.
Monitoring		Prior cannulation and catheterization.	VS q 8 hr.	HS monitoring per ICU. CVP. O₂ saturations. Temp. probe continuously for 24 hrs. Foley.	HS monitoring per pediatric ward. DC CVP, arterial line, Foley, central line.	HS monitoring q 8 hr.	
Extubation/Respiratory	Respiratory history.			Extubation within 1st 3 hrs., if possible. Nasal cannula or O₂ mask.	Inspiration spirometer q 30 min.	Inspiration spirometer q 15 min.	
Diagnostics	Blood typing and ABO/Rh compatibility. MRI/echo, if needed.		Chest X ray. EKG UA CBC Chem 23 Type and cross match	Arrival and 4 hrs. after arrival PICU: CBC, Chem 23, Ionized CA PT PLT and CK Chest X ray. EKG – arrival PICU.	CBC Chem 23 Chest X ray after CT removal.	Chest X ray.	
Treatments	Preop O₂. Change in medication.			Betadine shower or bath A.M. prior to OR.			

Critical pathway design of Kevin Turley, MD, chief of pediatric cardiovascular surgery, California Pacific Medical Center; and Consultant, Kaiser Permanente Medical Center, San Francisco.

Moment 6: Alimentation Early alimentation can interfere with the pain management protocol on postoperative day 1. Therefore, alimentation is usually begun late the first postoperative day or on postoperative day 2.

Moment 7: The Critical Question The question, What are we doing special for you today in the hospital that cannot be done at home? is asked of the family when appropriate. The family's response reflects their current feeling about their ability to manage the patient at home. On the standard pathway protocol (ROM 1), the question is asked on postoperative day 3.

Staff members understand the nature of the interventions because of their experience with the pathway plan. Issues identified at each critical moment alter the pathway in specific ways that caregivers must respond to. The CNC-CM is prominent in the proactive pathway process. This nurse is responsible for identifying the patient's plan, working with other nurses and physician implementers to promote their understanding of the plan, and communicating any changes from the surgeon planner to other members of the team. The CNC-CM is an intrinsic part of the pathway, identifying the pathway hinge points and, if appropriate, suggesting changes in the patient's ROM level.

Patient Assessment and Family Empowerment

The CV-ROM approach starts with helping the patient and family to understand the pathway design and their role in the process.[15] The patient and family are introduced to the pathway by the nurse coordinator on the day they are informed of their surgical date. Empowerment is an oft-used term, and there are many different definitions of the concept. In the CV-ROM process the term *empowerment* is used to describe the acquisition of new skills that enhance an individual's feelings of confidence, competence, and control. Patients and their families are empowered when they are recognized as equal partners in the health care system and when knowledge and skills are shared with them.[16] This empowerment permits the child's caretakers to render routine nursing care while also assuming the responsibility for it.

When the cardiovascular caregivers reviewed the literature on reactive pathway models, initial effectiveness studies for cardiac surgery patients showed that ambulation and spirometer usage were often not implemented. This was cited as one of the most common reasons for failure in meeting pathway goals.[17] This trend was reversed with the CV-ROM approach by involving patients and families in the health care delivery process.

Active and Accountable Family Participation To promote patient and family empowerment, the cardiovascular nursing staff adopted a new model of nursing care known as *active and accountable family participation*. This nursing process and associated intervention steps are described in two different research studies.[18,19] As an innovative nursing model, it transcends what the classic literature calls "general family nursing interventions," such as anticipatory guidance, role modeling, and preoperative teaching.[20] Through active and accountable family participation, the nursing staff gives family members new information and develops their skills as part of the health care team while making them accountable for performing those activities.

The family and patient expect to participate in the patient's care because they are taught recovery behaviors preoperatively. The nurse no longer advances the preconception that only a health care professional can fulfill this healing role for the patient. Because family members are viewed as equal and competent members of the team, they feel empowered, knowing that they are not completely dependent on professionals for their child's well-being and recovery. The result is an increase in the

FIGURE 9-3 Patient Progress Chart

Name:		
Walk Every Hour Designated Route ☺	Incentive Spirometer ★	Medications R
7:00 a.m.	7:30 a.m.	*Write in appropriate dose, route, and time interval—No "PRNs"*
8:00 a.m.	8:30 a.m.	**Tylenol**
9:00 a.m.	9:30 a.m.	
10:00 a.m.	10:30 a.m.	**Ibuprofen**
11:00 a.m.	11:30 a.m.	
12:00 p.m.	12:30 p.m.	
1:00 p.m.	1:30 p.m.	**Cefuroxime**
2:00 p.m.	2:30 p.m.	
3:00 p.m.	3:30 p.m.	
4:00 p.m.	4:30 p.m.	**Others:**
5:00 p.m.	5:30 p.m.	MS, Percocet, Digoxin, Lasix
6:00 p.m.	6:30 p.m.	

family's ability to solve problems and take responsibility for their own health care needs.

The active-and-accountable technique of working with families blends well with the CV-ROM methodology. The nursing staff tells the family what to expect on each day of the pathway and demonstrates how to hold and position the child postsurgery. Family caregivers are also taught the skills necessary to ambulate their children, assist them in the use of the incentive spirometer, and teach deep-breathing and coughing exercises. In more than 700 families of varied backgrounds, the child's caregivers in both the interactive and, subsequently, the proactive approach have become competent at performing hourly ambulation, spirometer use, and deep-breathing and coughing exercises.[21]

Patient Progress Chart Not only do family members assist in their child's recovery, they also become motivators and coaches. To encourage patient and family accountability, a simple patient progress chart was developed that shows the expected times for ambulation and spirometer usage. (See figure 9-3.) This chart is decorated with a heart and hung at the bedside.

Also included on the patient progress chart are the type and amount of medications ordered, the route for administration, and the time to be given. The chart reminds parents about when their child's ambulation and spirometer use needs to occur and also communicates important information about their child's medications and the plan of care.

The chart also fosters nursing accountability. Families and nurses find themselves collaborating in the child's recovery. The children respond well to motivational incentives such as rewards of stickers for a good job. Children and parents soon asked to take their patient progress charts home to place in scrapbooks and to bring to school for "show and tell." This request could be granted because the form was not designed to be part of the permanent record. The patient progress charts became a badge of courage and accomplishment. Even if there had been setbacks in the child's progress, because of the level of family involvement these were not viewed as defeats but merely events to be overcome as soon as the patient was able.

Role Modeling One of the most effective tools the CNC-CM has for teaching family and staff is role modeling. The CNC-CM actually walks with the child, the family, and the staff nurse on the child's first walk the day after chest tube removal. The child ambulates from the pediatric ICU to the elevators and into a room on the pediatric floor. The CNC-CM initiates the walk and stays with the child and family until they reach the elevators. Then with careful guidance and assistance from the CNC-CM and staff nurse, the family takes charge of the patient and ambulates from the elevators back to a bed on the pediatric ward. The family was taught preoperatively that, although the CNC-CM and staff nurses are always available for support, the responsibility for accomplishing tasks ultimately belongs to the family. In response to these empowerment techniques, patients progress quickly along the pathway and feel a sense of achievement.

Benefits to Nurses The patient and family are not the only ones who feel empowered. Staff nurses like the predictability that pathways bring to the episode of care. They can now feel assured that the information they give to families is reliable and accurate. Nurses have indicated that proactive pathways help them feel more in control of the patient's management and care, which in turn increases their authority. They are now active participants in determining how quickly patients progress through their hospital experiences.

By combining a proactive pathway model and the nursing intervention of active and accountable family participation, the CV-ROM approach has proved to be a success. This success is evidenced by recently collected data showing that 151 congenital heart surgery patients were discharged earlier than the pathway predicted, with no unexpected untoward outcomes.

Role of the Clinical Nurse Coordinator–Case Manager

A CNC-CM with master's-level preparation plays a pivotal role in communication and coordination of care. The CNC-CM is educated in the care of congenital heart disease and sensitive to case management issues. Figure 9-4 reproduces a job description of this position.

Under the CNC-CM's direction, the CV-ROM approach is a collaborative practice among doctors, nurses, and family and patient. These relationships are characterized by open communication, shared responsibility, problem solving, decision making, and commitment to the pathway plan for patient care. Such synergy actually creates a path for empowering nurses.[22] The relationships themselves are based on trust and the commitment of all the health professionals to the patient's successful recovery.

Prior to a patient's admission, the CNC-CM communicates with the family by telephone. In addition to gathering important information about the patient, the CNC-CM initiates preadmission teaching and begins the family empowerment process. One week before the child's operation, the CNC-CM is responsible for preparing the family for the postoperative phase. The preoperative education encompasses:

- What the family may expect their child to look like in the pediatric ICU, including chest tube and monitoring lines, and how to pick up the child without causing additional incisional pain
- How to ambulate their child
- How to coach their child in pulmonary exercises using an incentive spirometer

Parents and other family members who will be involved in the rapid surgical recovery also learn the rationale for keeping their child sitting up during the daytime hours.[23]

During the hospitalization the CNC-CM makes rounds frequently throughout the day to help staff and families maintain the aggressive activity program. Because the

FIGURE 9-4 Job Description for Clinical Nurse Coordinator–Case Manager (CNC-CM)

Professional requirements

CNC-CM must be an advanced practice nurse with graduate education in nursing and/or related field. Candidate must have 5 or more years of experience in cardiovascular nursing and be recognized by California Children's Services as a nurse specialist in pediatric cardiovascular nursing. This nurse should have superior verbal and written communication skills and be able to function independently and as part of a team. Good clinical skills are necessary as well as the ability to participate in research projects.

1. Communicate, facilitate, and educate the family and child preoperatively for a successful rapid recovery.
2. Coordinate patient admission and discharge. Evaluate and implement postoperative care in collaboration with the surgeon planner. Use advanced nursing skills to recommend patient advancement on pathway plan.
3. Assist surgeon planner with in-hospital and outpatient clinic procedures.
4. Provide consistent and continual telephone communication with families throughout all phases of care.
5. Collaborate with nursing and other disciplines in education, planning, and implementation of cardiovascular radical outcome method.
6. Provide information to all referring physicians regarding the patient's recovery and plan. Act as a liaison between tertiary and primary caregivers.
7. Participate in research activities and in professional nursing organizations at local and national level. Publish in peer-reviewed journals.

---

surgeon is often in the operating room during the day, the CNC-CM is accountable for carrying out the daily pathway plan with each postoperative patient. The CNC-CM, in collaboration with the surgeon planner, evaluates the patient's progress and the potential for advancement on the pathway plan. Simultaneously, the CNC-CM facilitates the plan and motivates the family. Preparation for discharge is accomplished by first removing the chest tube stitch, and then teaching the family:

- How to preventing incisional problems
- What the child's regime of discharge medications will be
- How to continue the child's activity program at home

Apprehension about leaving the hospital environment is relieved by the family's understanding of the child's problem and the in-hospital care they were able to provide.[24]

Following discharge the CNC-CM continues to provide support. The patient and the family have access to the CNC-CM 7 days a week via a message-taking beeper system. This communication tool allows the CNC-CM to give the follow-up assistance, advice, and reassurance necessary to facilitate patients' early discharge from the hospital. The CNC-CM also provides an important holistic approach by addressing patients' physical, psychological, and spiritual needs.

CV-ROM Information System

Clinical pathways were originally designed as a paper-based system. With the introduction of the CV-ROM process, it soon became apparent that a paper-based system was too inflexible. With a proactive critical pathway methodology, pathway recommendations and corresponding order sets change as patients move from one ROM level to another. This situation necessitated the development of a computerized system to achieve full CV-ROM operation. Flexibility was especially important for complex patient groups, to ensure consistent and reproducible acceleration of patient progress when such an accelerated response was appropriate. The information system software program is in the process of commercial development. A typical screen display of a simple pathway is presented in figure 9-2.

The computerized methodology closely parallels that described in previously published journal articles.[25,26] Both the surgeon planner and the CNC-CM input information into the system. As a team they evaluate patient response and the appropriateness of movement at the hinge points from one ROM level to another.

A proactive clinical pathway model such as the CV-ROM requires human and computer support to optimize the system. The interface between proactive, personalized, individual, humanized patient care and computer technology is the essence of this approach.[27,28] While the former provides for the milieu in which accelerated patient recovery is possible, the latter provides the tool by which optimization of this approach can be realized.

MEASURING SUCCESS

Experience with more than 500 patients has provided an opportunity to thoroughly study the effectiveness of the ROM. Effectiveness has been measured by comparing patients' actual versus expected hospital lengths of stay. Care has been taken in every study to closely match the comparison groups according to their diagnosis, comorbidities, and procedures. In addition to evaluating the impact of the CV-ROM on patients' hospital stays, patient outcomes have also been compared.

From their initial and now extensive experience with pathway design models and the CV-ROM, the authors are confident that the CV-ROM can be applied successfully to congenital heart surgery patients. Patients managed with the CV-ROM methodology exhibit uniformity of outcomes and significant decreases in average length of hospital stay and average length of ICU stay, and outcome data confirm both excellent quantitative and qualitative responses.

Detailed analyses of the CV-ROM methodology are available in several medical and nursing journal articles.[29,30] Only the highlights are presented in this chapter.

Length of Hospital Stay

Our initial experience demonstrated decreased average length of hospital stays for all groups of ROM patients over the standard interactive pathway group. The dynamic nature of the ROM process was demonstrated in 200 consecutive patients.[31] Patients having the same operating surgeon treated a single hospital were studied in two consecutive groups of 100, so patients with similar diagnoses and procedures could be matched. The following results were reported:

- 18 percent decrease in length of stay over time with atrial septal defects (ASDs)
- 10 percent decrease in length of stay with ventricular septal defects (VSDs)
- 21 percent decrease in length of stay with patent ductus arteriosus (PDA)
- 9 percent decrease in length of stay with coarctation of the aorta (CoA)
- 10 percent decrease in length of stay with more complex diagnoses
- In cardiopulmonary bypass, average length of stay was 3.4 days in the second group, as compared with 4 days in the first group.
- In noncardiopulmonary bypass, average length of stay was 2.7 days in the second group, as compared with 3.2 days in the first group.
- In the total group of matched patients, average length of stay decreased from 3.7 to 3.1 days, -16 percent, $p < 0.003$.

It was also noted that in the complex subgroups of patients, many of whom could not be matched because of differences in individual diagnoses, average length of stay was quite comparable with that seen in the matched patients. In addition, some complex subgroups, such as atrioventricular canals, aortic valve replacements, and bidirectional Glenn, had average lengths of stay well below their planned pathways.

To investigate the impact of the ROM on complex subgroups of patients and very heterogeneous groups of patients, a study was conducted on the next 100 consecutive patients. The goal of the study was to compare CV-ROM patients' actual lengths of stay with the planned estimated length of stay suggested by the standard pathway protocol. The 100 patients were divided into three categories:

1. 35 patients with simple lesions, PDAs, or secundum ASDs
2. 33 patients with intermediate lesions, such as VSDs, sinus venosus ASDs, primum ASDs with cleft mitral valves, and CoAs
3. 32 patients with complex lesions

When actual lengths of stay were compared with estimated length of stay, it was found that in the 73 patients who underwent cardiopulmonary bypass, a 15 percent decrease over standard pathway length of stay was encountered, $p < 0.0001$. In the 27 nonbypass patients, a 12 percent decrease was noted, although this was not statistically significant. Overall, in the 100 patients, a 14 percent decrease was noted, $p < 0.0005$. Thus, it was observed that it was in the more complex patients (those with cardiopulmonary bypass) that the greatest advantage of the ROM over the standard pathway length of stay appeared to occur.

The effect on the more complex patient becomes evident in an extensive study of 214 consecutive patients in which the current CV-ROM was uniformly employed.[32] There were 211 survivors (99 percent). Two hundred and one patients (95.2 percent), including 60 nonbypass patients (97 percent) and 141 bypass patients (95 percent), achieved their planned length of stay. Ten patients (4.7 percent) exceeded their estimated length of stay, 2 were nonbypass (3 percent) and 8 bypass (5 percent), while 127 patients (60.2 percent) had a length of stay less than estimated, 40 nonbypass (65 percent) and 87 bypass (58 percent). Statistical analysis revealed $p < 0.0001$ for the total and each subgroup and a negative change in length of stay of 156 days for the total group, 111 days for the bypass group, and 45 days for the nonbypass group. The average change in length of stay was −0.74 days per patient.

When the effect of comorbidities was examined, the following results were reported:

- Complicated cases including the VSD subgroup without comorbidities experienced 100 percent achievement of the estimated length of stay. No patients exceeded the estimated length of stay, and 82 percent had a length of stay less than estimated, with 61 percent achieving a 3-day length of stay.
- In complicated cases without comorbidities and without VSD subgroup, 100 percent achieved their estimated length of stay. No patients exceeded their planned length of stay, and 92 percent had stays shorter than planned.
- In the complex comorbidity cohort, 65 percent had a length of stay less than estimated, including 13 percent with a 3-day hospitalization and 3 percent with a 2-day hospitalization.

Cumulative results in table 9-1 demonstrate the actual length of stay (ALOS) for CV-ROM patients versus the estimated length of stay (ELOS) on the standard pathway protocol. On the diagonal, the denominator is the number of patients expected to achieve that ELOS. The numerator and the other reported values denote the number of CV-ROM patients achieving a particular ALOS for a given ELOS. Only eight patients

TABLE 9-1 Actual vs. Estimated Length of Stay: Cumulative Results for Total Bypass Patients

Estimated Length of Stay on Standard Pathway Protocol	\multicolumn{10}{c}{Actual Length of Stay on CV-ROM}
	2	3	4	5	6	7	8	9	10	>10
3	4	37/41								
4	2	28	12/42							
5		15	7	4/26						
6		3	6	4	0/15	1	1			
7		4	2	1	2	1/11		1		
8			4	1			1/7		1	
9							1	0/3		2 (13, 14)
10					2				0/4	2 (12, 31)
Total	6	87	31	10	2	4	3	1	1	4

exceeded the ELOS (eight is the sum of the numbers appearing above the diagonal). All eight of these patients were from the comorbidity group; however, 65 percent of the patients with comorbidities actually had an ALOS shorter than their pathway plan.

Outcomes

Outcome data demonstrated 3 deaths (1.4 percent) and 16 complications (7.6 percent), which are considered extremely low for congenital heart disease. Two patients had an unscheduled clinic visit within 14 days of discharge. One visit was for postpericardiotomy syndrome in a 14-year-old patient with sinus venosus ASD and partial anomalous pulmonary venous connection, and the other was for a superficial wound infection in a 10-month-old with VSD. Of note, four of the six readmissions or unscheduled clinic visits occurred in patients with ASDs or VSDs, and only two had more complex lesions (a subaortic stenosis and atrioventricular canal), with none occurring in our most complex subsets in whom early discharge had occurred. These incidences are comparable with and, in fact, less than the incidences per 100 patients in our previous studies of CV-ROM patients and interactive pathway patients. Family satisfaction surveys were completed by all patients in the study, and no negative comments related to the length of stay were received.[33]

Effectiveness in Very Complex Cardiac Surgery Patients

The CV-ROM approach was recently examined for adults with congenital cardiac disease, an extremely heterogeneous and complex patient group.[34] In this patient population, secondary changes due to the chronicity of the disease process alter anatomy and physiology and would appear to hamper attempted variance decreases. In 10 patients aged 18–58 years (mean 28 years), repair of congenital cardiac lesions was performed. Four of these patients were undergoing reoperations. ALOS was examined and compared with the planned length of stay for the entire cohort as well as the reoperation subset. For the total study group, the aggregate planned number of hospital days was 58 (5.8 days per patient, with a range of 4–7 days based on lesion and comorbidities). For the reoperation group alone, total number of planned hospital days was 25 days (6.25 days per patient, range 6–7 days). Of note, these planned lengths of stay were extremely conservative, with a maximum of only 7 days in these complex older patients.

Mortality, morbidity, readmissions, and unscheduled clinic and emergency visits were assessed, and patient satisfaction was measured. The total number of hospital days for this group was 40 (4 days per patient, range 3–5 days for the entire cohort). This represented a 31 percent reduction in length of stay (−18 days) when compared with the ELOS ($p < 0.003$). For the reoperation patient subset, total hospital days were 15 (3.7 days per patient, range 3–4 days). This represented a 40 percent reduction in length of stay (−10 days) when compared with the ELOS ($p < 0.003$).

There were no deaths, morbidities, readmissions, or unscheduled postdischarge clinic or emergency room visits. Patient satisfaction was excellent. This preliminary study demonstrates that adults with complex congenital heart disease can outperform even an aggressive pathway plan when the CV-ROM is used. The outcome measures confirm the effectiveness of the CV-ROM process, and patient feedback indicates their satisfaction.

CONCLUSION

The use of the pathway methodology for cardiovascular surgery patients has been a learning experience. It began with an interactive approach to provide effective pathway design for the very heterogeneous population of congenital heart disease patients. The interactive pathway model decreased variation while optimizing patient care.[35] The pathway initiative progressed to a proactive model, the CV-ROM, which, as noted, has improved results over time and continues to be a dynamic process.[36]

The CV-ROM provides a framework for proactive implementation of the pathway methodology. It can reduce negative variance as well as encourage positive variances, thereby markedly reducing the length of hospital stays.[37,38] The CV-ROM can be applied to all subsets of patients, even the most complex and heterogeneous groups, in which it seems to have its maximal effect.[39,40]

The CV-ROM method would not be as successful without the catalyst of patient and family empowerment and the oversight role of the CNC-CM. The nursing literature often discusses the importance of incorporating the family in the care of their child. However, the literature also cites nurses' fear of criticism from their peers if they invite family participation. In addition, with all their other tasks to complete, nurses find it difficult to include the family in the daily plan of care.[AQ12] The CV-ROM method of pathway implementation prevents criticism of nurses by other nurses because the parents are responsible for ambulation and spirometer use. It also relieves nurses of the task of bringing the family into their child's care because it is already done in the preoperative sessions by the CNC-CM. The family's participation in care continues to be reinforced postoperatively by all staff members.

Liability concerns about pathways are nonexistent when the patients and their families are treated with respect as equal members of the health care team. Patients and families feel a sense of satisfaction and pride, as substantiated in all of the family surveys regarding CV-ROM experiences. In examining the results of the proactive pathway model, caregivers found that accelerated patient recovery was possible. Further, a dynamic system was in place, one in which further improvements occurred over time.[42] This finding is common in a system where families are better prepared for the process, the staff understands the approach, and caregivers can make real-time changes in the plan of care to improve the process. These success stories were most evident in highly complex patients with heterogeneous congenital cardiac lesions and more recently in older patients with chronic congenital cardiac disease in whom secondary problems had occurred.[43,44]

Because of its interactive and proactive components, the CV-ROM can present daunting operational problems. Originally, paper pathways were designed for individual diagnoses. Once the CV-ROM hinge points were added to the paths it became apparent that paper-based pathways were no longer adequate. The varying ROM levels affected a number of individual pathways and altered the order sets for the patients. For example, when patients are extubated earlier than expected, ambulation and alimentation are accelerated. The decision made at the extubation hinge point causes a change in future order sets and within the ROM model, resulting in movement to a lower ROM level and a shorter hospitalization. Only a computerized pathway model could accommodate such a dynamic process.

Clearly, health care has entered a new era, and efforts at improving quality of care and cost containment will have major effects on the delivery system. Pathway methods such as the proactive CV-ROM methodology will allow clinicians around the world to meet these challenges. The combination of human intervention and computer technology offers caregivers an opportunity to pursue their cost reduction and patient outcome goals.

The ROM differs significantly from standard critical pathway methodologies. In the latter the power is in the plan: adherence to the plan results in reduced negative variance and success defined by statistical findings.[45] In the former the power is in the process.[36] The CV-ROM pathway model taps the power of the patient, and success is defined by the most important outcome measures: patient recovery and satisfaction.

References

1. Critical paths—a pre-existing tool ready-made for TQM implementation [Editorial]. *QI/TQM* 2:2–4, 1992.

2. Hofmann, P. A. Critical path method: an important tool for coordinating clinical care. *Joint Commission on Quality Improvement* 19:235–46, 1993.

3. Crummer, M. B., and Carter, V. Critical pathways—the pivotal tool. *Journal of Cardiovascular Nursing* 7:30–37, 1993.

4. Strong, A. G., and Sneed, N. V. Clinical evaluation of a critical path for coronary artery bypass surgery patients. *Progress in Cardiovascular Nursing* 6:29–37, 1991.

5. Strong.

6. Crummer.

7. Strong.

8. Turley, K., Tyndall, M., Roge, C., and others. Critical pathway methodology: effectiveness in congenital heart surgery. *Annals of Thoracic Surgery* 58:57–65, 1994.

9. Turley, K. M., Higgins, S. S., Archer-Duste, H., and others. Role of the clinical nurse coordinator in successful implementation of critical pathways in pediatric cardiovascular surgery patients. *Progress in Cardiovascular Nursing* 10(1):22–26, 1995.

10. Turley and others, 1994.

11. Turley and others, 1994.

12. Turley, K., Tyndall, M., Turley, K. M., and others. Cardiovascular-radical outcome method is effective in complex congenital cardiac lesions. *Annals of Thoracic Surgery* 62:386–92, 1996.

13. Turley, K., Tyndall, K., Turley, K. M., and others. Can adults with complex congenital heart disease outperform their critical pathway design? [Abstract]. Chicago: American Hospital Association, 1997.

14. Turley, K., Tyndall, M., Turley, K. M., and others. Radical outcome method: a new approach to critical pathways in congenital heart disease. *Circulation* 92(suppl. II):II-245–II-249, 1995.

15. Turley, K. M., and Higgins, S. S. When parents participate in critical pathway management following pediatric cardiovascular surgery: maternal child nursing. *American Journal of Maternal/Child Nursing* 21:229–34, 1996.
16. Malinski, V. M. Nursing science within the science of unitary human beings. In: V. W. Malinski, editor. *Explorations on Martha Roger's Science of Unitary Human Beings.* East Norwalk, CT: Appleton-Lange, 1987, pp. 25–32.
17. Strong.
18. Turley and others. Role of the clinical nurse coordinator.
19. Turley and Higgins.
20. Friedman, M. M. General family nursing interventions. In: M. M. Friedman, editor. *Family Nursing: Theory and Practice.* 3rd edition. East Norwalk, CT: Appleton-Lange, 1992, pp. 351–56.
21. Turley and Higgins.
22. Weinstein, R. Hospital case management: the path to empowering nurses. *Pediatric Nursing* 17:289–93, 1991.
23. Turley and others. Role of the clinical nurse coordinator.
24. Turley and Higgins.
25. Turley and others, 1996.
26. Turley and others. Radical outcome method.
27. Turley and others. Role of the clinical nurse coordinator.
28. Turley and Higgins.
29. Turley and others. Role of the clinical nurse coordinator.
30. Turley and Higgins.
31. Turley and others. Radical outcome method.
32. Turley and others, 1996.
33. Turley and others, 1996.
34. Turley and others, 1997.
35. Turley and others, 1994.
36. Turley and others. Radical outcome method.
37. Turley and others, 1994.
38. Turley and others. Radical outcome method.
39. Turley and others, 1996.
40. Turley and others, 1997.
41. Turley and Higgins.
42. Turley and others. Radical outcome method.
43. Turley and others, 1996.
44. Turley and others, abstract.
45. Turley and others, 1994.
46. Turley and others, 1996.

PART II
Information Technology Solutions

CHAPTER 10

Selecting an Automated Case Management and Clinical Path Information System

Sherry Lee

Much of the clinical and administrative information that flows through the health care system is still recorded on paper. More than 10 billion pages of patient records are produced in the United States each year.[1] Today, for instance, when home health nurses get new patient referrals they must visit the hospital if they wish to review the detailed patient care data contained in the inpatient record. Before today's managed care environment existed, providers had no incentive to design integrated information systems. This situation reflects the main task that patient records once served: a record of everything that happened to a patient during a particular episode of care. The development of a lifetime patient record accessible to clinicians at any site of care was not a priority. Today, however, the patient record has grown beyond the bounds of record keeping and communication within one provider site. With the advent of integrated health care delivery networks, clinical records have become information sources for analyzing patients' resource requirements and outcomes and the profitability of health care practices.

Managed care, case management, clinical pathways, outcomes management, and other recent healthcare phenomena are making health care informatics much more important.[2] All involved in patient care activities must have timely and accurate information to do their jobs. Case managers, as well as bedside clinicians, are constantly evaluating patients' level-of-care requirements and resource use. Never before have direct caregivers been so involved in evaluating costs and quality. The resulting demand for information is placing an enormous strain on health care's outdated information systems. What was once considered a freestanding hospital is rapidly becoming part of a larger health care network. Case managers are expected to coordinate patient care across provider sites. To do the job adequately, they must regularly discuss patient care requirements with physicians and other care providers in acute care facilities, skilled nursing and long-term facilities, hospice and home health agencies, and behavioral health facilities. The responsibilities of today's case manager span the continuum of care, where they are accountable for activities such as:[3]

- Determining patients' eligibility for health services (financial, medical, or other)
- Assessing patients' required levels of care and recommending a site for care
- Defining patients' needs and recommending a care plan
- Prescribing or arranging patient services
- Coordinating services patients receive from multiple providers
- Reassessing patients' needs throughout their episodes of care
- Monitoring completeness and quality of patient care services
- Supporting patients' families

Clinical paths have become an important case management tool. However, paper-based versions may not be readily accessible to caregivers and case managers during the process of patient care. Computerizing these tools would yield many benefits, including:

- Enhanced timeliness and availability of patient care information to care providers in multiple geographic locations[4]
- Point-of-care capture of data for clinical case evaluations to identify and reduce unnecessary variations in patient care practices and improve patient outcomes[5,6]
- Ease in designing data displays (graphs, charts, summaries, and so on) to assist in identifying areas where practice changes would be desirable[7]
- Integration of variance tracking with charting-by-exception documentation systems[8]
- Ability to link clinical path recommendations and physician orders[9]
- Computer prompts and edit checks to minimize omissions and data entry errors[10]
- Improved efficiency of patient record documentation for all caregivers[11]
- Patients' progression enabled based on their clinical needs[12]

This chapter focuses on the computerized information system requirements for case management activities. While working to fully integrate their data networks, organizations should be anticipating the case management components they will need and begin now to build the systems necessary to support these components.

THE IDEAL CASE MANAGEMENT SYSTEM FEATURES AND COMPONENTS

A computerized case management system must assist case managers in making decisions about patient care requirements and expected resource use. The system should also allow these managers to monitor the results of their care-planning choices. To accomplish these goals, the following elements should be in place.

Integration with the Financial or Claims Management System

The case management system should be integrated with the financial or claims management system for the following purposes:

- *Eligibility confirmation:* The case manager should be able to validate the patient's current insurance coverage.
- *Benefit plan limitations and coverage:* When planning for a patient's care requirements, the case manager will need to know the patient's current health plan benefit package and any out-of-pocket expenses to be incurred by the patient.
- *Referral access:* Patients enrolled in a managed care health plan may be required to receive care only from the plan's contracted providers. If the case manager has access to the names of participating providers in each health plan, posthospital discharge planning is streamlined.
- *Health plan authorization information:* Case managers should be able to validate the presence of necessary inpatient and outpatient admission certifications. If the admission or extended-stay health plan authorization process is performed by someone other than the case manager, communications between the provider and the health plan should be accessible to the case manager.
- *Second-opinion verification:* A patient's insurance plan may require a second physician's opinion prior to surgery or additional treatment. The case manager should be able to determine whether a second opinion was necessary and whether it was completed as required.[13]
- *Comparison of accrued costs or charges to expected reimbursement:* By having on-line access to charge and cost data, the case manager can quickly identify patients who are nearing their insurance coverage limits or who represent a potential financial liability for the organization.

Integration with the Administrative and Clinical Information Systems

The case management system should be integrated with the administrative and clinical information systems for the following purposes:

- *E-mail communication:* Case managers must converse daily with other care providers and health plans. Using E-mail, they can communicate with others efficiently and maintain documentation that contact was successful.[14]
- *Patient profile:* To complete an initial patient assessment, the case manager and direct-care providers will review the patient's history, demographic information, occupational history, past illnesses and surgeries, family history, and current health status. If these data are readily available in computer files, the care-planning process is more productive.
- *Predictive capabilities:* With access to information about a patient's severity of illness (using vital signs and other physical measures) and physiological reserve (age and comorbidities), the case manager can anticipate care coordination problems. Clinical pathways can be enacted to minimize complicating factors.[15,16]

Other Functions

Additional computerized functions that should be available to the case manager include the following.

- *On-line storage capabilities:* Case managers must be able to access current patient cases being managed, contacts at other provider sites, referral agencies, and other data vital to the care coordination function.
- *Report generation:* Information distillation tools are important for case managers to use in analyzing data in their system. Using database query techniques, the case manager should be able to generate nonstandard, customized reports. For example,

on-line analytical processing (OLAP) is a database query technique that supports decision making using information from complex, multidimensional data sets.[17] Using OLAP or other database query techniques, the case manager should be able to run standard and special reports without assistance from information system staff.

- *Discharge-planning notes:* The information system should include fields for discharge-planning notes to provide a central location for all care providers to document and update patient discharge plans.
- *Outcome documentation:* The progress of the patient toward achieving care plan outcomes should be charted by the case manager in the information system. The system should allow linkage of actual and expected outcomes.[18] Reasons for not achieving expected outcomes should also be documented.

Clinical Path Information System

An important component of a case management system is the clinical path module. The functionality of this component has a significant impact on caregivers' ability to monitor patient progress effectively and identify cost and quality improvement opportunities. The features to look for in a clinical path module are listed below.

Pathway Template The system should allow for the design of a standardized pathway template to meet the needs of multiple caregivers. If the software only supports the traditional day-to-day path format, clinicians will be frustrated should they wish to develop phase-oriented or outcome-driven paths.[19] Users should be able to define the patient care functions that will be listed down the left side of their pathways.

Do not expect the software vendor to provide predeveloped clinical pathways. Path development should be done internally by a interdisciplinary team composed of the organization's caregivers. The reason for this step is that predesigned paths are less likely to be accepted by all clinicians and even less likely to meet facility-specific case management objectives.[20] The paths that each facility develops will be unique to its clinical process improvement goals. For example, the path used at one hospital to resolve delayed discharge transport problems may be different from another hospital's path, which focuses on appropriateness of antibiotic use.

A standardized template also simplifies transfer of pathway recommendations into a computerized order entry system. Standard physician order sets increase the accuracy of the ordering process, minimize nursing time necessary to transcribe orders, and prevent omissions of critical interventions.[21]

Another pathway template that has been used successfully in many organizations is the patient and family pathway. This pathway describes the process of care in lay terms and is used for education and communication purposes.[22] The case manager and care team use the pathway to discuss with the patient and family expected progression stages, treatments and other interventions, and anticipated outcomes.[23] Both patients and families have reported greater satisfaction with the patient care process when they are educated with lay pathways.[24] These pathways also ensure that patients are provided uniform answers to their questions. For example, when the patient asks, "When will I get to eat solid food?" all members of the care team are referencing the same patient pathway in answering this question.[25]

If your facility does not have a computerized point-of-care documentation system, be sure that the clinical path module can print paper copies of pathways. When automated documentation is available, the templates can be integrated into the point-of-care system to eliminate duplicative charting.

Merger of Different Clinical Paths As the organization continues to mature in its pathway project, it may see the need to combine pathways for patients with two or more differing conditions (for example, hip replacement surgery and insulin-dependent diabetes). System programming capabilities to analyze duplicate orders, interventions, or outcomes and establish rule-based logic will assist with path mergers.[26]

Orders Generated Directly from the Clinical Path Physician orders are an important byproduct of a clinical path. When a patient is placed on a path, a computerized system can communicate admitting orders to various departments. Progression of the patient along a pathway can also be streamlined through automatic communication of new orders to relevant departments. For example, nurses can be prompted to advance the patient's ambulation routine if pathway documentation indicates the patient is ahead of schedule.

Documentation of Completed Tasks Interventions completed by nurses and other caregivers should be recorded on the path. Likewise, interventions not completed should be noted along with the reason for the variance. If such documentation can be accomplished through an exception-based documentation model, charting time is decreased because standard care is not written in narrative form and duplication of charting is eliminated.[27] In some case management computerized systems, caregivers can select a set of related items and indicate with one keystroke that all have been completed. If possible, invest in a system that does not require caregivers to select items individually.

Variances Variances are goals not met or interventions not performed according to the time frame suggested by the path.[28] When a variance occurs, the case manager or the involved caregiver documents the cause for the variance, immediate actions taken in response to the event, and any follow-up plans. Variance documentation for clinical pathways is crucial to the success of the case management initiative.

Look for an automated system that allows users to build a file containing the common reasons for variances. These standardized statements are automatically displayed when the nurse is charting the variance event. Nurses merely need to select the cause most suited to the immediate situation, rather than type in a statement in their own words. The case management system should provide users with an opportunity to develop similar standardized tables for other repetitive input tasks. Variances documented in the patient's automated medical record should not require an additional charting step for the path variance tracking system.

Aggregate Variance Analysis Variance analysis is important for evaluating the effectiveness of clinical paths, identifying areas needing change on existing paths, and determining compliance with important aspects of patient care.[29] The software system should provide a standard set of reports that answer common path-related questions posed by clinical and administrative staff. For example, monthly and quarterly reports showing reimbursement variances should be available. The system should be able to sort information about each category of patients on a path according to patient name, account number, medical record number, length of stay, physician, total charges, total costs, reimbursement, and cost-reimbursement variance. Another commonly used report shows length of stay, sorted by pathway diagnosis-related group (DRG), physician, nursing unit, and insurance provider. DRG length-of-stay and cost outlier reports can often indicate where new path development is needed. Variance reports that should be included in the software vendor's standard reporting package are shown in table 10-1.

TABLE 10-1 Standard Variance Reports

Report	Sort Capabilities
DRG outliers	Length of stay Cost
Cost to reimbursement variances	Physician Nursing unit Insurance provider
Actual length of stay versus length of stay target	Physician Nursing unit Cost variance Insurance provider
Patient- or family-related variances	Variance type Nursing unit Physician
Caregiver- or clinician-related variances	Variance type Nursing unit Physician Cost to reimbursement ratio
Hospital- or system-related variances	Nursing unit Cost to reimbursement ratio Length of stay
Number of minutes in operating room	Surgical procedure (first sort) and physician (secondary sort)
Use of critical care beds	DRG and physician
Use of appropriate diagnostic tests	DRG and physician

TECHNICAL ISSUES TO CONSIDER IN SYSTEM SELECTION

As impressive as some automated case management systems may seem, they still can be hampered by technology issues. In recent years several technological developments have occurred that can improve computer system capabilities and user friendliness. Some of the technology issues that should be addressed when purchasing a new system are described below.

System Interface Capabilities

An important consideration when selecting a system is its ability to interface with other existing information systems. Health Level Seven (HL-7) is one of the most widely used messaging standards for electronic interchange of health data. Messaging standards specify the syntax of an electronic message. A similar distinction exists for more familiar messages, such as postcards. The syntax of a postcard corresponds to the arrangement of its elements: the addressee's name appears in a standard position, the city in another; the message is placed in a box on the left half and the stamp in the upper right; and so on. The arrangement is set by international postal conventions. Similarly, HL-7 and other messaging standards specify the order of the many discrete elements that make up a message and indicate which elements are required and which are optional.[30]

Windows™ Technology

Windows™-based technology is becoming widely used within all industries. Health care is one of the last industries to adopt Windows™ and part with lackluster green screens and flashing cursors. Windows™ environments use a graphical user interface with icons and point-and-click steps for navigation through the system. As a result, employees having little previous computer experience find it easier to use a Windows™-based system.[31]

Be sure to find out whether the software package being considered for purchase is Windows™ based or Windows™ front ended. If the product was not originally designed for the Windows environment, the developer may have simply added a Windows™ interface to allow the product to run within the Windows™ operating system. If this is the case, the software will not have standard Windows™ features such as pull-down menus or the ability to move one window on the screen while working on another. A Windows™ front-end product can be opened from within the Windows™ environment, although when performing everyday tasks it has no relationship to Windows™. Some software vendors may indicate they are moving to a totally Windows™-based product. If this is the case, ask for a specific release date and consider including it as part of your contract.

Relational Database

The case management information system should be a relational database in order to provide the performance, control, and connectivity required for integrated applications. In addition, it can accommodate a multitude of data and users as well as a high rate of information retrieval and updates.[32] For example, if you want to determine the impact of a specific medication on a certain age group of people who live in a particular ZIP code area, a relational database can provide the information you need.

Hardware

Handheld computers are becoming increasingly popular. Be careful to consider the weight of the device; it may be asking too much of nurses to have a 5-pound laptop computer strapped to their shoulders all day long! However, bear in mind that as devices get smaller (2 pounds or less), functionality becomes more limited.

Wall-mounted documentation screens are also available. Be sure to evaluate the stability of these products if permanent placement in patients' rooms is planned. One hospital decided not to place wall-mounted screens on the pediatric unit because of breakage concerns. Consider the cleaning issues involved with wall-mounted units, especially in isolation rooms and high-traffic areas. Personal computers on customized rolling tables are becoming popular. This allows bedside documentation without the expense of placing a computer at every bed.[33]

If handheld or wall-mounted computer terminals are being considered, be sure to check the screen's visibility. In other words, if it is relatively dark in the patient's room, can the nurse view the information on the screen? Can data be entered in a darkened room, or must the room lights be turned on each time data are entered?

The Human-to-Computer Interface

There are numerous ways for humans to interact with computers: keyboard, mouse, trackball, touch screen, and light pen. In selecting your system, choose the human-to-computer interface that will be most efficient for your circumstances. If staff lack proficient keyboard input skills, consider purchasing a mouse- or pen-based system. Touch screen technology is rapidly improving, although two obstacles remain: dirty screens and faulty touch interpretation.[34]

SELECTING A CASE MANAGEMENT AUTOMATED SYSTEM

Before examining the capabilities of different case management software packages, the organization must clearly define what it hopes to gain from an automated case management system. This needs analysis should be done by a multidisciplinary system evaluation team. Ideally, this team includes a representative from the organization's management information system (MIS) department, key staff involved in case management and clinical path initiatives, and representatives from other departments that may have a secondary relationship with case management (health information management, social services or discharge planning, quality management, and so on). To fully realize the goals of automation, some team members should have had experience using the organization's paper-based case management or pathway system.

Establish System Goals

Start by asking the team to establish clear goals for the case management system. By writing down the primary goals, the selection of necessary system features becomes much easier. The goals may be specific reports that are needed, data manipulation capabilities, automated patient care documentation using exception-based charting, predictive capabilities, or the ability to interface with existing information systems to minimize duplicate data entry. To illustrate how information system goals will vary slightly among facilities, the goals established by the managed care system evaluation team at Richland Memorial Hospital in Columbia, SC, and those developed by the Point-of-Care Project team at Mount Carmel Health System, Columbus, OH, are listed in figure 10-1.

Identify Desirable System Functions

After defining the goals, identifying desirable automated case management system functions is much easier. Ask the team to brainstorm a "wish list" of anything and everything it can think of. Practicalities should not get in the way of listing every possible feature. Examples of desirable system functions or features, which are discussed throughout this chapter, are listed below:

- HL-7 compliance
- Windows™-based system
- Relational database
- On-line, user-friendly report writer
- Exception-based and legend charting
- Physician order sets for clinical pathways
- Handheld device weighing less than 2 pounds for data entry
- Portable personal computers (PCs) on customized rolling tables for data entry
- Color PCs on each nursing unit and ancillary department and in physician offices
- Access to system from all health care system geographic locations
- Variance documentation as a byproduct of routine patient care documentation
- Option for additional variance-related documentation
- Standard variance reports interfaced to hospital information system and cost-accounting system
- No duplicate data entry

FIGURE 10-1 Two Organizations' Goals for Automated Information Systems

Organization A

Hospital Goals for Automated Managed Care Information System
- Create unified approach to automation, eliminating fragmentation
- Offer totally integrated solution
- Coordinate automation across continuum of care
- Enhance cost-effectiveness of patient care
- Support multidisciplinary team approach to patient care
- Decrease documentation time
- Enhance quality of care
- Provide on-line, user-friendly report writer for nonprogrammers
- Create central database repository
- Assist with the Joint Commission on Accreditation of Healthcare Organizations (JCAHO) survey process
- Provide fast and thorough means for patient assessment
- Help to identify areas of care needing enhancement
- Enhance predictive capabilities
- Create paperless environment

Organization B

Health System Goals for a Point-of-Care Automation Project
Improve productivity by:
- Decreasing documentation time
- Aiding recruitment and retention
- Eliminating redundant data entry
- Choosing an easy-to-use, user-friendly system, considerate of nontypists
- Decreasing paper management tasks
- Improving information consolidation and presentation flexibility
- Providing caregivers with empirically based clinical decision support capabilities

Enhance quality of health care delivery by:
- Providing consistent, structured quality documentation
- Satisfying regulatory requirements (such as JCAHO and Medicare requirements) for clinical information and research
- Increasing direct care time, maximizing patient and staff interaction
- Supporting data access for quality outcome measurement
- Allowing real-time authentication with electronic signatures

Manage health care costs through:
- Timely access to accurate data
- Reductions in loss of revenue due to incomplete documentation
- Access to patient profiling information
- Decreased exposure to medical liability or litigation

Support integrated health care by providing:
- Appropriate data standards
- Multiple, simultaneous access to patient records from any location
- Critical elements of the computer-based patient record
- Required information to third-party payers
- Data access by secondary users of the patient record
- Full integration with the hospital information system and future information technology
- Confidentiality and security

Sources: Organization A—Reprinted, with permission, from Richland Memorial Hospital, Columbia, SC. Organization B—Reprinted, with permission, from Mount Carmel Health System, Columbus, OH.

- Ability for caregivers to document against clinical path recommendations and expected patient outcomes
- Standard template for clinical path, physician orders, and patient and family path
- Ability to customize pathway templates
- Multiple time frame options for pathways
- Ability to merge multiple pathways
- Automatic notification of case manager when variances occur that may delay discharge
- Automatic notification of physician and case manager when patient reaches "risk range" for costs or length of stay

Once all possible system features are listed, team members should rate each item on the "wish list" by priority as follows:

1. Necessary
2. Need now, but could wait for future release
3. Nice to have

A sample priority-setting form is shown in figure 10-2. It is unlikely that the entire list of desirable functions will be available in one software package. By ranking the importance of each feature, the team can pinpoint the system or systems most likely to meet the necessary requirements.

The case management system evaluation team should keep in mind that other computerized information systems within the organization may already have features that the team considers necessary. The MIS department team member should be able to suggest duplicative functions that can be eliminated from the case management system if it can easily interface with these other systems.

Develop a Request for Information

Convert the list of desired system features into a request for information (RFI) to be sent to all potential vendors. This document asks vendors to indicate if they currently have each feature or have plans to develop the feature in the future. A sample RFI is shown in figure 10-3. Mail the RFI to vendors with a cover letter asking them to complete the form and return it within a specified time frame (usually 3 to 4 weeks). There are several ways to identify vendors who should receive your automated case management program RFI:

- Contact case management colleagues who have computerized systems.
- Review articles and advertisements in case-management-related journals.
- Research vendor names in available publications.[35]
- Visit vendor demonstration booths at case management or informatics seminars.
- Attend informatics sessions at case management seminars.
- Participate in local, regional, or national case management professional organizations.
- Ask vendors to identify their major competitors.
- Obtain students' vendor research from university-based medical or nursing informatics programs.
- Review seminar brochures for vendor display listings.
- Watch informatics journals for vendor comparison research articles.[36]

FIGURE 10-2 Software Package Feature Priority-Setting Form

Feature	Necessary	Need now, but could wait	Nice to have
HL-7 compliant			
Windows based			
Relational database			
On-line, user-friendly report writer			
Exception-based charting			
Legend charting			
Order sets for paths			
Handheld device weighing < 2 lb.			
Portable PC on rollable table			
Color PC on units, ancillary depts., physician offices			
Access to system from all geographic locations			
Variance documentation a routine byproduct of path documentation			
Option for additional variance documentation			
Standard variance reports interfaced to HIS and cost accounting			
No duplicate data entry			
Documentation against path interventions and outcomes			
Standard path template with customized categories			
Physician orders template			
Patient/family path template			
Customized templates			
Multiple time frame options for paths			
Multiple path merger capabilities			
Auto notification of case manager of variances which may delay discharges			
Auto notification of physician and case manager when patient reaches "risk range" for cost or LOS			

FIGURE 10-3 Sample Request for Information

	(Please check appropriate box)			
Desired Feature	**Currently Installed**	**Currently in Development** (provide expected release date)	**Future Development Planned** (provide expected release date)	**No Plans to Develop This Capability**
On-line, exception-based documentation				
User-defined pathway templates				
Variance reporting on demand: Sorted by patient				
Sorted by nursing unit				
Sorted by attending physician				
Sorted by cause of variance				
Multidisciplinary patient care plan can be incorporated into pathway				
Allows development of patient copy of pathway in lay terminology				
Maintains audit trail of documentation corrections				
HL-7 compliant				
Windows™ based				
Provides two-level security				

Review RFI Responses and Finalize Top Vendor List

Once the RFIs have been returned, the evaluation team can eliminate those vendors least able to provide necessary system features. When the list of potential vendors is narrowed to no more than three, it is time to delve more deeply into the capabilities of the remaining systems and the companies offering them. This is usually done through the distribution of a more formal request for proposal (RFP) to inquire about key vendor issues, and through site visits and product demonstrations.[37]

Key Vendor Issues

Any time you are planning to purchase an expensive product and want to be certain the vendor will back its product claims, there are several issues that should be evaluated. Tips for obtaining accurate and complete vendor evaluation information are listed below.

Company Stability   Look at the vendor's stability: employee size, history, age of company, stock patterns, headquarters, and financial status. Determine where the corporate headquarters is located—is it in someone's garage or in a reputable section of the business district? Do there seem to be enough employees? Is the company rumored to be for sale, or is it in the process of purchasing other software vendors? If a change in the company's status is anticipated, some of its products may be discontinued. If it is a publicly owned company, a recent financial statement should be available. Another indicator of stability is the CEO's length of tenure and success of the company during this time.

New System Development Because of the rapidly changing information needs in health care, new system development should be an important part of a software vendor's strategy. Ask questions such as:

- How much of the company's annual net profits are channeled into new software development?
- Do current system users have input into setting priorities for new system development?
- How much do customers' needs influence the design of new software?

Future Product Releases If some of the software features your organization is particularly interested in purchasing have yet to be developed by the company, ask about future availability. If the vendor indicates that the feature "will be ready soon" or "is almost ready for release," ask for the specific release date and have this documented in the RFP response. Many organizations now include a statement in their software vendor contracts indicating that all promises made in the RFP are included as part of the contract.

Customer References Request a customer reference list from the vendor. Ask for organizations that are similar to yours based on annual discharges, number of internal information management support staff, staffing, and so on. Call several customers and ask to speak to actual system users, not just the information systems staff, and get their answers to the following questions:[38]

- How responsive are the people who staff the vendor's customer service line?
- How much input, if any, have you had in new software development?
- Have promised upgrades and other items been delivered promptly?
- Have you been pleased with the functionality of the system?
- Do you have any plans to replace your current system with another vendor's product?
- What new systems on the market today would you consider purchasing to replace your current system?
- What other products were evaluated before you chose this one?
- Would you purchase this software product again?
- What is your relationship to the vendor, if any (in other words, do you or your organization own stock in the company)?
- How satisfied were you with the software implementation and go-live process?
- What do you think is the most positive aspect of this vendor and its product?
- What do you think is the most negative aspect of this vendor and its product?
- What has been your most frustrating experience with this vendor?

Live Product Demonstrations

The evaluation team or its key members should conduct site visits to view the software in action and talk with end users. Frequently, the vendor will accompany a prospective customer on the visit. However, it is advisable to arrange some time to talk to system users outside of the formal demonstration. This will allow for more candid discussions of system advantages and disadvantages.

Arrange for a product demonstration within your organization. Invite members of the system evaluation team as well as other potential system users. Request that the vendor provide a "live" software demonstration because a preconfigured demonstration may not be representative of actual system performance. Some of your organization's evaluation team members should get a hands-on feel for the system during the demonstration. While they will not have time to become familiar with the system's functionality, they will have an opportunity to judge ease of use and basic system design.

Before the software demonstration, determine important questions to be asked of the vendor and assign the questions to different team members. Following the demonstration, have the team members submit the vendor's responses to their questions in writing to the team coordinator for distribution to all team members. Important questions to ask during the product demonstration include the following:

- For each system feature, ask for the names of organizations in your area that have that feature installed.
- If any system feature or module is in beta testing (being tested for the first time in a live environment), find out the name of the organization involved in the testing. You will want to talk to people at the beta test site to find out whether they are satisfied with their experience.
- When a feature is identified as "in development" or "scheduled to be released soon," ask for specific dates. These dates may be included in the contract you sign with the vendor, together with a defined penalty for delays.
- Is the hardware used during the demonstration the same equipment you are planning to purchase? If not, ask to evaluate the product on the hardware you will be using. If this request is made prior to the demonstration date, the vendor should be able to accommodate you.

Provide the vendor with sample scenarios from actual case management situations in your facility and ask that these situations be made part of the demonstration. Although these scenarios can be provided to the vendor in advance, you may wish to make an "on the spot" request during the demonstration to evaluate the program's flexibility and ease of use.

Enter data into the system during the demonstration and request on-screen reports. You will be able to observe report response times and readability. If the vendor connects the vendor system to a printer during the demo, ask for printed reports also.

System Selection

After the RFP is returned and on-site and off-site product evaluations are complete, the system evaluation team must make a decision. It should return to its original "wish list" of system features and priorities when making the final choice. Ideally, the team has found a company that offers a case management software package that currently includes all the necessary features and a few of the "nice to have" elements. If not, the organization may decide to relax its criteria or continue with its paper-based case management process until the right automated product comes along.

SUMMARY

Selecting an automated case management system can be an exciting learning experience. It is especially important to coordinate a multidisciplinary system selection process, with all team members having input into system selection. The organization's MIS department has valuable expertise in the field of informatics and technology.

Patient care providers offer worthwhile input regarding software and hardware functionality and usability. Health information management professionals are skilled in data security and quality control issues. Developing a cohesive team that recognizes the value each discipline brings to the system selection process will ensure success.

The selection team starts by establishing goals for the system. It then makes a lengthy "wish list" of features and identifies "must have" components. Key features to look for in a case management system are flexibility, ease of use, a on-line report writer, HL-7 interface, insurance data for verification, cost and expected reimbursement data, clinical paths with standard templates and customization capabilities, standard variance reports with a report writer feature, graphics capabilities, and a relational database. Once the required features are defined, the team is ready to contact software system vendors.

Gather data about vendors and schedule on-site demonstrations for the selection team. Be sure to do your homework when evaluating the vendor's software and hardware. It is also important to consider the vendor's general level of professionalism and sophistication. Make site visits to analyze the finalist vendors further. During the site visits, obtain candid opinions from current users of the software product. It is often reassuring to have one or more of the vendors return for a second demonstration and discussion of unanswered questions.

The future challenge for health care providers is to manage a scattered and diverse patient population across multiple settings for numerous episodes of care. To succeed, data must be integrated across all encounters to allow case managers to optimize patient health status in the most cost-effective manner. The ideal case management information system provides real-time decision support for longitudinal outcomes analysis across multiple patient populations, physician groups, direct care providers, and facilities.

References

1. U.S. Congress. *Automated Medical Records: Leadership Needed to Expedite Standards Development.* Washington, DC: U.S. General Accounting Office, 1993.
2. Brandt, M. Clinical practice guidelines and critical paths roadmaps to quality, cost effective care. *Journal of the American Health Information Management Association* 65(2, pt. 2):54–57, Feb. 1994.
3. Williams, J. K. *Case Management: Opportunities for Service Providers.* Syracuse, NY: Haworth, 1992.
4. DiJerome, L. The Nursing Case Management Computerized System: meeting the challenge of health care delivery through technology. *Computers in Nursing* 10(6):250–58, 1992.
5. Berkey, T. Benchmarking in health care: turning challenges into success. *Joint Commission Journal on Quality Improvement* 20(5):277–84, May 1994.
6. Nugent, W. C., and Schults, W. C. Playing by the numbers: how collecting outcomes data changed my life. *Annals of Thoracic Surgery* 58(6):1866–70, Dec. 1994.
7. Maehling, J. A., and Badger, K. Information system tools available to the case manager. *Nursing Case Management* 1(1):59–61, 1996.
8. Ashworth, G. B., and Aubrey, C. Collaborative care documentation by exception system. *Proceedings of the Annual Symposium on Computer Applications in Medical Care* 16:109–13, 1992.
9. New, K. W. Parallel MD orders keep critical paths in physicians' view daily. *Hospital Case Management* 2(11):177–78, 181–82, Nov. 1994.
10. Gardner, R. M., and others. Real time data acquisition: experience with the medical information bus (MIB). *Proceedings of the Fifteenth Annual Symposium on Computer Applications in Medical Care* 15:813–17, 1991.
11. Gwozdz, D. T., and Del Togno-Armanasco, V. Streamlining patient care documentation. *Journal of Nursing Administration* 22(5):35–39, May 1992.

12. Spath, P. L. *Mastering Path-Based Patient Care.* Forest Grove, OR: Brown-Spath and Associates, 1995, pp. 113–19.
13. Saba, V. K., and McCormick, K. A. Practice applications. In: *Essentials of Computers for Nurses.* New York City: McGraw-Hill, 1996.
14. Kedrowski, S. M., Munk, S. J., and Leung, E. Computers in case management advancing health care delivery through technology. *Nursing Case Management* 1(2):59–61, 1996.
15. Zimmerman, J. E., Knaus, W. A., and Seneff, M. Outcome prediction in intensive care. *Intensive Care Rounds* (no. 10125). Abingdon, England: Medicine Group (Education), Ltd., Jan. 1993.
16. Knaus, W. A., and others. The SUPPORT prognostic model: objective estimates of survival for seriously ill hospitalized adults. *Annals of Internal Medicine* 122(3):191–203, Feb. 1, 1995.
17. Radding, A. Blue Cross climbs mountain of data with OLAP. *Infoworld,* p. 64, Jan. 30, 1995.
18. Ignatavicius, D. D., and Hausman, K. A. *Clinical Pathways for Collaborative Practice.* Philadelphia: Saunders, 1995, p. 362.
19. Gardner and others.
20. Graybeal, K. B., Gheen, M., and McKenna, B. Clinical pathway development: the Overlake model. *Nursing Management* 24(4):42–45, 1993.
21. Language, order sets, progress notes. Three physicians share leadership strategies. *Issues Outcomes* 1(1):8–9, Jan.–Feb. 1995.
22. Baptist Hospital (Nashville, TN). Patient care pathway: total hip replacement. *Inside Case Management* 1(5):4, Aug. 1994.
23. De Jong, R. L. This path has pictures. *RN* 58(9):44–45, Sept. 1995.
24. Shulkin, D. J., and Ferniany, W. The effect of developing patient compendiums for critical pathways on patient satisfaction [Abstract]. *Journal of General Internal Medicine* 10(4):81, Apr. 1995.
25. Doherty J., and Coleman, J. Using critical pathways as a patient/family teaching tool. *Oncology Nursing Forum* 22(1):149, Jan.–Feb. 1995.
26. Nugent and Schults.
27. Eggland, E. T., and Heinemann, D. S. *Nursing Documentation: Charting, Recording, and Reporting.* Philadelphia: Lippincott, 1994, p. 193.
28. Zander, K. Critical paths. In: M. M. Melum and M. K. Sinioris, editors. *Total Quality Management: The Health Care Pioneers.* Chicago: American Hospital Publishing, 1992, p. 310.
29. Mateo, M. A., and Newton, C. Managing variances in case management. *Nursing Case Management* 1(1):45–51, 1996.
30. U.S. Congress. Information technologies for transforming health care. In: *Bringing Health Care Online: The Role of Information Technologies.* Washington, DC: U.S. General Accounting Office, 1995.
31. Schneider, P. The windowful world of healthcare. *Healthcare Infomatics* 13(4, special section):ss4–ss15, 1996.
32. Transition Systems, Inc. The information requirements of total quality management. *The Quality Resource* 11(4):3–4, July–Aug. 1993.
33. Grimm, C. B. Wireless winning wider appeal. *Healthcare Informatics* 13(4):26, Apr. 1996.
34. From 1996 comments offered by Dr. Thomas Naegele, a physician who was trained as a computer systems analyst prior to entering medical school. Dr. Naegele has given more than 400 hours of lectures and workshops in the field of computerized medical records, clinical decision making, and total quality management to numerous managed care companies and state medical societies. He lives in Albuquerque, NM, and can be reached at (505) 275-7267 or by E-mail at tanman@caswcp.com.
35. Software vendor information sources:

    - Health Management Technology publishes an *Annual Market Directory* journal issue that includes more than 50 companies offering health care information systems. Single copies of the directory are available from Inter Tech Publishing, 6151 Powers Ferry Road NW, Atlanta, GA 30339; (770) 955-2500.
    - Medical Group Management Association (MGMA) publishes a computer system search package and a directory of vendors. For information contact MGMA at (303) 799-1111.

- The Healthcare Computing Publications *Directory of Medical Office Management Computer System Vendors with Satisfaction Ratings* and *Directory of Medical Software* are available from the American Medical Association.

36. For example:

    - Hughes, S., and Andrew, W. Calling all nurses: report to Jericho STAT. *Healthcare Informatics* 13(4):52–60, Apr. 1996.
    - Dorenfest, S. The healthcare informatics top 100: stepping around the pitfalls. *Healthcare Informatics* 12(6):81–100, June 1995.

37. Resources for developing an RFP are available from the following sources:

    - *The Guide to Successfully Automating Your Home Health Organization.* Available from Home Health Business Resources, Los Altos, CA; (415) 903-9494.
    - Medical Group Management Association has a computer system search packet available for purchase. To order, phone (303) 799-1111.

38. Hannah, K. J., Ball, M. J., and Edwards, M. J. Selection of software/hardware. In: K. J. Hannah, M. J. Ball, and M. J. A. Edwards, editors. *Introduction to Nursing Informatics*. New York City: Springer, 1994.

CHAPTER 11

Building a Cost-Efficient Path Variance Database

Darice M. Grzybowski

Hinsdale Hospital, a 462-bed, acute care hospital in the Chicago metropolitan area, began its clinical path initiative in 1993 following an intensive reengineering effort in patient care services. The paths, known at Hinsdale Hospital as *care guides,* were designed to reduce resource use, increase patient and provider satisfaction, and maintain or improve quality of patient care. To help achieve these goals, nurse case managers were hired to implement the care guides for various patient populations.

An overriding goal of the care guide initiative was to enhance the patient care process. It was clear to medical staff and administrative leaders at the hospital that even the best-intentioned clinical path program can fail if it is not carefully integrated into the system of care. For this reason steps were taken to ensure that the care guides were actually used and clinicians provided with the information management support necessary to achieve their goals.

One of the challenges encountered by case managers was the collection of care guide variance and outcome indicator data. As the number of paths increased, so did the information management demands. However, the facility did not have the resources to purchase a software program dedicated to collecting data specific to the care guides. Through innovative solutions, caregivers at Hinsdale were able to use their existing computerized order entry information and decision support system to capture path variance and outcome data. With minimal modification, a clinical and financial data repository was created within the order entry system. The repository eliminated system interfaces and duplicate data entry, which would have been necessary if a freestanding path variance software product had been purchased.

This chapter focuses primarily on the information management components of Hinsdale Hospital's care guide initiative. To understand the path documentation and automated data-tracking system, a brief discussion of the care guide initiative at Hinsdale Hospital is necessary.

This chapter is dedicated to the memory of Jan Ridder, RN, former coordinator of case management at Hinsdale Hospital.

HISTORY OF HINSDALE HOSPITAL CARE GUIDES

In 1993 hospital leaders committed to developing care guides for 80 percent of Hinsdale's patient population. To achieve this goal, clinicians needed to design approximately 40 different guides. The guides were not to be used for patients who have complex diagnoses or whose care needs are unpredictable (anticipated to be 20 percent of the inpatient population).

From 1993 through 1994 administrative and medical staff leaders spent considerable time planning the care guide process, including the development of procedures for designing care guides and variance tracking, selecting the care guide patient populations, creating documentation tools, and defining success measures. The guiding principles established for the program are as follows:

- Each care guide will be developed by a multidisciplinary team consisting of, at a minimum, the following members:
  — Key physicians
  — Key nursing staff
  — Appropriate ancillary staff (such as laboratory and pharmacy)
  — Finance representative
  — Health information management department representative
  — Case manager (serving as team chairperson)
- Each team is charged with designing an outcome-oriented, evidence-based care guide using clinical practice guidelines and other literature sources, comparative external data, and data about internal "best practices." The goal of the team's care guide is to improve or maintain quality while stabilizing processes and potentially reducing resource utilization.
- Each team will follow the recommended steps when developing their care guide. (See figure 11-1.)
- Standardized care guide formats (figure 11-2) will be used throughout the organization. On each care guide the outcome goals (OCGs) defined for the patient population are listed in the first column, at the top of the form. The interventions necessary to achieve these goals are illustrated in the remaining columns on the path.
- A standardized path variance reporting form (figure 11-3) will be used by the case managers and staff.
- The use of care guides will be optional for physicians.
- Care guides will not duplicate traditional patient record documentation and will not be maintained as a permanent part of the patient record.
- Where possible, care guide variance and performance measurement data collection, aggregation, and reporting will be automated.

Between 1994 and 1995, multidisciplinary teams met and designed care guides for approximately 80 percent of the inpatient population and several key outpatient patient groups. As of October 1996, 32 care guides were under development or completed, covering pediatric asthma, bone marrow transplant, and other topics. Clinician members of the teams varied according to topic; however, support department members (that is, health information management, finance, and ancillary services) remained fairly constant. Each team met weekly for 1 to 2 hours, with each care guide development taking approximately 2 months.

In 1996 the care guide initiative evolved to the next phase: interfacing the care guide with patient record documentation and standardizing data collection techniques. These efforts are described in greater detail in the next two sections.

FIGURE 11-1 Care Guide Development Process

1. Identify
   — Topic (including identified population of patients)
   — Team leader (case manager)
   — Team members (including, at a minimum, a case manager, nurse, physician, and representatives from the health information management and finance departments, and ancillary departments, as needed)

2. Establish meeting time and date (schedule and reserve rooms)

3. Prepare basic "kick-off" handout, including:
   — Mission statement or charter
   — Charge-versus-cost information
   — Description of care guides
   — Examples of relevant paths from other organizations
   — Literature search of "best practices"
   — Other pertinent historical data about the topic

4. Develop care guide (using subgroup for detail work)
   Note: It is important to have a defined patient population at this point either based on patient types, service, International Classification of Diseases codes, charge codes, or diagnosis-related group (or a combination of these elements)

5. Develop standardized physician orders (including standardized pick lists, formulary choices, and lab choices as necessary)

6. Determine performance measures (process and outcome) with approval and implementation through health information management and finance departments

7. Implement care guide (packets):
   — Get any new forms approved for pilot use by forms committee
   — Work through nursing services for any new on-line documentation requirements

8. Collect data and monitor system

9. Trend and analyze data each quarter

10. Improve processes where necessary

THE PATIENT RECORD–CARE GUIDE INTERFACE

Every organization implementing clinical paths must determine whether the path will be used in place of traditional patient record documentation. If the answer is yes, clinicians must determine which record elements the path documentation will replace. Because the use of care guides at Hinsdale Hospital is considered optional, the guide could not be used to uniformly replace documentation found in all patient records. However, there was a strong desire to minimize duplicative record and care guide documentation.

To operationalize the care guide and assure appropriate documentation, two changes were made in the way nurses and physicians document. Since 1994 the nursing staff at Hinsdale Hospital has used Clinicom™, an automated point-of-care documentation system. To bridge the care guides with this automated system, traditional nursing care goals were replaced with the OCGs on the care guides. To illustrate this relationship, the Clinicom™ system "active care plan" screen for cardiac catheterization or percutaneous transluminal coronary angioplasty (PTCA) patients is shown in figure 11-4. Each OCG from the care guide (see figure 11-2) is listed on the active care plan used by the nursing staff. In some instances, such as in this illustration, slight modifications in the care guide OCGs may be necessary when individualizing the care plan for a particular patient's needs. Each active care plan is designed around the needs of the patient but is based on the predetermined standardized protocol of care

FIGURE 11-2 Standard Care Guide Format for Cardiac Catheterization or Percutaneous Transluminal Coronary Angioplasty

Diagnosis/Procedure: Cardiac Cath / PTCA	Physician:	Case Manager:
OUTCOME GOALS	**PRE-PROCEDURE**	**POST-PROCEDURE**
Minimize post procedure discomfort		
Patient/family able to verbalize understanding of teaching plan		
Vital signs and rhythm are stable		
Absence of complications related to access site		
Interventions will be performed in a timely manner		
Patient Location (circle one)		· 3 S · CCU · Cath Lab Recovery · Intermediate Care · No EKG monitor an option
Consults	· Notify primary MD. · Notify Case Manager.	· Cardiac Rehab (for PTCA) · Nutrition Assessment/Dietary (for PTCA)
Diagnostics: Lab	As indicated by MD on standing orders.	CKMB, Hgb, Hct 8 hours after procedure (for PTCA)
Radiology	CXR (if indicated)	
Other	EKG (if ordered)	EKG STAT for chest pain and after procedure as ordered by physician.
Treatments	Have consent signed & witnessed.	· For hypotension (as indicated), open IV to run @ 100 cc/hr. Place in trendelburg. · Foley if unable to void (unless documented valve disease) · Sheath removed as per order
Assessments	· Notify cardiologist of abnormal tests or chest discomfort. · Vital signs per unit protocol and PRN	· Vital signs and assessment per unit policy. · Notify cardiologist as indicated. · Strict I/O · If bleeding, apply pressure for 30 minutes; notify physician. open IV to 100cc/hr. & monitor vital signs every 15 minutes.

OUTCOME GOALS		PRE-PROCEDURE	POST-PROCEDURE
Medications	IV's	• Continue all infusions unless otherwise ordered by physician.	IV 0.9% NS as ordred.
	Other	• Administer all meds scheduled during procedure unless otherwise ordered by physician.	Heparin drip as ordered.
		• ASA, CA channel blocker (if indicated)	Ca channel blocker, ASA (if indicated).
		• Benadryl & Valium pre-procedure.	PRN's: Restoril, Vicodin, Tylenol, Compazine, Ativan
		• PRN's Restoril, Ativan, Tylenol.	O2 2-4 L per NC prn.
		• O2 2-4 L per NC prn.	
Nutrition/Diet		NPO(except meds) or Clear liquid breakfast, then NPO	Push clear liquids; advance to low fat, low cholesterol 4 hours after PTCA. Advance diet as soon as tolerated for cath.
ADL	Activity	Activity as tolerated or previously ordered prior to procedure.	Bedrest. HOB only elevated 15-30 degrees & PTCA leg straight until 6 hours after sheath is removed. May use soft restraints/knee immobilizer to keep leg straight. Patient may be log rolled but not to side of sheath insertion.
			Ambulate (first time w/assistance) if no bleeding and v.s. are stable 6 hours after sheath is removed.
Teaching		Review items #1-6 on Teaching Plan for PTCA.	Complete teaching plan for PTCA. Notify pharmacy for teaching as needed.
Discharge Planning/Coordination		Old chart to Cath Lab with patient.	Cardiac rehab to asses need for Phase II.

Adherence to the careguide is voluntary. Except where a statement herein explicitly indicates otherwise, these parameters should not be considered inclusive of all proper methods of care of exclusive of other methods of care reasonably directed to obtaining the same results. The ultimate judgement regarding the propriety of any specific procedure must be made by the physician in light of the individual circumstances presented by the patient

Source: Hinsdale Hospital.

203

FIGURE 11-3 Standardized Care Guide Variance Reporting Form for Cardiac Catheterization or Percutaneous Transluminal Coronary Angioplasty

HINSDALE HOSPITAL CARE GUIDE CQI/VARIANCE REPORT FOR CATH/PTCA

Please return to Case Manager

A. Please indicate on each shift whether variance occurred. If yes, complete section B.

DAY 1 DATE ___	DAY 2 DATE ___	DAY 3 DATE ___	DAY 4 DATE ___	DAY 5 DATE ___	DAY 6 DATE ___	DAY 7 DATE ___
Yes No Initials	Yes No Initials	Yes No Initials	Yes No Initials	Yes No Initials	Yes No Initials	Yes No Initials
N ☐ ☐	N ☐ ☐	N ☐ ☐	N ☐ ☐	N ☐ ☐	N ☐ ☐	N ☐ ☐
D ☐ ☐	D ☐ ☐	D ☐ ☐	D ☐ ☐	D ☐ ☐	D ☐ ☐	D ☐ ☐
E ☐ ☐	E ☐ ☐	E ☐ ☐	E ☐ ☐	E ☐ ☐	E ☐ ☐	E ☐ ☐

B.

Date	Variance Code	Variance Description	Action Taken to Resolve Variance	Affected Outcome
				☐ Y ☐ N ☐ NA
				☐ Y ☐ N ☐ NA
				☐ Y ☐ N ☐ NA
				☐ Y ☐ N ☐ NA
				☐ Y ☐ N ☐ NA
				☐ Y ☐ N ☐ NA
				☐ Y ☐ N ☐ NA
				☐ Y ☐ N ☐ NA
				☐ Y ☐ N ☐ NA
				☐ Y ☐ N ☐ NA
				☐ Y ☐ N ☐ NA
				☐ Y ☐ N ☐ NA

C.

Please address the following variances.	
1. Did the patient have a bleed/hematoma post CATH/PTCA?	☐ Y ☐ N
2. Was the time from arrival to balloon inflation < 90° for PTCA?	☐ Y ☐ N
3. Was the sheath pulled w/i 4 hours post PTCA?	☐ Y ☐ N
4. Was the teaching plan completed?	☐ Y ☐ N
5. Was the teaching plan completed and signed?	☐ Y ☐ N

Variance Code Key

Patient/Fam	Careprovider	System	Community
A1. Condition	B5. Doctor order	C9. Bed/appt	D13. Place HC
A2. Decision	B6. Decision	C10. Info delay	D14. Trans del
A3. Availability	B7. Response time	C11. Suppl/equip	D15.
A4.	B8.	C12.	E16.

Source: Hinsdale Hospital

FIGURE 11-4 Screen Display of Active Care Plan

```
                    HINSDALE HOSPITAL              07/18/96 11:32
                                                        Page: 1
                      ACTIVE CARE PLAN
                From 07/17/96 11:31  To 07/18/96 11:31
                ---------------------------------------

     - Name: PRACTICE, MIA L.     MD: AGOSTINO,GUY J
       Sex: F Age: 43Y Adm: 12/01/95 09:37 Patient Id: 1234567 Med Rec No: 1234567

  Date           Freq  NURSING DIAGNOSIS
  07/18(DSD)     7114.CG: PTCA
                      Goals:
  07/18(DSD)  BY DISCH   -  OCG: Absence or minimalization of pain
  07/18(DSD)  BY DISCH   -  OCG: Hemodynamic stability and Dysrhythmia stability
  07/18(DSD)  BY DISCH   -  OCG: Affected extremity will maintain good perfusion
  07/18(DSD)  BY DISCH   -  OCG: Pt verbalizes understanding of procedure and possible
                                 complications
  Care Providers:
  Davis,Deborah Sue (DSD) RN
```

Source: Hinsdale Hospital.

within the care guide. It is anticipated that greater consistency will be gained over time as the use of care guides becomes more prevalent.

A patient's progress toward achieving his or her goals and any necessary modifications of the plan of care are noted in the automated nursing documentation system. (See figure 11-5.) When a specific goal is reached, that part of the care guide is discontinued and the patient progresses to the next set of goals or problems. At the present time, support services staff (for example, respiratory therapy, dietary, and social workers) do not use the automated point-of-care documentation system. These caregivers must refer to a paper copy of the care guide in the front of the hospital chart binder. When all caregivers begin using the automated point-of-care documentation system, the paper copy of the care guide will no longer be necessary. The active care plan (on line) can also be documented on a manual (paper) form for multidisciplinary input.

The second step in implementing the care guide was to develop sets of standardized preprinted physician orders. (See figure 11-6.) For cardiac catheterization or PTCA patients, preprocedure and postprocedure order sets were created to correspond to the two phases of care illustrated on the care guide. Currently, the preprinted orders are kept on the nursing units and initiated when necessary. Physicians may modify orders by crossing them out and initialling the changes or by adding an addendum. Hinsdale Hospital plans to create standing order templates in the automated order entry system.

Physicians have found the preprinted standing orders an ideal method for handling their care guide responsibilities. The benefits of preprinted orders for physicians include:

- Saves time—it is no longer necessary to write out the orders
- Eliminates unnecessary practice variation
- Reduces excess documentation in patient records
- Creates a more legible record

Clinicians view the care guide as the "cookbook," the active care plan as the "recipe," and the physician orders as the "ingredients." This simplified perspective has increased caregiver buy-in and helped everyone appreciate the value of the care guide tool.

FIGURE 11-5 Screen Display of Admission, Discharge, or Transfer Care Plan

```
                    HINSDALE HOSPITAL                    07/18/96 11:36
                        ADT/CARE PLAN                         Page: 1
              From 07/17/96 11:35   To 07/18/96 11:35
              -----------------------------------------

       - Name: PRACTICE, MIA L.    MD: AGOSTINO,GUY J
       Sex: F Age: 43Y Adm: 12/01/95 09:37 Patient Id: 1234567 Med Rec No: 1234567

ADDITIONAL CHARTING
         NO DATA FOR THIS SECTION

ADMISSION/DISCHARGE/TRANSFER
         NO DATA FOR THIS SECTION

CHART AGAINST CARE PLAN
Dx #7114. CG: PTCA
   Diagnosis Evaluation
   Reviewed by Davis,Deborah Sue on 07/18/96 at 11:22. Diagnosis remains appropriate for
   patient. No Changes made.
07/18/96
11:32   OCG: Hemodynamic stability and Dysrhythmia stability
           Not achieved, will continue current plan. (DSD)
        OCG: Absence or minimalization of pain
           Not achieved, Target Date extended. (DSD)
        OCG: Affected extremity will maintain good perfusion
           Not achieved, Interventions revised. (DSD)
        OCG: Pt verbalizes understanding of procedure and possible complications
           . (DSD)
Care Providers:
Davis,Deborah Sue (DSD) RN
```

Source: Hinsdale Hospital.

THE INFORMATION MANAGEMENT COMPONENT

A variety of information management functions are necessary to support a successful clinical path initiative. While the care guides are beneficial in improving the process of patient care, it is also important to provide clinicians with feedback about the effectiveness of the tool and its impact on patient outcomes. Health information management professionals play an important role in this phase of clinical path implementation. They can provide specialized assistance in four key areas: selection of data elements, collection, reporting, and analysis. The information management staff and caregivers at Hinsdale Hospital dealt with these issues using a variety of technological support tools. Most important, they were able to accommodate the information management requirements of the care guides using their existing computerized data system. Hinsdale's experiences in care guide measurement data selection, collection, reporting, and analysis are detailed in this section.

Selection of Data Elements

Identification of the data elements necessary to evaluate the effectiveness of the care guides was an essential first step. The care guide teams relied heavily on health information management staff to acquaint them with the data already being collected in the facility and to retrieve information from existing databases. The care guide teams selected measures they believed important to report to hospital committees involved in performance improvement. For example, the PTCA care guide team chose to measure the time between the PTCA procedure and the removal of the sheath. They believed the timeliness of sheath removal is an important predictor of length of stay and

FIGURE 11-6 Preprinted Physician Orders for Cardiac Catheterization or Percutaneous Transluminal Coronary Angioplasty Patients (Excerpt)

Date	Time		NOTED BY NURSE/HR
\multicolumn{3}{l	}{**CARDIAC CATH/PTCA CAREGUIDE PRE-PROCEDURE PHASE INTERVENTIONS/ PHYSICIAN SUGGESTED ORDERS** (Page 1 of 2)}	
\multicolumn{3}{l	}{Unless otherwise indicated, all orders will be implemented. Complete spaces as appropriate.}	

1. **SCHEDULING:**
   a. Schedule case for cardiac cath/PTCA with Cardiac Cath Lab.
   b. Notify primary care physician.
   c. Notify case manager.

2. **DIAGNOSTICS-LAB/RADIOLOGY:** Please indicate Yes or No

	Yes	No		Yes	No
CBC	__	__	Protime	__	__
Chem 7	__	__	PTT	__	__
HCG	__	__	Fibrinogen	__	__
Chest X-ray	__	__	EKG	__	__ (on admit)

   Type Screen ___ ___ (if scheduled as definite PTCA, do prior to going to cath lab - all others to be done in cath lab at time of PTCA)

   Other _____

   (Lab tests should be done no greater than 5 days before. CXR should be within one month. Obtain test results and have copy on chart.)

3. **TREATMENTS:** Have consent signed by patient and witnessed by RN for:
   ____ cardiac catheterization
   ____ percutaneous transluminal angioplasty and possible additional therapies as indicated
      (i.e. intra-aortic balloon pump, stent placement)
   ____ coronary artery bypass surgery
   ____ receiving blood/blood products
   or _____
   Physician performing procedure _____

4. **ASSESSMENTS:**
   a. Notify cardiologist on call for any abnormal tests or chest discomfort occurring within the last 24 hrs.
   b. V.S. per unit protocol and prn.

5. **MEDICATIONS:**
   a. Prior to procedure, administer <u>all</u> medications scheduled during procedure and continue all IV infusions <u>unless</u> instructed otherwise by physician.
   b. Diuretic/K+ supplement: _____ hold _____ give as scheduled
   c. Aspirin (non-enteric coated) dose _____ frequency _____
   d. Ca channel blocker: _____

(Continued on page 2)

ADDRESSOGRAPH

Physician Signature _____

Hinsdale Hospital
PHYSICIAN'S ORDERS

WHITE   - CHART
YELLOW - PHARMACY
PINK   - NURSE
GOLDENROD - IV PHARMACY

SP 2215 1/96, pg. 1 of 2

Source: Hinsdale Hospital.

catheterization success. By reviewing sheath removal times and other PTCA-specific measures, the medical staff identified practice patterns that achieve desirable outcomes.

An inventory of performance measures used for each care guide is maintained by the health information management department. This inventory includes the data definitions for the measures, the population to whom the measures are applied, and the start dates for data collection. An excerpt from the care guide data inventory is illustrated in figure 11-7.

Data Collection

One phenomenon that seems to occur with the implementation of clinical paths is the proliferation of manual data collection tools. At Hinsdale Hospital it quickly became apparent that manual data collection would become increasingly burdensome as the number of care guides increased. Several options for maximizing data collection activities were discussed, such as hiring an additional person to collect and aggregate the data or purchasing an automated clinical path and outcomes management software program. However, expending the resources necessary to support these choices could not be justified. A team of representatives from the finance, health information management, and nursing departments evaluated less costly choices and arrived at a solution that involved Hinsdale's existing computerized information system. The hospital's order entry system, which was already being used by nursing staff to enter charge information, was reconfigured to capture care guide variance and performance measurement data.

The care guide measures were incorporated into the order entry system's charge master table and associated with a "zero dollar" amount. This functionality was already being used for nonbillable services, such as counseling. In the HBOC Trend-Star™ system used at Hinsdale Hospital, this order entry application is termed a "statistical" charge. By including noncharged items in the system and entering "quantity" data, information about the frequency of an activity can be gathered, although no billing charges are generated.

Clinical path performance measures were input into tables in the order entry system as zero-dollar, statistical charges. A cost center was established for case management, and all care guide measures were linked to this charge master category. Because the measures have a zero-dollar amount, they do not appear on the patient's bill.

Data for each care guide performance measure had to be coded for entry into the computerized system. It was important to document the coding scheme used to ensure that accurate comparative rates could be calculated later. Some of the care guide indicators are time based (for example, time to first respiratory treatment), some are continuous measurement data (for example, the patient's level of postprocedural pain compared with 48 hours postdischarge), and others refer to outlier situations (for example, patient refused smoking clinic consultation). To accommodate these various types of performance measures, rules had to be established for entering coded data. Examples of these rules and the coding scheme include the following:

- For the measure "time from PTCA to sheath removal," the datum entered in the charge quantity field for each patient is "number of hours."

- For the measure related to the patient's level of pain, a sliding scale (1–4) was established. The patient's immediate postoperative pain score is recorded in one charge quantity field, and the score reported during conversations with the patient at the postdischarge follow-up contact is recorded in another charge quantity field.

- When an outlier exists, such as a patient refusal, the value 1 is recorded in the charge quantity field. If no outlier exists, the quantity field is left blank.

FIGURE 11-7 Care Guide Data Inventory (Excerpt)

CARE GUIDE DIRECTORY
APRIL 28, 1997

CARE GUIDE	CASE MANAGER	ABBRV.	C.G. CHARGE CODE	CLINICAL POPULATION	STATISTICAL CHARGES	CHARGE CODE	CLINICAL INDICATORS	CHARGE CODE	PCC
CEREBROVASCULAR ACCIDENT	N. BEVAN	CVA	6010-9094	ICD INPT CODES - 43600, 43311, 43321, 43331	NEURO DEFICIT AT DC>ADM	6010-0172	DVT ALL COMPLICATIONS DVT	ICD P OR S 99700, 45100-45390 ICD P OR S 99600-99990 ICD P OR S 99720, 45100-45390	NEURO
				43000, 43100, 43200, 43290 43381, 43391, 43401, 43491 DRG's 424-432-INPT				ICD P OR S 99750, 99664, 99665, 59000-59090, 59500-59590, 59700-59789, 59389, 60130, 5990 ICD P OR S 70700	
DEPRESSION	J. HUBACEK	DEP	N/A						MEDICAL
DIABETES KETOACIDOSIS	?J. CHILSON	DKA	6010-9014	ICD 25010-25013	KETONES IN URINE AT DC SMBG > 150 AT DC	6010-0191 6010-0192	UTI DECUB ULCER		MEDICAL
DEEP VEIN THROMBOSIS	J. CHILSON	DVT	6010-9010	ICD INPT: 99720, 45100-45390 ICD 9929-OTPT			WARFARIN BEGUN <48 HOURS DAYS OF HEPARIN	7070-2002-2007 7070-3065	SURGICAL
HIP FRACTURE	N. BEVAN	HFX	6010-9002	ICD INPT: 82000-82090 82100, 82110, 73314, 73315 ICD INPT: 7935	HRS ADMIT TO OR	6010-0211	ALL COMPLICATIONS UNITS OF PACKED CELLS DVT WOUND INFECTION	ICD P OR S 99600-99990 7025-4503 ICD P OR S 99720, 45100-45390 ICD P OR S 99851, 99859	
OUTPATIENT INOTROPE	D. DAVIS	INO	6010-9015	ICD 9929-INPT ICD 42540, 42800-INPT ICD 9929-OTPT ICD 42540, 42800-OTPT	INPT ADMIT PAST 30 DAYS	6010-0231	UTI	ICD P OR S 99750, 99664, 99665, 59900, 59000-59090, 59500-59590, 59700-59789, 59389, 60130	NON-INTERVENTIONAL CARDIOLOGY
LUMBAR LAMINECTOMY	N. BEVAN	LAM	6010-9004	ICD 309, 8051-INPT	NEURO DEFICIT DC>ADM	6010-0172	ALL COMPLICATIONS WOUND INFECTION DVT	ICD P OR S 99600-99990 ICD P OR S 99851, 99589 ICD P OR S 99700, 45100-45390	SURGICAL
LAPROSCOPIC CHOLECYSTECTOMY	T. CARLSON	LCH	6010-9007	ICD 5123-INPT ICD 5123-OTPT	LAP CHOLE CONVERT TO OPEN H-LAP CHOLE CONVERT TO OPEN	6010-0411 7181-5001			SURGICAL
MYRINGOTOMY	T. CARLSON	MYR	6010-9008	ICD 2001, 2009-INPT ICD 2001, 2009-OTPT	OPS-NAUS/ VOMIT POST OP OPS- PAIN >3 POST OP OPS- NAUS/VOMIT HOME OPS- PAIN >3 HOME	6010-0251 6010-0252 6010-0253 6010-0254			
NORMAL NEWBORN	?M. GRETEMAN	NWB							
OVERDOSE/ INTOXICATION	C. SELLERGREN	OVD	6010-9030	ICD 96000-98999-INPT	HRS. TO PSYCH EVAL ALGORHTYHM NOT FOLLOWED NO P&C ON CHART	6010-0273 6010-0271 6010-0272			ICU
PANCREATITIS	?J. CHILSON	PAN	6010-9013	ICD 57700, 57710-INPT	PAIN SCORE >3 >24 HRS ENZYMES > INITIAL AT DC	6010-0451 6010-0452			
PEDIATRIC ASTHMA	?M. GRETEMAN	PAS	6010-9028	ICD 49300-49391-INPT AGES 0-17 ICD 49300-49391-OTPT AGES 0-17-OTPT HH PTTYPE:ER	PEAK FLOW >80 AT DC ADM ASTHMA SCORE DC ASTHMA SCORE	6010-0071 6010-0072 6010-0073			PEDIATRIC

Source: Hinsdale Hospital.

FIGURE 11-8 Average Length of Stay Comparison for Percutaneous Transluminal Coronary Angioplasty Patients, 1995

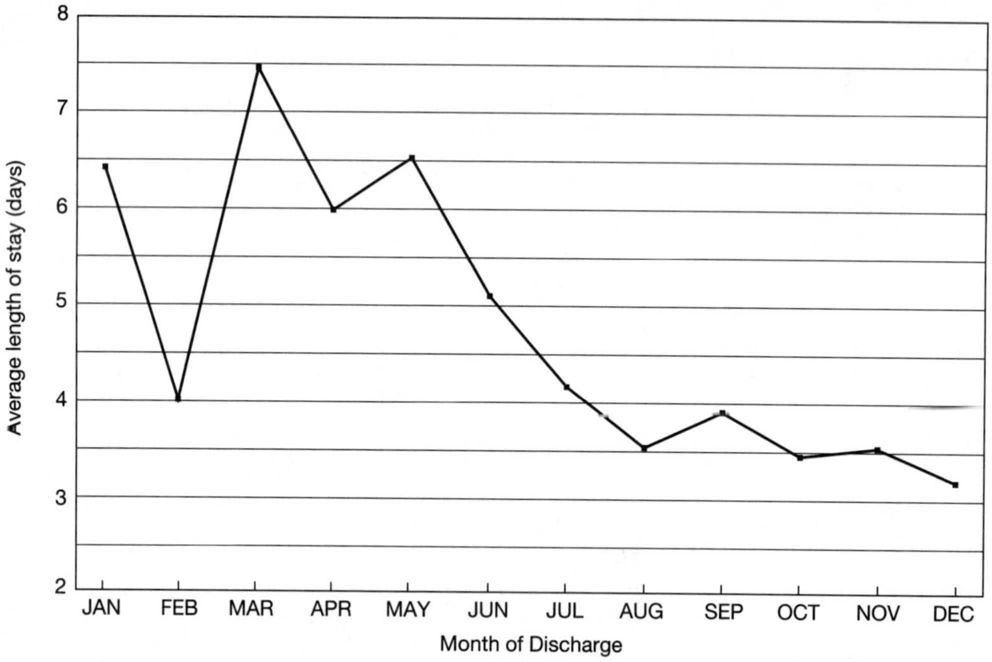

Source: TrendStar™.

Case managers are primarily responsible for concurrently entering care guide performance measurement data as part of their care coordination role. Total amount of entry time averages 1 minute per case per day. In those instances where a case manager is not directly involved in a patient's care, the nursing staff documents information on the variance report form for later data entry by coding staff in the health information management department. Eventually, this two-step data collection process will be eliminated as more bedside caregivers assume the responsibility of on-line documentation.

In those hospitals where path variance data are recorded on paper forms, an order entry information system solution could also be used. The variance data could be recorded by bedside caregivers and then later entered "batch" style by staff in data processing or the health information management department. The disadvantage to this approach would be the need to establish some controls to ensure that all paper forms reach the data input staff.

Data Reporting and Analysis

Reporting aggregate information is simplified because care guide variance and performance measurement data are readily available in a computerized information system. Using the report writer and decision support system already built into the clinical and financial information system, the data elements relevant to care guide variance can be extracted and stratified by any number of categories, including:

- Variances for a defined time period
- Variances for specific practitioners
- Variances sorted by patient characteristics such as age or sex
- Variances sorted by patients' principal diagnosis or comorbidities

FIGURE 11-9 Average Charge Comparison for Percutaneous Transluminal Coronary Angioplasty Patients, 1995-96

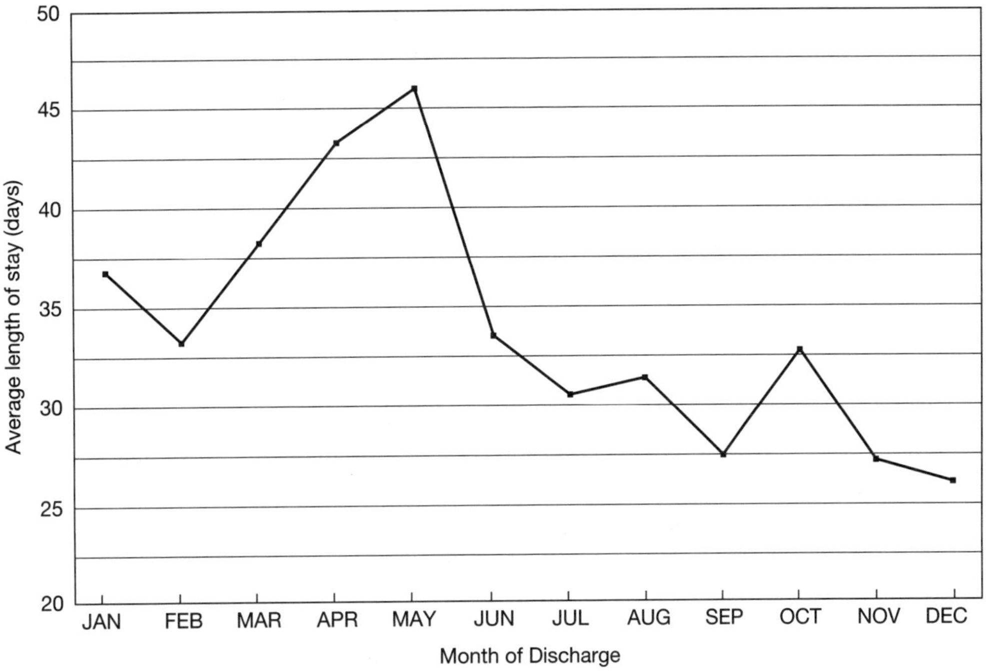

Source: TrendStar™.

The care guide data for each patient can be easily matched to any of the data elements contained in the clinical and financial information database.

With input from case managers and other providers, standard care guide performance measurement reports are produced each quarter. To answer unexpected questions that may come up, ad hoc queries are run. Using a spreadsheet, case managers can sort, manipulate, report, and analyze all data elements within the system. A special benefit is the hospital's link to comparative data. Hinsdale utilizes the 3M All Patient Refined-Diagnosis-Related Groups risk adjustment system to assign severity level codes to each patient, and the HBOC TrendStar™ decision support system allows caregivers to establish a benchmark for their mortality rates.

The health information management department is responsible for extracting the care guide data from the clinical and financial information system. The data files are then provided in paper format or transferred in ASCII format via E-mail to the case management department, where further analysis takes place. The staff in each area is able to create a variety of graphical reports to help providers analyze the effectiveness of the care guide tool and measure its impact on outcomes. Shown in figures 11-8 and 11-9 are general reports showing pre–care guide and post–care guide length of stay and cost data for PTCA patients. More detailed PTCA variance data allow analysis at the patient level. (See figure 11-10.) Although the examples of data displays included in this chapter are quite basic, advanced analyses can be performed using statistical process control charts, cross-tabs, and various data sorts.

FIGURE 11-10 Care Guide Data Report for Percutaneous Transluminal Coronary Angioplasty, June 1996 (Excerpt)

Account No.	Patient Name	Age	Severity Level	Discharge Date	Length of Stay (days)	Nursing Unit at Discharge	Sheath Duration	Vessel Closure (sentinel event)	Unable to Open Vessel (sentinel event)
9626600414	P. Jones	72	0	06/19/96	5	ICC	3 hrs	1	0
9616500173	S. Smith	81	1	06/20/96	7	3S	9 hrs	0	1
9617000691	F. Brown	41	0	06/21/96	3	3S	12 hrs	0	0
9617100163	C. Young	61	0	06/23/96	1	CCU	0 hrs	0	0
9617800187	M. List	65	0	06/27/96	1	ICC	5 hrs	0	0

Note: Fictitious data for demonstration purposes only.

CONCLUSION

The success of any clinical path initiative must be measured by the opportunities realized to improve patient care efficiency and effectiveness. However, burdensome path-related data collection can quickly deflate caregivers' enthusiasm. To minimize the challenges of data collection, only gather information about critical elements of care that clinicians believe impact patient outcomes. Another hint is to use data that already exist in a database—such as *International Classification of Diseases* diagnosis or procedure codes, or medications—to track resource use or complications. Before purchasing a PC-based clinical path information system, be sure to check out the capabilities of your existing automated information systems. Your internal systems may not have the "bells and whistles" of a computerized product dedicated to pathway data collection, but the trade-offs may make it worth pursuing. It is important for clinicians to work with health information management professionals in designing efficient clinical path data management systems. These professionals have a deep understanding of their organization's information systems and are a valuable resource for clinical path teams.

Some organizations have the luxury of on-line clinical decision support systems, with paths and other reminder tools built into the system and integrated with their financial systems. When caregivers document patient care activities in these organizations, path variance and other performance measurement data are automatically captured. Other organizations have purchased dedicated PC-based clinical path software packages to be used by case managers or other staff for recording path variance data. However, these systems may not be linked to financial or clinical databases, and interfaces must be built.

Caregivers at Hinsdale Hospital wanted to be fiscally responsible in designing a clinical path information management system. By using their existing computerized clinical and financial information system, they were able build a comprehensive care guide database without spending additional resources. Hinsdale Hospital was able to create a miniclinical and financial data repository without the need for duplicate data entry or additional software. Further, the order entry system was already being used by caregivers, so very little additional training was necessary. It is hoped that by learning about the Hinsdale Hospital experience, other organizations will realize that they, too, may be able to provide low-cost computerized support for their clinical path initiatives.

CHAPTER 12

Automating Clinical Pathway Variance Analysis

Beth Weber, Linda Ratzlaff, Tom Hearn, and Joan McCanless

Bristol Regional Medical Center, a 377-bed, not-for-profit tertiary facility in Bristol, TN, is an exciting example of what can be accomplished with automated clinical path variance analysis. Serving an eight-county area in Tennessee and Virginia, Bristol is committed to improving patient outcomes. Frequent analysis of data, coupled with open and honest communication among path team members, has enabled Bristol to achieve significant, quantifiable improvements in clinical outcomes while reducing costs, improving teamwork, and increasing patient satisfaction. One critical factor in this success is Bristol's automation of path variance data. Computerization of patient outcomes and path variances has enabled case managers and clinical pathway teams to accelerate the evaluation of clinical pathways and the implementation of improvements.

Led by its director of case management, Bristol's clinical pathway effort began in 1993 as an integral component of its case management model. To date the medical center has 14 clinical pathways in place, including paths for:

- Congestive heart failure (CHF)
- Myocardial infarction (MI)
- Pneumonia
- 23-Hour chest pain
- Cerebrovascular accident (CVA)
- Total hip replacement
- Coronary artery bypass graft (CABG)
- Upper gastrointestinal bleed
- Small bowel resection
- Chronic obstructive pulmonary disease (COPD)
- Percutaneous transluminal coronary angioplasty (PTCA)
- Total abdominal hysterectomy

- Anterior and posterior laminectomy
- Spinal fusion

This chapter describes the role of computerization in support of Bristol's case management and clinical path initiatives. Decision Support Systems' PathPlan 2000 product played an important role in helping Bristol Regional Medical Center physicians and staff achieve their quality improvement and cost reduction goals.

A NEW FRAMEWORK FOR IMPROVED PATIENT OUTCOMES AND REDUCED COSTS

In the early 1990s Bristol initiated many strategies in response to cost containment pressures and rapid changes in the health care environment. The most significant of those strategies involved a collaborative effort between physicians and administration. Physicians in the Bristol area had begun to feel the effects of tougher contract negotiations with payers, and most recognized the need to focus on resource utilization and collaboratively planned patient care. The medical center, its physicians, and its medical director created a program that provided physicians with profiles of their resource utilization as compared with their peers. By studying physician practice variation in a confidential and anonymous environment, physicians and administrative leaders positioned the medical center to focus on reduced resource utilization and improved patient outcomes. One of the many new initiatives that came out of these discussions was a case management strategy that included the development of multidisciplinary clinical pathways.

Case Management

Bristol defines *case management* as the "collaborative coordination of care for patients across the continuum of care, from admission to discharge, and often prior to admission and beyond discharge." Case managers ensure a smooth transition for patients upon discharge and play an especially important role in the care of high-risk patients who have a multitude of care requirements following discharge from acute care. Bristol's case managers are responsible for the following activities:

- Concurrent and retrospective utilization review
- Quality assurance and quality improvement data collection
- Clinical pathway design, implementation, and analysis
- Social work services
- Resource utilization studies and physician practice pattern analyses via clinical paths
- Discharge planning

Integrating these responsibilities into the case management department has allowed the medical center to increase efficiency by streamlining many patient care processes. Prior to the implementation of this integrated case management model, the six activities were somewhat fragmented, resulting in less-than-optimal communication among disciplines. Today each case manager is responsible for functions that were previously managed by three different disciplines representing three different departments (utilization review, discharge planning, and social work). Case managers evaluate each admission to determine whether the patient's condition meets acute care admission criteria. By identifying the special discharge needs of patients at the

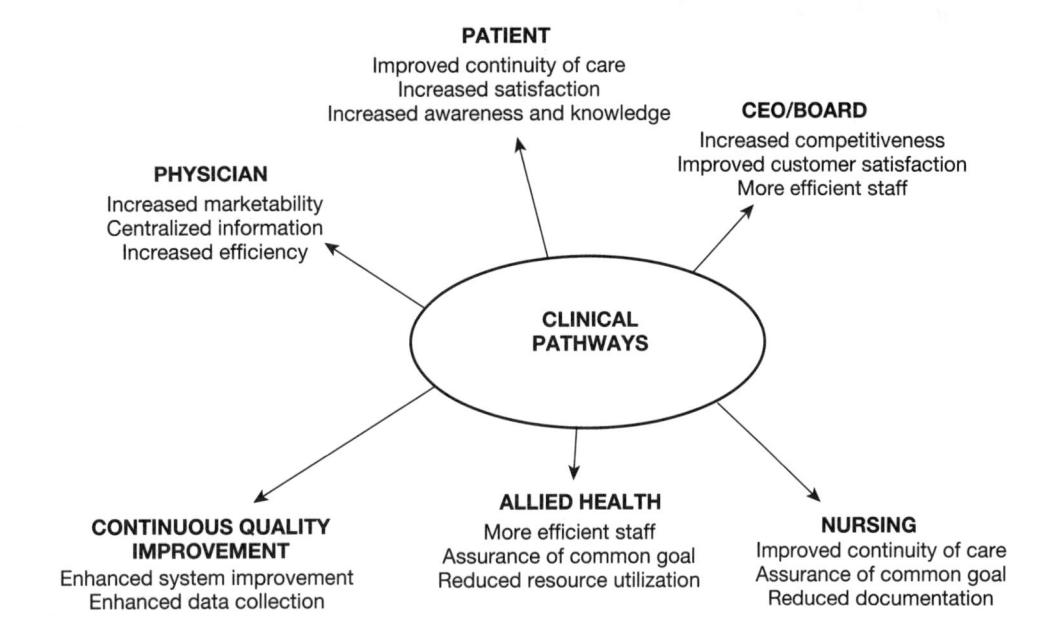

FIGURE 12-1 Stakeholders in the Clinical Path Process

PATIENT
Improved continuity of care
Increased satisfaction
Increased awareness and knowledge

CEO/BOARD
Increased competitiveness
Improved customer satisfaction
More efficient staff

PHYSICIAN
Increased marketability
Centralized information
Increased efficiency

CLINICAL PATHWAYS

CONTINUOUS QUALITY IMPROVEMENT
Enhanced system improvement
Enhanced data collection

ALLIED HEALTH
More efficient staff
Assurance of common goal
Reduced resource utilization

NURSING
Improved continuity of care
Assurance of common goal
Reduced documentation

---

time of their admission, case managers can intervene where necessary to help avoid or reduce discharge delays.

Bristol's case managers possess strong clinical backgrounds and are self-directed professionals. They are centrally located on each nursing unit and are positioned to intervene quickly and effectively with multidisciplinary team members to improve patient outcomes. In general, their caseloads average 26 to 30 patients at any one time. The director of case management provides leadership and guidance for the case manager team.

In addition to tracking patients' progress along their clinical paths, a typical day for the case manager includes:

- Patient referrals to long-term care facilities and home health agencies
- Verbal and written correspondence with insurance companies
- Concurrent utilization review
- Meetings with patients and families to assist with postdischarge needs
- Multidisciplinary team meetings

This consolidation of functions has greatly reduced operating costs and helped ensure high-quality, efficient patient care.

Clinical Pathways

After completing the restructuring necessary to support the integrated case management model, Bristol began its clinical pathway initiative. Bristol defines a *clinical pathway* as "a coordinated plan of care for an individual procedure or diagnosis that promotes collaboration among all caregivers." The path specifies which caregiver is accountable, the time frame for completion, and the expected patient outcomes to be achieved. Bristol has recognized several stakeholders in the clinical path process, all benefiting in many ways from improvements generated by the clinical path. (See figure 12-1.)

FIGURE 12-2 Clinical Path Variance Report

PATHWAY: _____						
Date	Path Day	Category	Procedure	Variance Code	Comment/Action	Initials

Initials   Signature   Initials   Signature   Initials   Signature

Variance Source Codes (Select All Applicable Codes):

1. Patient condition
2. Patient/family decision
3. Patient/family availability
4. Patient/family cognition
5. Physician's order
6. Caregiver decision
7. Caregiver action
8. Information/data availability
9. Supplies/equipment availability
10. Department overbooked/closed
11. Bed availability
12. Placement/home care delay
13. Transportation delay
14. Other

RETURN TO CASE MANAGEMENT WHEN PATIENT IS DISCHARGED

THIS IS NOT A PERMANENT PART OF THE MEDICAL RECORD

In 1994 a clinical pathway steering committee was created to oversee the medical center's clinical quality improvement efforts, including the development, implementation, and analysis of clinical pathways. This committee was composed of representatives from the administration, medical staff, quality management, and various clinical departments. After making a careful analysis of length-of-stay and cost data, the steering committee selected five initial patient populations on which to pilot clinical paths: MI, CHF, pneumonia, CVA, and total joint replacement. Multidisciplinary teams, co-chaired by a case manager and a physician, were formed to evaluate the care provided to each of these patient populations.

The most difficult task for these teams was not the pathway design process, which proceeded very quickly. What the teams found most frustrating was data management after pathway implementation. During the pathway pilot phases, case managers were responsible for gathering information about path variances using the variance reporting form. (See figure 12-2.) The case management department had promised the path teams that they would periodically receive data about the effectiveness of the pilot pathways. However, the information management component of pathways overwhelmed the case managers.

The case management department lacked the resources necessary to analyze all the variance data adequately, and it could not provide detailed feedback to the pathway teams. Broad measures of success indicated that the paths were effective in achieving overall reductions in length of stay and cost. However, without more sophisticated information management capabilities, the case management department could not pinpoint improvement opportunities or effectively illustrate the impact of paths on clinical outcomes. Without an automated variance analysis system, investigating variances became even more labor intensive than developing the paths.

AUTOMATION OF CLINICAL PATHWAY ANALYSIS

About the time that Bristol was struggling with evaluating its paths' effectiveness, it was approached by Decision Support Systems of Charlotte, NC, to serve as a site for beta testing (being tested for the first time in a live environment) of Decision Support's automated clinical path information system, PathPlan 2000. Opportunity knocked at a perfect time! Bristol realized that computerization of path variance and patient outcome data would reduce paperwork and allow for more detailed analysis of pathway effectiveness.

PathPlan 2000 is a Windows™-based software application that allows users to manage clinical paths and associated information effectively. The system provides more than 40 standard reports designed to help answer common questions from physicians, nurses, case managers, quality improvement staff, and management. Many types of graphical analysis can be created, including control charts to help identify special- and common-cause variation.

One benefit of this clinical information system, which streamlined Bristol's pathway process, was its ability to support clinical path development and revision activities. Rather than designing paths only on paper and then redesigning the entire document every time a revision is necessary, the PathPlan 2000 system stores all versions of all paths in a database. When new paths are created the computerized path template can be entered quickly. (See figure 12-3.) Updates of already implemented paths can also be performed very quickly.

Integrating the computerized variance tracking portion of PathPlan 2000 into Bristol's existing data collection process required some decisions about how to input data into the system. It was determined that the case management department would be responsible for data entry, with one clerical employee entering information from the variance reports completed by case managers. Someday the case managers may concurrently input variance data using laptop computers or workstations located at each nursing unit.

Variance data are entered into the clinical information system by viewing the path and highlighting the interventions or outcomes that were identified as variances. The system automatically prompts users for the variance codes (for example, patient condition or caregiver decision), which are selected from a user-defined table. Additional information, such as the action taken or patient response to the action, can also be captured. Any and all variances are reported because automation of analysis does not require clinicians to limit data entry. (See figure 12-4.)

Not long after PathPlan 2000 was installed, detailed clinical pathway analysis reports were available. Computerization of the data elements eliminated many of the frustrations caused by manual data collection. Data could be sorted easily according

FIGURE 12-3 Variance Tracking Screen Display

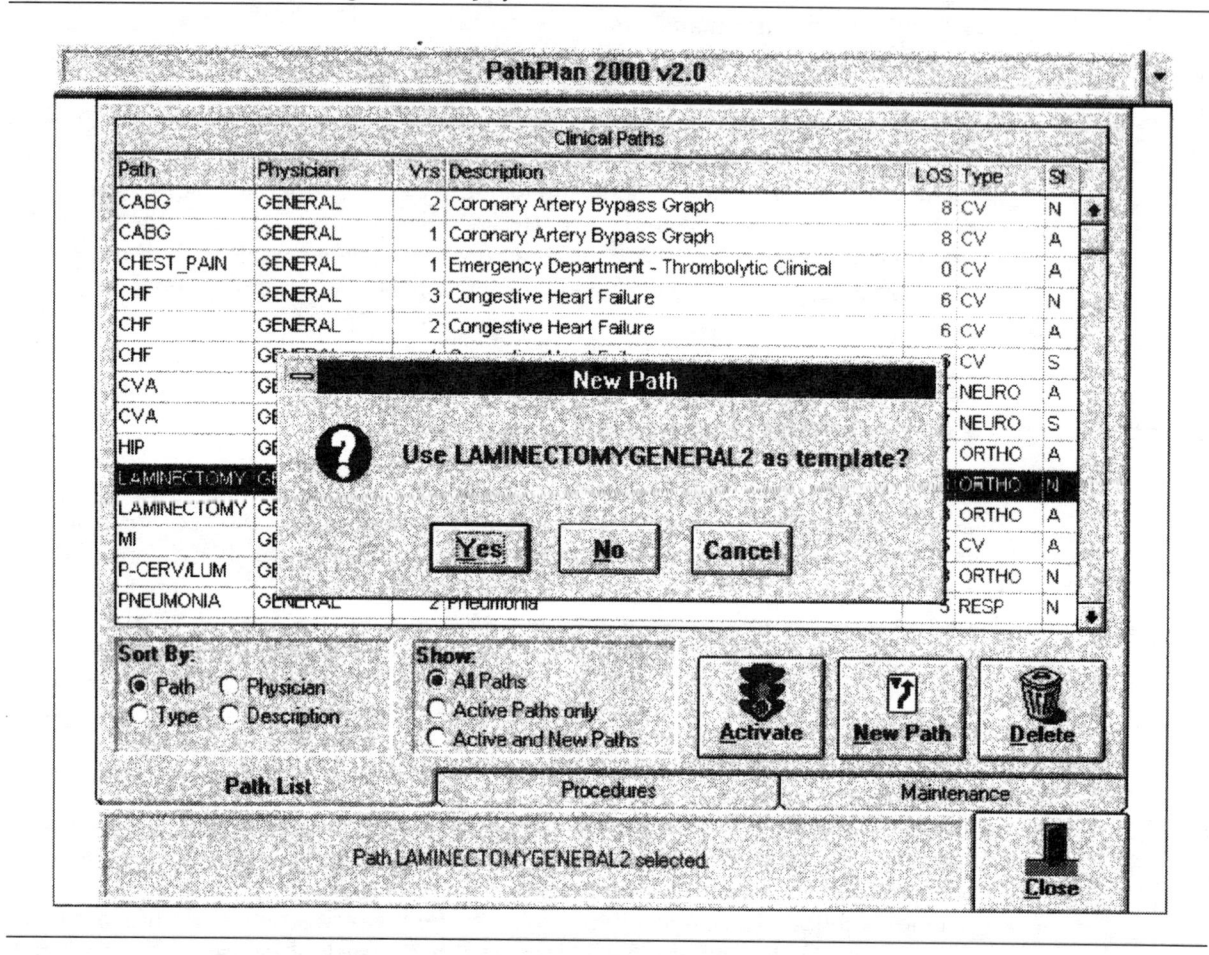

to predefined parameters without shuffling and reshuffling paper! The case management department could efficiently study variance data in multiple ways—by patients, physicians, paths, or variance categories. Prior to automation, Bristol had very shallow variance analysis capability. It was only able to track the percentage of patients on and off the paths in addition to length of stay and charges. Through automation, the medical center was able to analyze detailed variance data regularly and identify opportunities for improvement. (See figure 12-5.) In addition, it was able to accelerate the identification of improvement opportunities that were not readily apparent when data were collected and reported manually.

AUTOMATION ENHANCES IMPROVEMENT ACTIVITIES

The clinical path teams meet regularly to review pathway variance reports and to identify improvement opportunities. The teams agree that the ability to sort clinical data and probe deeper and deeper into key variances is critical to their successful identification of additional improvements. With the addition of automated data analysis, even teams that had been reviewing manually collected data for several months detected new improvement opportunities. Pathway variance data helped, in some instances, to confirm case managers' suspicions and, in others, to dispel mistaken beliefs. Several examples of how patient care has been improved by enhanced automated path variance reporting are listed below.

AUTOMATION ENHANCES IMPROVEMENT ACTIVITIES 219

FIGURE 12-4 Variance from Expected Outcome (VEO) Pop-Up Table

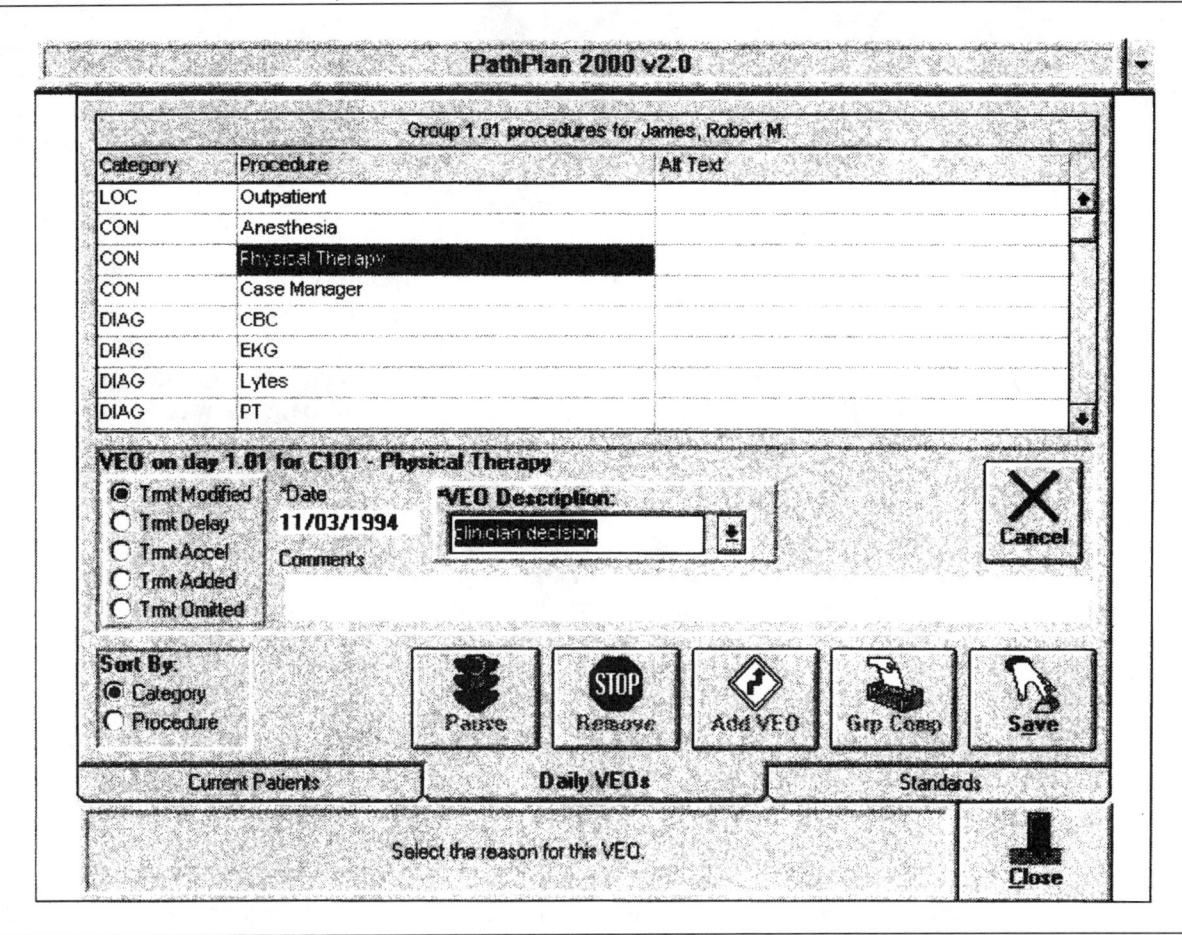

FIGURE 12-5 Sample Variance Report

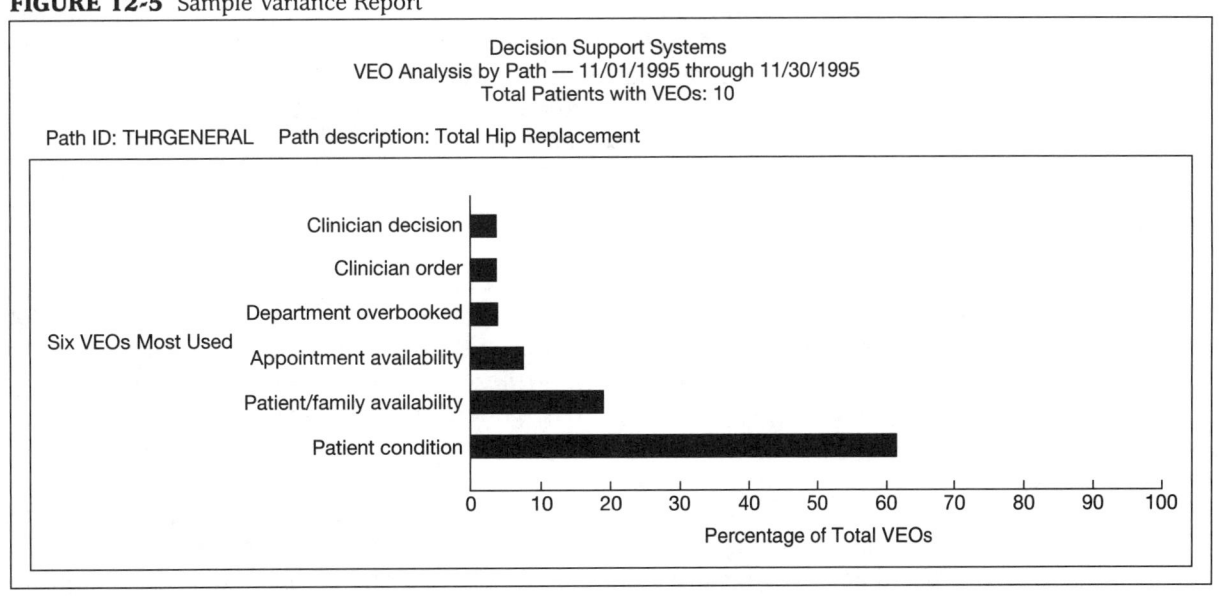

Decision Support Systems
VEO Analysis by Path — 11/01/1995 through 11/30/1995
Total Patients with VEOs: 10

Path ID: THRGENERAL   Path description: Total Hip Replacement

Six VEOs Most Used:
- Clinician decision
- Clinician order
- Department overbooked
- Appointment availability
- Patient/family availability
- Patient condition

Percentage of Total VEOs

Congestive Heart Failure

As part of the CHF path analysis, Bristol found two critical areas that needed improvement: patient education and diet compliance. Because approximately 85 percent of all CHF patients were discharged to home health care, the path teams extended the path to include the home health component. Home health agencies are now supplied with baseline weights for all patients prior to discharge from the medical center. Bristol works with families and home health agencies to ensure that each patient has an accurate scale for recording daily weights. In some cases Bristol provides the scale. As a result of the clinical path and case management interventions, the medical center significantly reduced readmissions for CHF patients. To illustrate, in 1995 CHF represented 18 percent of all readmissions for Bristol. One year later, CHF represents less than 2 percent of all readmissions. Before the implementation of case management and clinical paths, the average length of stay for CHF patients was 8.1 days. One year later the length of stay dropped to 5.2 days. In addition, costs have been cut by 20 percent.

Initially, the decision whether to place a CHF patient on a pathway was left to the admitting physician's discretion. Because of the overwhelming success of the CHF pathway, in 1996 the medical staff agreed that all patients with an admitting diagnosis of CHF should be automatically assigned to the CHF path.

Pneumonia

In analyzing pneumonia pathway data, the path team discovered that the path had produced very limited reductions in length of stay and mortality. It knew from its analysis that the majority of the patients were admitted from long-term care facilities and had multiple health problems. This information helped to explain why mortality rates were not reduced by the original path: Bristol was treating a high-risk population. Consequently, the team revised its initial path to address the problems of a typically sicker population.

Variance analysis also revealed a delay in the administration of the first dose of antibiotics. Before the automated variance analysis, only 60 percent of patients were able to meet the standard of "antibiotics administered within 90 minutes of admission." After carefully reviewing the variance data and realizing there were barriers within the system, the path team began initiating the pathway in the emergency department and subsequently changed the standard to "initiate antibiotic in the emergency department prior to transfer to nursing unit." Today, 95 percent of all patients are able to meet this standard. (See figure 12-6.)

Myocardial Infarction

MI was Bristol's first clinical path and has resulted in a 21 percent reduction in costs and a 3.5-day reduction in length of stay. Because this path served as the initial pilot project, a significant amount of variance trending data have been available to the path team. The initial variance analysis revealed opportunities to reduce unnecessary resource utilization. For example, many patients received arterial blood gases as opposed to less expensive pulse oximetry, and creatine phosphokinase tests were overutilized.

The path team noticed that as few as 17 percent of patients at one point were able to attend the cardiac nutrition class. The variance analysis revealed that the class was scheduled at an inconvenient time for patients and families, and some improvement was achieved when the class was rescheduled from the afternoon to the morning. However, the team was not satisfied and sought additional ways to increase class

FIGURE 12-6 Sample Outcomes Analysis Report

PathPlan 2000		Decision Support Systems Outcomes Analysis All Path Treatment Groups									
Report Period: Nov 1995											
Path ID: THRGENERAL	Description: Total Hip Replacement										
		Current Month				Previous success rates					
Procedure ID and Description		Met		Not Met		Oct 1995		Sep 1995		Aug 1995	
ED105	Pain management	0	0.00%	0	0.00%	0	0.00%	0	0.00%	0	0.00%
ED106	Ambulation & exercise	14	100.00%	0	0.00%	0	0.00%	0	0.00%	0	0.00%
ED107	Reinforce preop teaching	17	100.00%	0	0.00%	1	8.33%	0	0.00%	0	0.00%
ED108	IS/CDB	32	100.00%	0	0.00%	0	0.00%	0	0.00%	0	0.00%
ED109	Review pain management	32	100.00%	0	0.00%	0	0.00%	0	0.00%	0	0.00%
ED110	Review TED's	32	100.00%	0	0.00%	0	0.00%	0	0.00%	0	0.00%
ED111	Reinforce PT education on ambulation & exercise, sitting/standing	29	100.00%	0	0.00%	0	0.00%	0	0.00%	0	0.00%
ED112	Review home equipment ordered	14	100.00%	0	0.00%	0	0.00%	0	0.00%	0	0.00%
ED113	Review medications	14	100.00%	0	0.00%	0	0.00%	0	0.00%	0	0.00%
ED114	Review DC instructions	14	100.00%	0	0.00%	0	0.00%	0	0.00%	0	0.00%
L CBC	CBC	30	100.00%	0	0.00%	0	0.00%	0	0.00%	0	0.00%
L EKG	EKG	15	100.00%	0	0.00%	0	0.00%	0	0.00%	0	0.00%
L K	K	15	100.00%	0	0.00%	0	0.00%	0	0.00%	0	0.00%
L LYTES	Lytes	15	100.00%	0	0.00%	0	0.00%	0	0.00%	0	0.00%
L PT	PT	73	100.00%	0	0.00%	1	1.67%	0	0.00%	0	0.00%
L PTT	PTT	15	100.00%	0	0.00%	0	0.00%	0	0.00%	0	0.00%
L T&C	Type & cross	15	100.00%	0	0.00%	0	0.00%	0	0.00%	0	0.00%
L100	Outpatient	32	100.00%	0	0.00%	0	0.00%	0	0.00%	0	0.00%
L101	Operating Room	17	100.00%	0	0.00%	0	0.00%	0	0.00%	0	0.00%
L102	Recovery Room	17	100.00%	0	0.00%	0	0.00%	0	0.00%	0	0.00%
L103	Orthopedic Unit	75	100.00%	0	0.00%	0	0.00%	0	0.00%	0	0.00%
O200	Ambulate 60–80 ft with walker	12	85.71%	2	14.29%	0	0.00%	0	0.00%	0	0.00%
O DC	Discharge per plan	0	0.00%	0	0.00%	0	0.00%	0	0.00%	0	0.00%
O100	Pt verbalizes preop instructions	15	100.00%	0	0.00%	0	0.00%	0	0.00%	0	0.00%
O101	Pt verbalizes postop activity & dc plans	15	100.00%	0	0.00%	0	0.00%	0	0.00%	0	0.00%
O102	Pt demonstrates use of IS, CDB, & turning with abduction pillow	61	100.00%	0	0.00%	3	6.25%	0	0.00%	0	0.00%
O103	Pt verbalizes hip precautions	61	100.00%	0	0.00%	3	6.25%	0	0.00%	0	0.00%
O104	Pt verbalizes pain relief with prescribed meds	78	100.00%	0	0.00%	0	0.00%	0	0.00%	0	0.00%
O106	Dressing dry & intact	61	100.00%	0	0.00%	0	0.00%	0	0.00%	0	0.00%
O107	No ss & sx of dislocation	61	100.00%	0	0.00%	0	0.00%	0	0.00%	0	0.00%
O108	Ambulates 10–20 ft with moderate assistance	15	100.00%	0	0.00%	5	41.67%	0	0.00%	0	0.00%
O109	Ambulates 20–40 ft with moderate assistance	15	100.00%	0	0.00%	1	8.33%	0	0.00%	0	0.00%
O110	Ambulates 40–60 ft with moderate assistance	14	100.00%	0	0.00%	0	0.00%	0	0.00%	0	0.00%
O201	Ambulate 80+ ft independently	0	0.00%	0	0.00%	0	0.00%	0	0.00%	0	0.00%
O202	Pt verbalizes home care	0	0.00%	0	0.00%	0	0.00%	0	0.00%	0	0.00%

attendance. Patients and families are now asked to come back to the hospital for the class after discharge, when life settles down for them. This change has dramatically improved class attendance, and as of August 1996, 75 percent of patients participate in the cardiac nutrition class.

Through careful study of the cause of variances, the team was able to significantly reduce length of stay and eliminate unnecessary treatments. In addition, the team adopted a more systematic, prospective approach to patient education and developed a corresponding patient education pathway. This "patient-friendly" version of the clinical path has been so successful that all path teams now design patient education pathways in addition to clinical versions. By having their own pathways, patients have a better understanding of what to expect each day during their hospital stays. In addition, patients and their families can participate more fully in their care.

23-Hour Chest Pain

In response to managed care pressures, Bristol developed a 23-hour chest pain path (figure 12-7), which begins in the emergency department and ensures a definitive diagnosis within 11 hours of admission. Bristol's path includes new, state-of-the-art diagnostic tests (myoglobin and troponin I) that facilitate earlier diagnosis. Patients with a confirmed MI are automatically "bridged" to the MI path. For patients without a positive MI diagnosis, the path provides additional time for testing to determine whether the patient has another diagnosis requiring inpatient admission or discharge. After implementing this pathway, Bristol significantly reduced payment denials for unnecessary chest pain admissions.

Total Hip Replacement and Fractured Hip

With the implementation of the hip path, Bristol determined that the 5-day length-of-stay objective was achieved. However, the path team found delays in scheduling surgery for hip patients admitted through the emergency department. It discovered that orthopedic surgeons were often busy in the operating room, and lab tests for newly admitted patients were not ordered until the physician was available to order them. Having identified this improvement opportunity through path variance analysis, the team developed preoperative orders that are now initiated in the emergency department.

Anterior and Posterior Laminectomy

Bristol caregivers learned about the importance of strategic variance analysis when studying the orthopedic procedures of anterior and posterior laminectomy. The path team started with one combined path for both procedures. However, reviewing a quarter's worth of variance data, it was obvious that the team could not expect the same outcomes from both types of surgery. There were simply too many justifiable variances. As a result the team created two separate paths, which has allowed outcomes specific to each procedure to be developed and tracked.

CONCLUSION

The most important lesson learned by Bristol Regional Medical Center in developing its case management and clinical pathway initiatives was the importance of data in determining the effectiveness of these initiatives. Most caregivers agree that one of the benefits of paths is the ability to capture information useful for identifying and

FIGURE 12-7 Chest Pain Pathway

PathPlan 2000	BRMC Data 6/96 and After Clinical Path: CHEST PAINGENERAL1	
Path Description: 23 Hour Chest Pain		
Category	0–12 Hours	12–23 Hours
LOCATION	- PCCU - 4 WEST	- PCCU - 4 WEST
ASSESSMENT & EVALUATION	- VS q 4 hr	- VS
CONSULT	- Cardiology, if desired - Cardiac Rehab nurse	
DIAGNOSTICS	- Chem 10 - CBC w/o diff - EKG on adm & repeat in 2 hr - CXR - R/O MI Panel	- Treadmill per order - Echo per order - Cardiolyte scan per order
DIET	- AHA	- AHA
ACTIVITY	- Bedrest with BRP	
EDUCATION	- Signs & Sx to report - Cardiac Rehab	
TREATMENT	- RT protocol	
MEDICATION	- Per MD order	- Per MD order
DISCHARGE PLAN/ EXPECTED OUTCOME	- Results of 3 hr Myoglobin & Troponin on chart within 3 hrs. - Pt/SO verbalize S&S to report, F/U care EXCLUSIONS 1) BLUNT TRAUMA 2) AGE LESS THAN 18 3) ACUTE MI – AORTIC DISSECTION; RHYTHM DISTURBANCE; PE (OTHER MAJOR DX) 4) FEVER GREATER THAN 100 5) NEW CHANGES ON EKG 6) HYPOXEMIA PO$_2$ LESS THAN 60, O$_2$ SAT LESS THAN 90% 7) NURSING HOME PATIENT WITH DNR 8) TRANSFER FROM ANOTHER FACILITY	- Pain free

Clinical pathways do not represent a standard of care. They are guidelines for consideration which may be modified to the individual patient's needs.

assessing quality issues. However, it was not until the case management department was able to computerize its clinical path development and analysis process that it was able to advance beyond simple length-of-stay and cost-of-care analyses. Automation of clinical paths and variance analysis has accelerated Bristol's ability to analyze path variance data frequently.

The caregivers at Bristol also learned the importance of establishing administrative liaisons for the path teams. When a team identifies the need to expend capital or human resources to make necessary improvements, it is crucial that administration make resources available. For example, Bristol's chest pain path called for the addition of new diagnostic tests. Although they require a capital expenditure, the tests will improve the timeliness of diagnosis. Improved timeliness should result in fewer payment denials for chest pain admissions. Early administrative involvement in the chest pain path team's recommendations clearly helped in securing the necessary capital.

Bristol has also learned the importance of accurate data collection. Rather than ask many different bedside caregivers to gather variance information, data quality is improved by delegating all data collection responsibility and analysis to case managers.

Clearly, Bristol's integrated case management model, supplemented by clinical pathways, is positively influencing clinical quality improvement efforts. The improvement opportunities identified through sophisticated computer analysis of path variances are acted upon by quality improvement teams. To provide the most effective and appropriate patient services throughout all levels of care, Bristol foresees the development of additional paths that span the continuum. A team is currently designing a pathway for patients with chronic obstructive pulmonary disease, a condition that often results in hospital admissions. The path will incorporate pre- and posthospitalization needs as well as a home health care component. The ultimate goal is to improve collaboration among all health care organizations, which should result in more efficient, patient-focused care and increased patient satisfaction.

Bristol may already lead the way for best practice in some clinical areas. It was recognized in 1996 for its improvement activities by the Baltimore-based company HCIA. One of the nation's largest health care data companies, HCIA provides comparative data for thousands of health care organizations. During a recent meeting with Bristol Regional Medical Center leadership, HCIA officials noted that the medical center is already the benchmark facility in some clinical areas.

Improved patient outcomes will continue to be the mission of the medical center's case management and clinical pathway efforts. The PathPlan 2000 system will provide the framework for gathering and analyzing process and outcomes data in hopes of achieving even higher levels of patient care effectiveness.

CHAPTER 13

Designing Information Systems for Disease Management

Dianne J. Anderson, Christine W. Freire, and Patricia Hale

Glens Falls Hospital (GFH) is a 442-bed sole community provider located in upstate New York. It serves a large, predominantly rural geographic region having a population base of 200,000. The hospital provides a wide range of inpatient and outpatient services and like many of its counterparts has seen a significant decline in its inpatient discharges, from 15,203 in 1992 to 13,307 in 1995. Outpatient programs and services continue their upward trend. GFH serves a predominantly geriatric population and generates 42 percent of its total revenues from Medicare. Managed care is gaining a slow but steady presence in the region with about 20 percent penetration.

THE ORIGINAL PATHWAY INITIATIVE

Clinical pathway implementation had begun at the hospital in 1991 as a result of a state-funded demonstration project but was found to be relatively ineffective in achieving managed care goals. Although the original pathways were designed through a multidisciplinary process, the implementation component was weak. For example, methods for variance tracking and ongoing data analyses had not been established. Paper pathways were not well integrated into the process of care delivery, and in these early years, there was no case management process to supplement the pathway system. Although some positive results were reported, staff, physicians, and managers agreed that the original pathway initiative had not met all its intended goals. The pathway program was discontinued in 1994, when funding ended.

The authors acknowledge the following individuals for their many contributions to the Glens Falls guidelines and pathway project: Richard P. Leach, Jr., MD; Surendra Nevatia, MD; Stephen Monn, MD; W. Bruce Armstrong III; K. Cantiello, MT/ASCP; I. Fischer, RN; D. Garcia, RN; K. Hodge; K. McMore; S. Perry, RN; J. Hathaway; K. Sumner; J. Vadnais; P. Bachman; and D. VanLoan, RN.

In late 1995 there was growing interest among a small number of senior physician leaders and hospital senior management to reestablish the clinical pathway initiative and explore the concept of an organized approach to disease management across the entire continuum of care. This resurgence of interest was caused by several factors, which occurred simultaneously:

- Recognition by the physician community, hospital leadership, and home care agencies that managed care in the region would increase significantly
- A desire by all providers to retain as much of the premium dollar as possible within the region to reinvest directly in health care for the local communities
- Recognition by the hospital and physicians that hospital length of stay and readmission rates could be decreased
- Recognition by all parties that creative and innovative programs would be needed in the community to decrease lengths of hospitalization, including increased focus on home care programs
- Recognition of the need to improve and develop more outreach, prevention, and health education in the community

PREPARING FOR A MANAGED CARE ENVIRONMENT

The changing marketplace, strong community support, and new leadership heightened the health care system's commitment to and enthusiasm for positive change. Adirondack Medicine, Inc. (AMI), is a large, independent physician alliance (IPA) comprising all primary care providers and specialists in this region. AMI leadership realized that preparation for a managed care environment was critical and in 1995 entered into a joint venture agreement with the hospital and an insurance partner to enable them to contract for managed care services. GFH is working with AMI to develop an integrated delivery system with a goal of establishing regional health care standards. Opportunities for enhancing the quality and cost efficiencies of the multiple health care services provided in the community have been identified. The primary goal of this collaborative effort is developing the systems and tools needed to facilitate the current delivery system's transition into a health care environment committed to regional wellness and the seamless delivery of patient care and services. Underlying this transition are clinical practice guidelines that enhance disease management in hospital and outpatient settings. An integrated, automated information system will be the primary mechanism for operationalizing the guidelines.

The rapid growth of medical information and technological advances in computerization over the past few years have left most physicians struggling to keep pace. In addition, payers, consumers, and physicians have become concerned about the increased cost of health care, issues of cost-effectiveness, and quality of care. These changes have required a major shift in how physicians make clinical decisions and how they implement care. Physicians must be concerned about managed care issues, cost of care, and scrutiny of their practice by many entities. Clinical decision-making processes that were based on personal experience and methods learned during training are increasingly being replaced by continuing medical education and medical literature filled with various practice guidelines and treatment recommendations.

As practice guidelines become more prevalent, physicians and other caregivers need to be aware of "accepted practices" and either utilize the guideline suggestions or document information to explain exceptions and/or help modify the guidelines. The major problems with implementing the more than 2,000 clinical practice guidelines available include:[1-12]

FIGURE 13-1 Components of the Regional Disease Management Model

◄──────────────── Patient Care across the Continuum ────────────────►

Adirondack Medicine, Inc.	Glens Falls Hospital	Home Care
Clinical guidelines	Case management	County public health agencies
Physician office-based information system	Clinical pathways Clinical information system	Hospital-based IV therapy and durable medical equipment Oxygen therapy

- Difficulties in making the guidelines available and easy to use at the time of physician-patient contact
- Inability to adjust to regional variations in clinical practice
- Inability to update the guidelines frequently to match the continuous flow of new scientific information
- Exacerbation of the already overwhelming paperwork required for medical documentation
- Lack of integration into a continuum of patient care in both the inpatient and outpatient settings
- Lack of methods for evaluating outcomes resulting from using guidelines in a community setting (especially "end-point" outcomes, such as the day the patient returned to work and full functional status)

To overcome these guideline implementation barriers, physicians and other caregivers in the GFH community are designing a computerized patient record system to augment their deployment of clinical practice guidelines. The move away from paper-based medicine will no doubt require a significant effort by physicians, hospital staff, and others involved in patient care to achieve a seamless flow of information through the continuum. The process will be influenced partly by the challenge to utilize the vast and growing number of clinical practice guidelines. By involving all caregivers throughout the continuum it is hoped that the information system will greatly enhance community health care services.

GFH and AMI have jointly committed to a number of strategic initiatives related to the integration of clinical practice guidelines into health care delivery. These major initiatives include: case management, guideline-based disease management, clinical pathway implementation, and automated, integrated information system design. Each initiative is a separate project lead by representatives from GFH and AMI. Together, all of these initiatives are creating the framework for a community-based disease management model. (See figure 13-1.) This chapter describes these initiatives and how they are helping GFH and AMI achieve their regional health care goals.

CASE MANAGEMENT

GFH introduced case management as its first disease management initiative in 1996. The case management model adopted at GFH combined the functions of social work, discharge planning, and utilization review into an integrated process. This model was chosen because of the growing demands of managed care and GFH's commitment to eliminate system redundancies. The primary focus of case management was to promote integrated delivery of quality-focused, cost-effective patient care. During its first year of implementation, case management goals included:

TABLE 13-1 Length-of-Stay (LOS) Comparative Data for Top 10 Ranked Medicare DRGs, Jan. 1–June 30, 1996 (Includes Outliers)

DRG	Title	No. of Cases	HCFA Mean LOS	GFH Mean LOS
127	Heart failure and shock	197	6.7	8.78
89	Simple pneumonia and pleurisy, age > 17 w/CC	172	7.6	12.62
88	Chronic obstructive pulmonary disease	134	6.6	9.43
209	Major joint and limb reattachment procedure of lower extremity	94	7.6	9.89
14	Specific cerebrovascular disorders except TIA	73	8.2	12.08
182	Esophagitis, gastroenteritis, and miscellaneous digestive disorders, age > 17 w/CC	71	5.4	7.87
132	Atherosclerosis w/CC	71	4.0	5.90
138	Cardiac arrhythmia and conduction disorder w/CC	66	5.0	5.97
121	Circulatory disorders w/acute myocardial infarction and CVC, discharged alive	57	8.4	10.75
296	Nutritional and miscellaneous metabolic disorders, age > 17 w/CC	48	7.0	9.08

Note: HCFA = Health Care Financing Administration, GFH = Glens Falls Hospital, CC = Comorbidities/complications, TIA = Transient ischemic attack.

- Improve physician and patient satisfaction.
- Develop and implement 10 multidisciplinary clinical pathways in targeted diagnosis-related groups (DRGs).
- Reduce total inpatient service days by 38,844.
- Reduce the number of per-patient contacts by discharge planning, social work, and utilization review staff.

These goals were designed to meet several quality and financial needs. GFH recognized that the average length of stay for many of its high-volume DRGs was longer than the Medicare mean length of stay. (See table 13-1.) A successful case management process could reduce the GFH lengths of stay. Facility leaders also identified duplicative data collection activities among the utilization review, social work, and discharge planning staff. This situation caused patients to be contacted by several professionals who were gathering essentially the same information. Further, physicians perceived that many patient discharge delays stemmed from bureaucratic hospital systems that could be streamlined with case management activities.

At the start of the case management program a commitment was made to use currently employed, interested staff as case managers. GFH discharge planners, social workers, and utilization review staff brought with them a wealth of knowledge and skills from their specific areas of expertise. A case management training program (figure 13-2) was designed to enhance the staff's knowledge base, thereby facilitating its transition into the new patient care delivery system.

Case management staff was actively involved in the development and implementation of the program. Staff subgroups were created to develop case management product lines, plan the educational curriculum, and integrate the program throughout the health care delivery system. The subgroups' input formed the framework for the program's implementation plan.

The GFH case management department consists of 1 director, 11 case managers, 2 clinical social workers, and 1.5 full-time equivalents of clerical support staff. The job description and eligibility requirements for the case manager position are detailed in figure 13-3.[13] While employed by the hospital, each case manager works collaboratively with a specific group of physicians and is responsible for following select pa-

FIGURE 13-2 Case Manager Education Topics

- The prospective payment system and managed care reimbursement systems
- Overview of case management — state of the art
- The role of the case manager
- Case management tools and their applications
- Outcomes, variances, and continuous quality improvement
- Case management application in various health care settings
- Case management steps
- Documentation issues for case management — case studies
- How to identify high-risk patients — criteria
- Choosing a case management tool
- Continuous quality improvement
- Evaluating a case management model
- Creating case management tools
- Identifying outcomes
- Variances
- Change and chaos theory
- Nine steps toward case management implementation

tients through inpatient, outpatient, and community-based settings.[14] Clinical social workers focus their efforts primarily in the outpatient renal and oncology settings.

Each case manager is responsible for approximately 25 patients, with approximately 50 percent of these patients under active follow-up. As case managers develop a better understanding of their role and case management tools such as clinical paths are developed for direct caregivers, the percentage of patients under active follow-up is expected to decline to 25 percent.

Case management referral criteria (figure 13-4) have been developed to assist multidisciplinary staff, physicians, and physician office staff in identifying patients who can benefit from case management services. As the case management program continues to evolve, these criteria will be refined further according to the needs of various patient populations.

One of the most critical roles of the case manager has been that of change agent. Case managers are actively involved in educating all caregivers, including hospital-based and physician-office-based staff. They are a vital bridge throughout the continuum of care to promote regional disease management. They also play an important part in the development and implementation of clinical pathways that will promote multidisciplinary care planning and disease management. Case managers serve as team leaders for the GFH clinical implementation teams charged with designing pathways.

GUIDELINE-BASED DISEASE MANAGEMENT

Until recently the health care environment in upstate New York had not experienced a high penetration of managed care. This situation is expected to change rapidly over the next few years. Consequently, the advantages of guideline-based patient care have become apparent to many physicians and administrators only lately.

Once health care providers acknowledged that changes were needed, the stage was set for creating a community-wide, guideline-based disease management model. The model, which is still under development, combines guidelines, pathways, case management, home care, and patient education to meet the community's health care needs. Implementation of these initiatives involves the cooperation of the three health care providers in the community: AMI, GFH, and the regional public health home

FIGURE 13-3 Case Manager Job Description

The case manager is responsible for:
- Integrating, facilitating, and coordinating patient care across the health care continuum
- Ensuring the delivery of cost-effective, outcome-oriented, quality care within an appropriate length of stay
- Managing patient care to prevent fragmentation and duplication of services
- Working in collaborative practice with the physician and other members of the health care team to meet patient-specific and age-related needs, linking cost and quality to patient care.

Primary Duties and Responsibilities

Time Spent Performing This Duty, %

Clinical Role   35%

- Completes a comprehensive assessment of patient and family before or at visit, treatment, or admission and throughout hospitalization to include:
  - Previous precipitating health factors associated with present hospitalization or visit
  - Previous and current levels of physical and psychosocial functioning as well as coping abilities
  - Availability of resources and support systems
  - Identification of patient's actual and potential problems relating to continuing care needs
- Develops and utilizes the multidisciplinary care plan, guidelines, and clinical pathways in collaboration with members of the health care team, identifying key tasks or events to be accomplished relating to specific patient outcomes.
  - Identifies variances from the standard protocol of care (clinical pathways, guidelines, and maps)
  - Works with other health care professionals to resolve identified variances
  - Reviews and evaluates the effectiveness of the pathway
- Arranges for timely consultation with specialist or specialized services
- Facilitates patient transfer to appropriate care area, setting, or program
- Initiates and follows through on continuing care needs as identified in the plan of care in collaboration with the health care team in both in- and outpatient settings

Collaboration Role   45%

- Integrates, facilitates, and coordinates patient care to ensure timely patient outcomes across the health care continuum
- Negotiates the care provided with members of the health care team and the patient and family to prevent duplication or fragmentation of services
- Establishes the desired patient outcomes before or at visit, treatment, or admission; plans length of stay (when applicable) as it relates to the DRG, clinical path, or guideline; initiates and formulates a plan for continuing care needs
- Acts as a patient advocate by strategizing and negotiating with the multidisciplinary team, patient and family, providers, and payers about the care provided and the best course of action
  - Promotes self-care activities, autonomous decision making, and active patient and family participation in treatment and care planning and health promotion
- Conducts concurrent and retrospective quality reviews to identify and improve clinical, resource, and systems problems, utilizing the continuous improvement process
- Initiates or participates in unit rounds
- Acts as a resource person to the health care team
- Acts as a health care team facilitator to promote an integrated, multidisciplinary approach to patient care throughout the health care continuum
- Initiates modifications to the delivery of a product line to improve service and patient outcomes

Financial/Resource Role   20%

- Demonstrates competency related to DRGs and allocated length of stay and applies established utilization criteria
- Identifies and takes action based on utilization review issues: admit denies, extended length of stay, and delays in discharge
- Demonstrates knowledge related to cost of resources, reimbursement procedures, and resource allocation related to an identified product line

Job Specifications

Education/Experience: RN or Baccalaureate prepared social worker. Two years of acute care or case management experience preferred. Computer literacy and data analysis skills are preferred.

Skills/Abilities: Able to function autonomously, maintaining a high level of clinical and professional accountability. Demonstrates skill in creative problem solving, facilitation, collaboration, coordination, and critical thinking. Committed to promoting excellence in customer service. Functions as a team player. Maintains professional image by demonstrating strong verbal and written communication skills. Applies continuous improvement principles and practices in all areas of professional involvement. Demonstrates ability in self-starting, self-directing, and clear decision-making behaviors.

Licenses/Certificates/Registrations: Maintains current licensure or certification in appropriate professional affiliation.

FIGURE 13-4 Case Management Screening Criteria

Complex Medical Needs
- Multiple physicians caring for patient
- Drastic changes in patient's condition
- Multiple admissions for patient
- Patient with multiple comorbidities

Complex Psychosocial Needs
- Patient has compromised support systems

Complex Functional Needs
- Patient has impairments in activities of daily living

---

care agencies. Working together, these partners will develop clinical guidelines that embrace the continuum of care. They will also design tools, such as pathways and protocols, to disseminate guideline recommendations. The model is continuing to evolve and develop as clinicians gain more insight into the data management and patient care processes necessary to support disease management. While many obstacles still exist, administrative and medical staff leaders believe that the disease management model has established an important framework for designing an innovative health care approach for the community.

Initial Disease Management Initiatives Undertaken by the Physician Practice Community

To design an internal physician-driven disease management system, AMI organized two committees to develop clinical guidelines: the utilization review committee and the quality improvement committee. Both committees are chaired by physicians and include physician members having primary care and specialty backgrounds. Key hospital personnel, including the vice president for patient services, the director of case management, and the executive director of the hospital-based home care agency, also serve on these committees. The goals established by AMI for the clinical practice guideline initiative include:

- Develop regional standards of care.
- Decrease use of resources.
- Reduce the inpatient length of stay.
- Decrease hospital readmission rates.
- Decrease use of ancillary services.

In support of these goals, the AMI utilization review committee was charged with:

- Providing input into the clinical pathways initiative at the hospital
- Identifying operational problems that might impact one or more providers along the continuum of care
- Participating in the development of creative, cost-efficient health care delivery solutions (such as a "fast-track" day surgery program or an asthma day care center)
- Developing clinical guidelines that encourage high-quality, cost-effective patient management throughout the continuum of care with a focus on preventive as well as sickness care

The primary responsibility of the quality improvement committee is to monitor the quality of care delivered by the physicians in the community. It was charged with evaluating:

- Access-to-care issues
- Risk management issues

- The peer review process
- Physician credentialing
- Preventive health services
- The medical record review process
- Condition-specific or diagnosis-specific care improvement opportunities

Initial Disease Management Initiatives Undertaken by the Hospital

The GFH senior management team recognized that managed care penetration was on the rise in the region and took proactive steps through the strategic plan process. In 1996 a new strategic plan was created and key strategic goals were identified, including:

- Implement integration strategies with physicians and other providers to improve service, quality, and economic value.
- Enhance financial viability.
- Build new information systems.
- Create an environment at GFH that will foster change through innovation.
- Develop or enhance programs that demonstrably improve and sustain the health of the community.

To accomplish these goals, a number of initiatives were identified as being important, including support of the disease management model.

AMI-GFH Collaboration to Implement the Disease Management Model

In 1996 GFH formed a clinical pathways steering committee (CPSC). This committee included senior leaders from clinical, financial, and information services. This leadership-driven approach had been missing in the first clinical pathway initiative in 1991. GFH believed that high-level teamwork was necessary to bolster the importance of guidelines and disease management throughout the organization.

The hospital's vice president for patient services and the chief of neurology, a senior member of the medical staff, cochaired the committee. The physician chosen to serve as cochair had expressed personal interest in the disease management initiative and had significant credibility within the medical community. He was successful in securing other key physicians as CPSC members and pathway advisors.

Initial CPSC membership included representation from: specialty and primary care physicians, staff nurses, case management, rehabilitative services, finance, information systems, clinical specialists, quality assurance, medical records, senior management, pharmacy, and the vice president for managed care. Later the group added representatives from the home health agency and two nearby public health departments. The final link was to add members from AMI administration. This collaboration helped to ensure that AMI's guideline development plans were integrated with the hospital's pathway initiative. By including AMI representatives on the CPSC, the hospital caregivers also hoped to identify ways to decrease hospital utilization.

CLINICAL PATHWAY IMPLEMENTATION

The CPSC then defined the following mission statement, goals, and pathway implementation plan.

Mission Statement

To develop the process and format for implementation and evaluation of guideline-based clinical pathways.

Goals

- Identify key patient groups for pathway development, focusing on opportunities for improving quality and decreasing costs.
- Coordinate the hospital's pathway design process with AMI guideline development projects to streamline care across the continuum
- Examine current pathways already implemented within the hospital to determine their level of use and effectiveness.
- Establish a process of pathway development that is user friendly, efficient, and meaningful to clinicians.
- Develop a method of tracking pathway variances and measuring patient outcomes.

Pathway Implementation Plan

A work plan was established. (See figure 13-5.) After drafting the implementation plan, the committee sought outside consultation to be sure all issues were being addressed. The hospital engaged a consultant from the Healthcare Association of New York State to provide support and direction for the first pathways that would be developed.

After analyzing volume and length-of-stay data for GFH's top 15 Medicare DRGs in 1995, the CPSC chose to start the pathway development process for patients with chronic obstructive pulmonary disease. This group of patients was chosen because it presented a unique challenge to develop systems spanning the hospital and the community to provide better, more efficient care. For example, home care and patient education initiatives are required to improve quality of care and decrease hospitalizations and length of stay.

Patients admitted for major total joint replacements were also chosen for pathway development because a pathway had been designed for this group earlier, during the 1991–94 initiative. Revisiting this patient population would provide caregivers with the opportunity to examine the effectiveness of the original pathway and discuss ways to further streamline the process of care.

Finally, the CPSC chose to develop a clinical pathway for patients with community-acquired pneumonia (CAP). This patient category was selected because AMI physicians were interested in developing CAP practice guidelines for outpatient care. By linking the GFH's clinical pathway with the guidelines being designed by the physicians for their practices, the visionary disease management model could be realized.

The following section describes the complete guideline and pathway development process for patients with CAP. This project includes designing a computerized information system to enhance guideline compliance and support continuity of care among all involved providers. The CAP project is evolving because of growing interest and experience with practice guidelines, clinical pathway development, and computerized medical records. Project enthusiasm, as well as technical and management expertise, has come entirely from within the local medical community. Many physicians in the area are actively participating in the project design and early implementation plans.

FIGURE 13-5 Clinical Path Work Plan

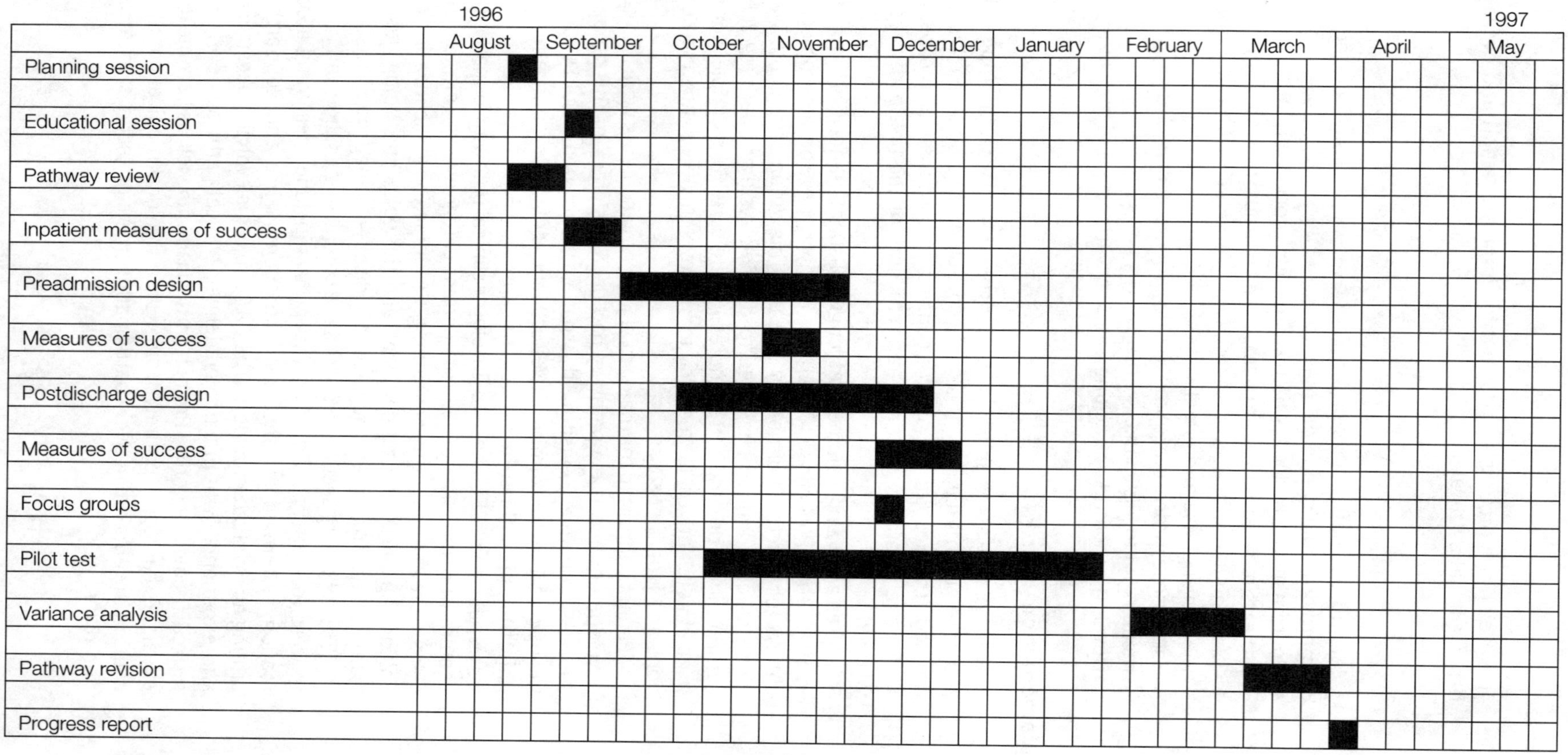

Community-Acquired Pneumonia Disease Management Project

The goal of the CAP project was to enhance the quality of care provided for patients in the region who are diagnosed with CAP. To accomplish this goal, five objectives were established:

1. Design clinical practice guidelines for managing patients in the region with CAP.
2. Design and implement a CAP clinical pathway for patients who require hospitalization.
3. Encourage physician utilization of CAP clinical practice guidelines through the use of a computerized information system.
4. Collect process and outcome data so physicians can compare their practice with regional and national norms.
5. Examine local outcome trends to determine whether any refinements of the guideline or pathway are appropriate.

The project was initiated by an infectious disease consultant and an internal medicine physician, who was primarily responsible for developing the computerized information system and managing the software programming efforts. As the project progressed, interest in participating grew to include a cross section of the community's physicians. Internal medicine and family practice groups are involved, as are specialists in pulmonary medicine. These specialists have also been involved in refining GFH's physician order set and clinical pathway. The project is being coordinated with the AMI computer initiative and the hospital's department of medicine and CPSC. The CAP project initiators, acting as joint project coordinators, work closely on program design and data analysis.

Development of Community-Acquired Pneumonia Practice Guidelines The CAP guidelines were derived from those of the American Thoracic Society (ATS).[15] Based on the disease consultant's observations of infection patterns in the GFH geographic area and on a literature review, modifications were made to the ATS-recommended antibiotic choices for each category of illness severity.[16–19]

Ultimately, the CAP guidelines were intended to serve as a module within PatRec, the computerized patient record program discussed later in this chapter. To permit computerization of the guidelines, it was necessary to break the process down into discrete logical steps to create programmable flowcharts. These flowcharts were built using condition-based (branching) logic, in which the condition encountered at a decision node, or point of branching, determines the next pathway.[20] This was not a straightforward process, as the ATS CAP guidelines consist of narrative lists of factors that should be taken into consideration when managing patients. For example, patients with severe pneumonia are defined as having at least one of the following symptoms:[21]

- Respiratory rate > 30/min
- $PaO_2/FiO_2 < 250$
- Mechanical ventilation required
- Bilateral or multiple lobe involvement
- Increasing infiltrate by more than 50 percent in 48 hours
- Presence of shock, oliguria, requiring pressors

Each of the factors had to be reworded into questions that would lead to a yes or no decision. The order in which decisions were to be made had to be sequenced into individual flow paths. Weighting factors were assigned to those clinical findings that the ATS guidelines indicate should be considered when making a decision

FIGURE 13-6 Preliminary Statistical Analysis of Patients with Community-Acquired Pneumonia, June 1, 1994, to May 31, 1995

Data Source: Hospital information system

Patient Selection: Pneumonia as principal diagnosis

494 Total Cases Identified:
- 373 compromised cases*—not analyzed
- 121 uncompromised cases—analyzed
- 50 physicians involved in caring for these patients
  - —4 surgeons with 4 cases (deleted from analysis)
  - —2 pediatricians with 3 cases ≥ 17 years of age (included in analysis)
  - —44 Department of Medicine physicians

117 Cases Evaluated:
- Length of stay range = 1 to 85 days
- Median length of stay = 5 days
- Mode length of stay = 5 days

Length-of-Stay Distribution:

≤5 days:	62 cases (53%)
>5 days ≤10 days:	29 cases (25%)
>10 days ≤15 days:	13 cases (11%)
>15 days ≤85 days:	13 cases (11%)

*Compromised patients are those with a principal diagnosis of pneumonia and a secondary diagnosis representing any of the following conditions or situations: cancer, congestive heart failure, chronic obstructive pulmonary disease, renal failure requiring dialysis, receiving cytoxic therapy, HIV, AIDS, diabetes with immunosuppression. Compromised patients are also those who are institutionalized and whose pneumonia is considered nosocomial.

to hospitalize patients. Numerous combinations of findings were evaluated to arrive at weighting factors that reasonably reflected accepted practices for hospitalization.

Design Clinical Pathway for Hospitalized Patients In late 1995 the GFH medical care review committee addressed problems relative to management of patients admitted with CAP. The ATS CAP guidelines were used as a benchmark to analyze the care being provided to hospitalized patients. A retrospective review of patient records (figure 13-6) revealed variations in medical treatments with corresponding differences in hospital lengths of stay. The recommendations on the CAP clinical pathway that GFH ultimately developed (figure 13-7) were derived from ATS guidelines, with local modifications approved by the pulmonary specialists and the infectious disease consultant.

Encourage Physician Utilization of Community-Acquired Pneumonia Guidelines Physician use of the CAP guidelines is encouraged through an automated medical record system locally designed especially for this project. The system is tailored to the needs of physicians practicing in the region and allows guidelines to be instantly available at the point of care. To be successful, the AMI leaders knew that the automated system had to have several key attributes:

- It must promote the utilization of guidelines by providing instant access to them.
- It must provide an automatic system to evaluate patient risk factors and test results so the management approach suggested for the patient is appropriate for the severity of the illness.
- It must be able to gather performance measurement data.
- It must be able to correlate outcome data with any selected clinical or treatment variable and provide physicians with immediate feedback on the results of different patient management choices.

FIGURE 13-7 Emergency Care and Inpatient Community-Acquired Pneumonia Clinical Pathway

Emergency Care Phase

PREADMIT	ARRIVAL MODE	NURSE TRIAGE OUT FRONT	REGISTRATION		ECC MD OR PA	TESTING	DIAGNOSIS CAP CATEGORY (CLINICAL/RADIO-GRAPHIC)	CASE MANAGER/ PUBLIC HEALTH INTERVENTION	DISPOSITION	TREATMENT PLAN
? Assess & Rx started in field	Ambulance	No (ECC room)	> Later	>	Yes	CXR (ECC/MI) Blood work • CBC • Pulse O$_2$ • Blood culture (fever) • SMA 6 (>60 or comorbidity)	I	prn	Home	**Therapeutics** • Antibiotics (see guidelines) • Tylenol prn • Bronchodilators prn • Mucolytics prn **Patient Education** • Antibiotic directions • Activity level • Nutrition/hydration • MD office appointment • Failed treatment warnings *TEAM recommends:* • Case management follow-up process to measure outcome • Preprinted patient CAP instructions
MD Office	Ambulatory	Yes	> Now	>	Maybe		II	Yes	OAP	
MD Phone Referral	Ambulatory	Yes	> Now	>	Yes		III	prn	General nursing unit	
Nothing	Ambulatory	Yes	> Now	>	Yes		IV	prn	Special care unit	

Vitals
Health history
Pulse O$_2$
EKG prn
O$_2$ prn
IV prn
? Isolation

Assess
History and physical
Testing
Initiate Rx

I. <60 and no evidence of comorbidity
II. Comorbidity or ≥60; can be treated in outpatient setting
III. Requires admission but not to intensive care
IV. Severe CAP; generally requires intensive care

FIGURE 13-7 *Continued*

Inpatient Phase

	DAY 1	DAY 2	DAY 3	DAY 4	DAY 5
Diagnostic Studies	CBC SMA6/60 Blood C&S if febrile Pulse oximetry ABG prn Chest X ray Sputum gram stain	Oximetry or ABG	CBC and CXR if not improving Oximetry		Discharge Criteria: • CXR clearing • WBC down • Temperature down • Respiration easier
Oxygen	Oxygen assessment protocol	->	->	->	
Medications	• Begin antibiotic therapy (see attached guideline) • Tylenol prn • Bronchodilators prn • Mucolytics prn	Continue IV antibiotics	Continue antibiotics Consider oral antibiotics If not responding, SEE**	Consider oral antibiotics after 72 hrs if meets criteria, SEE***	Consider discharge. To complete 10- to 14-day course of antibiotics.
Discharge Planning	• Nurse assess for discharge needs • Case management consult	Discharge services/Community resources in place	->	->	->
Nutrition	• Nutrition screen	Nutrition Assessment (if indicated by screen)			
	• Regular diet (unless ordered otherwise)	->	->	->	->
Activity	As tolerated	->	->	->	->
Education	Specific antibiotic Rx Nutrition and hydration Pneumonia education Breathing exercises Infection control Smoking cessation prn	Continue reinforcement	->	->	->

**If not responding after 48–72 hours, consider:
- Not pneumonia (other dx: PE, CA, inflammatory lung disease)
- Unusual pathogen (PCP, TB, Legionella virus, fungus, anaerobes)
- Pneumonic or therapeutic complication: empyema, meningitis, drug fever, antibiotic-associated colitis
- Antibiotic choice inadequate
- More extensive diagnostics for unusual pathogen
- Assess for swallowing dysfunction
- Pulmonary or infectious disease consult
- Change antibiotic

***Oral antibiotics if:
- Afebrile 24–48 hours
- Clinical improvement
- Able to take po and gut functioning
- Blood culture is negative

FIGURE 13-7 *Continued*

Antibiotic Therapy

Exclude patients who are immunosuppressed, institutionalized, diagnosed with AIDS, oncology patient ≤6 months of Rx, or on dialysis

Severity of Illness

Category I:
Outpatient

18–60 years with no comorbid conditions
Empiric Therapy
Macrolide

    Drug
> Erythromycin 500 mg q6h

Category II:
Outpatient

Greater than 60 years or a comorbid condition
Empiric Therapy
Second- or third-generation cephalosporin

    Drug
> Cefuroxime 750 mg IV q8h
    or
    Ceftriaxone 1 Gm qday

± Macrolide IV or po (if Legionella is a concern)
Add Rifampin if Legionella is documented

> ± Erythromycin 500 mg q6H
    ± Rifampin

If penicillin allergy: Consider floxin and erythromycin

Category III:
OAP inpatient

Hospitalized patients with CAP
Empiric Therapy
Macrolide (add Rifampin if Legionella is documented)

    Drug
> Erythromycin 0.5–1 Gm IV q6h
    plus
    Ceftriaxone 1 Gm qday

Third-generation cephalosporin

> If penicillin allergy: Consider floxin and erythromycin

Category IV:
Inpatient
ICU

Severe hospitalized CAP
RPM > 30, respiratory failure, mechanical ventilator, CXR with bilateral/multiple lobe involvement, shock, oliguria
Empiric Therapy
See Category III

    Drug
See Category III

Source: American Thoracic Society Guidelines, July 1993; formulated Sept. 1995; revised Mar. 12 and 14, 1996.

240 CHAPTER 13 DESIGNING INFORMATION SYSTEMS FOR DISEASE MANAGEMENT

INTEGRATED INFORMATION SYSTEM DESIGN

The computer system is undergoing constant refinement and, as of this writing, has yet to be fully implemented. The ultimate goal of the clinical information system is to provide for free flow of patient data across all health care delivery sites and with relevant external groups. (See figure 13-8.) To support this free flow of information, structural and technological impediments to information exchange will need to be minimized. In addition, adequate security and confidentiality mechanisms will need to be put in place so that all participants will trust the system and input their information.

FIGURE 13-8 Plans for Information System Links

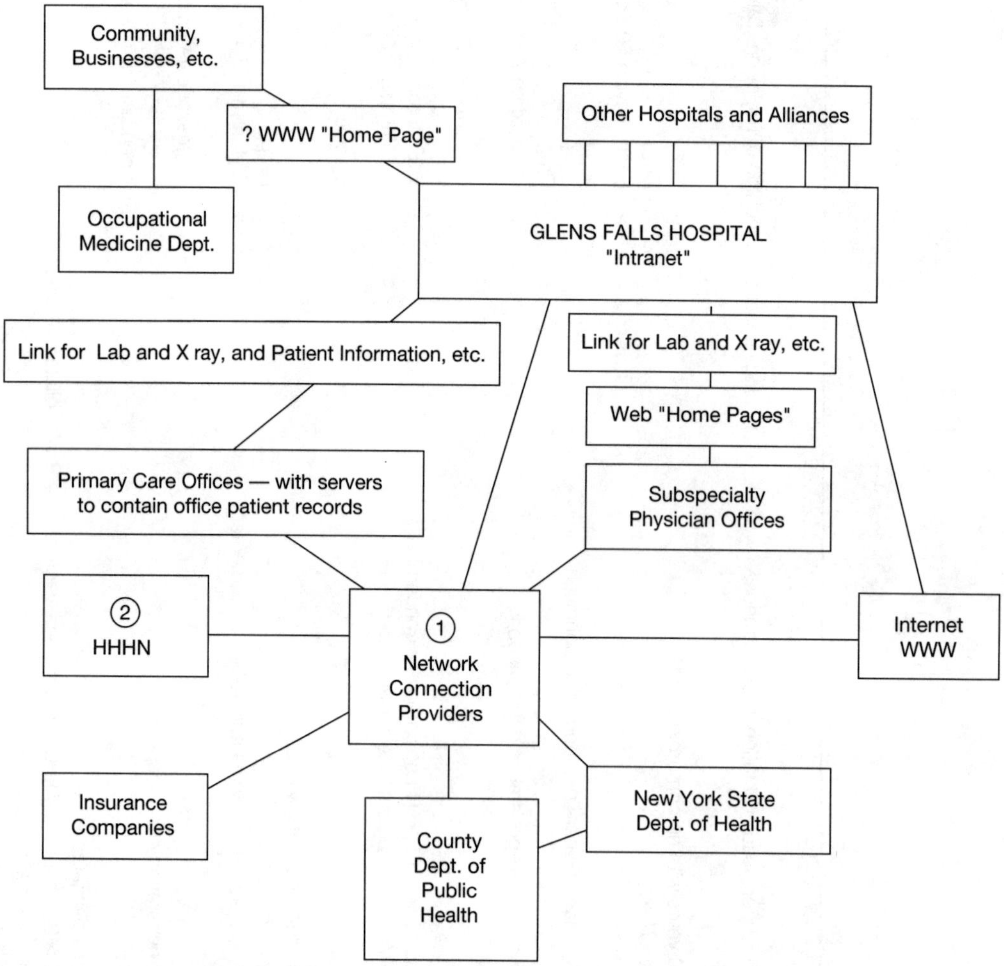

Recent advancements in computer networking technologies and multiple parallel computer network initiatives have allowed the hospital, physician's offices, and "mobile" laptop computer "offices" to all participate in joint data collection and information processing. Connections may occur by a number of methods, including closed networks, open networks, dedicated lines, and dialup modems. (1) "Medserv" is a local medical information server sponsored by our independent physician alliance (Adirondack Medicine, Inc.) and a state initiative for childhood immunization data collection. Members of the medical community, health service providers, and the hospital are joining together in a network of connections through this service via "dedicated" 56 kb lines and dialup modems. (2) Hudson Headwaters Health Network (HHHN) is a network of rural primary care health centers in our region.

Although not yet complete, system installations are planned for all key providers. A brief description of the system architecture and components is included in the following section to illustrate its potential for operationalizing the CAP guidelines as well as other disease management guidelines developed in the future.

The Medical Computer Network

The computer program is written with Microsoft Access™ 7.0 as the database program. It has been named PatRec, which stands for "patient records." Input screens are provided for physician office progress notes, hospital history and physical reports, and hospital discharge summaries. The history and physical input screen is shown in figure 13-9. Information is keyed in to the fields by the physician or an assistant. Pull-down menus of common data entries are available for some fields to minimize keyboard input time. In addition, a central data repository known as "KIT" (key information transfer) has been built into the system. This database includes key patient information that multiple providers can access at their points of service. All links have yet to be established; however, the final systems integration plan is expected to look similar to the diagram shown in figure 13-10.

At the time information is entered into a diagnosis field in any screen, the physician has immediate access to a list of guidelines relevant to the management of that patient. For example, when the physician enters a diagnosis of CAP, the CAP guidelines can be reviewed prior to making treatment decisions. The first screen available to the physician offers a choice of guidelines. For example, if the CAP protocol is selected for viewing, the next screen provides the physician with advice about types of patients who are *not* candidates for CAP protocol management. If the patient does not meet any of these exclusion criteria, the physician proceeds along the CAP protocol, which leads from the CAP diagnosis through a series of steps, such as accounting for the severities and comorbidities of the patient, deciding whether to manage as an inpatient or outpatient, and so on.

The CAP protocol begins with a calculation of the patient's illness severity. The physician may not need to key in additional data to calculate the patient's severity score if the necessary information has been entered into the system during the initial history and physical, from progress notes, or as a data transfer from the KIT. If there is not enough information in the system to evaluate patient illness severity, further information can be added in the appropriate fields. (See figure 13-11.) The physician is also prompted to flag any abnormal lab findings or vital signs. The data entered on this screen encompass all the factors that the ATS guidelines suggest should be considered when establishing the patient's severity of illness.

The next screen (figure 13-12) shows CAP guideline recommendations for hospitalization based on the weighting factors for comorbidities. If the decision is made to admit the patient, the next screen shows the reweighted factors relevant to the level-of-care categories. For example, Category 4 represents the severely ill patient for whom intensive care unit admission and mechanical ventilation is recommended. Category 3 represents the mildly to moderately ill patient who may be admitted to a general nursing unit for less intensive care.

If the physician elects to treat the patient as an outpatient, the outpatient protocol screen (figure 13-13) is displayed. Patients are categorized according to the severity of their illness, with corresponding CAP protocol recommendations. Subsequent screens offer further protocol details for inpatient and outpatient treatment choices. To enhance continuity of care for hospitalized patients, the physician can choose to print out a treatment plan, which is used as an admitting physician order sheet. (See figure 13-14.) Antibiotic orders are automatically transferred from the choices made on

FIGURE 13-9 Input Screen in PatRec for Hospital History and Physical (H&P)

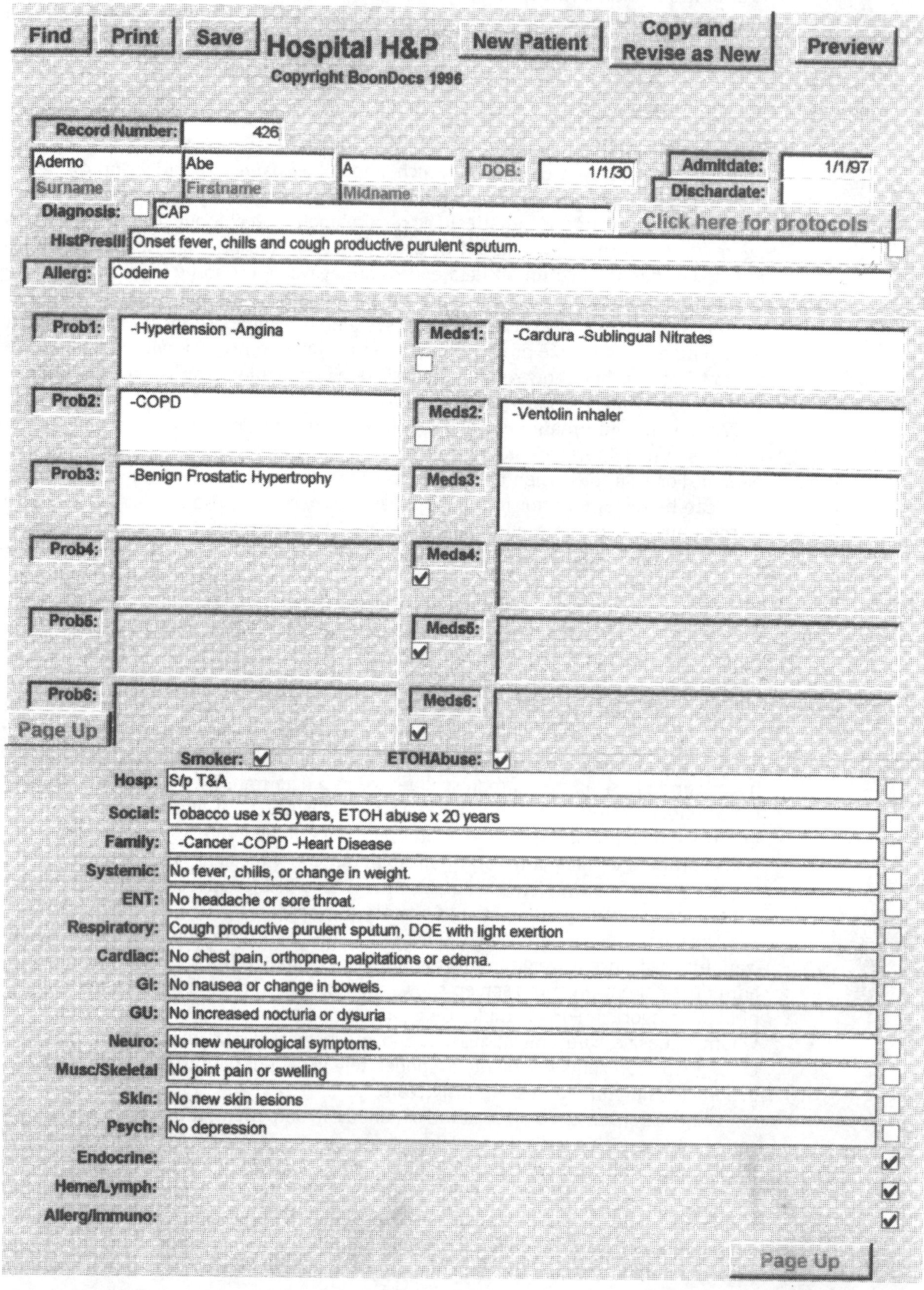

```
[Find] [Print] [Save]  Hospital H&P   [New Patient]  [Copy and Revise as New]   [Preview]
                      Copyright BoonDocs 1996

  Record Number:   426
  Ademo           Abe           A              DOB:    1/1/30    Admitdate:   1/1/97
  Surname         Firstname     Midname                          Dischardate:
  Diagnosis: ☐ CAP                                              Click here for protocols
  HistPresIll  Onset fever, chills and cough productive purulent sputum.
  Allerg:  Codeine

  Prob1:  -Hypertension -Angina          Meds1:  -Cardura -Sublingual Nitrates
                                           ☐
  Prob2:  -COPD                          Meds2:  -Ventolin inhaler
                                           ☐
  Prob3:  -Benign Prostatic Hypertrophy  Meds3:
                                           ☐
  Prob4:                                 Meds4:
                                           ☑
  Prob5:                                 Meds5:
                                           ☑
  Prob6:                                 Meds6:
  Page Up                                  ☑

              Smoker: ☑           ETOHAbuse: ☑
       Hosp:  S/p T&A
     Social:  Tobacco use x 50 years, ETOH abuse x 20 years
     Family:  -Cancer -COPD -Heart Disease
   Systemic:  No fever, chills, or change in weight.
        ENT:  No headache or sore throat.
 Respiratory: Cough productive purulent sputum, DOE with light exertion
    Cardiac:  No chest pain, orthopnea, palpitations or edema.
         GI:  No nausea or change in bowels.
         GU:  No increased nocturia or dysuria
      Neuro:  No new neurological symptoms.
Musc/Skeletal: No joint pain or swelling
       Skin:  No new skin lesions
      Psych:  No depression
  Endocrine:                                                                      ☑
 Heme/Lymph:                                                                      ☑
Allerg/Immuno:                                                                    ☑

                                                                         [Page Up]
```

FIGURE 13-9 Continued

OBJECTIVE FINDINGS:

BPSYST:	140	BPDIAST:	60	Pulse:	114	Resp:	38	Temp:	104

Gen:	WDWNWM in mild to moderate respiratory distress
Skin:	No lesions or rash
HEENT:	NCAT PEERL EOMI OC/OP: Clear, TMs: R: Clear L: Clear
Neck:	No JVD, adenopathy or thyromegaly. Carotids 2+ without bruit.
Chest:	Lungs: decreased breath sounds and increased volumes bilaterally with scattered rhonchi increased LLL
Heart:	RRR without murmur, gallop, or rub, and nl S1 and S2 PMI nondisplaced.
ABD:	Soft, nontender, no HSM or masses, BS+
Pelvic:	NA ☑
Back:	☑
Rectal:	WNL, stool heme negative
Extrem:	No cyanosis, clubbing or edema. Distal pulses intact bilateral.
Neurol:	No focal deficits. Oriented X 3.
LabResults:	WBC 22000
XRAYS:	LLL infiltrate
EKG:	WNL
Assess:	CAP
Plan:	As per CAP protocol#3

Examdate: 1/1/97

Philip J. Gara, Jr. MD

Screen shot of hospital H&P input form. Any information previously obtained in the physician office can be viewed within the form and used without re-input of information. Clicking on the Diagnosis field results in a "pop-up" button for protocols. Screen format can be customized to physician style.

---

previous screens. The physician order sheet can be sent to the hospital with the patient; the orders match those contained on the inpatient CAP pathway. Such integration has helped to promote physician acceptance of the inpatient pathway.

For hospitalized patients the PatRec system provides for creation of a discharge summary. (See figure 13-15.) The next screen gathers final outcomes data at the patient's last clinic follow-up visit. Summary printouts are available for the physician to use as office notes and for the hospital history and physical and discharge summary.

Variations in patient response are inevitable, and contingencies are built into the protocol to allow for such variation. A screen can be accessed as needed to view recommendations from local pulmonology and infectious disease experts for those patients not responding as expected.

The entire computerized CAP patient management process, including inpatient and outpatient care, is conceptualized in figure 13-16.

Refining the PatRec System in the Future

As physicians and hospital caregivers have familiarized themselves with the PatRec system, they have suggested several improvements. Plans are under way to incorporate some or all of these elements into the next system revision:

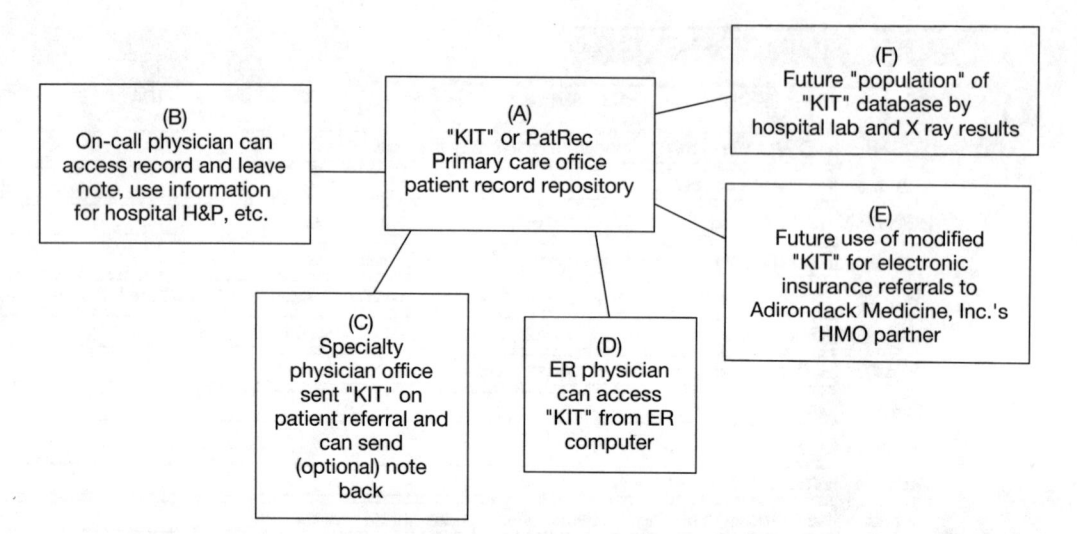

FIGURE 13-10 Information Flow Using Computerized Patient Records

(A) "KIT" or PatRec Primary care office patient record repository

(B) On-call physician can access record and leave note, use information for hospital H&P, etc.

(C) Specialty physician office sent "KIT" on patient referral and can send (optional) note back

(D) ER physician can access "KIT" from ER computer

(E) Future use of modified "KIT" for electronic insurance referrals to Adirondack Medicine, Inc.'s HMO partner

(F) Future "population" of "KIT" database by hospital lab and X ray results

Information gathered in the primary care office server allows access for specific database queries for multiple uses. (A) The primary care physician office computer server houses a database of outpatient clinical office records and selected inpatient information including an up-to-date medical problem list and medication list. (B) On-call covering physicians can have access to this information even during off hours. Information can be used for H&Ps, etc., without re-entering the data. (C) Referrals to specialty physicians include electronic transfer of a "KIT" of up-to-date key information on the patient. After seeing the patient the referring physician can then send back any changes and recommendations. Duplication and error in information as well as tests is limited. (D) ER physicians can access limited key information on patients during off hours. Primary care physicians will choose what information is to be available with the patient's permission. ER physicians can also leave notes with return notification of receipt for the primary care physician to allow better continuity of care. (E) Modified queries can electronically transfer appropriate information to insurance carriers to facilitate the referral process. (F) Eventual "population" of this program or a more complete clinical record system would further complete information flow.

- Transfer the recommended medications from the guideline protocol to the hospital record. Ultimately the patient's medication will be transferred automatically from the PatRec system to the "plan" area of the admission assessment note or the history and physical, as well as to the hospital physician order sheet. All of these forms can then be printed out on paper and included in the patient's hospital chart.
- Modify the outcomes reporting screen to obtain further detail.
- Develop a module that will allow assignment of patient identifiers (in place of names) so that data can be downloaded for research purposes without compromising patients' privacy.[22]
- Develop a module to allow electronic data transmitted from the hospital or other sources (lab results, X-ray reports, and so on) to be integrated with the patient's PatRec file.
- Add a report writer to allow user-friendly database queries for reporting purposes.
- Add other software enhancements to enhance physician acceptance of the system.

Automating the Pathway Variance Reporting Process

To evaluate data accumulated through the computerized guideline process and implementation of hospital clinical pathways, variances will need to be measured. Some of these data are obtainable from the clinical follow-up data fields in the CAP computer program. Methods for tracking inpatient CAP pathway variances have yet to be designed. Options currently being discussed include:

FIGURE 13-11 Community-Acquired Pneumonia Data Summary Screen

	Mild to Moderate	Boundary (Severe if)			Mild to Moderate	Boundary (Severe if)	
Systolic Pressure	140	<90	**Severe**	PaO2	66	<60	**Severe**
Diastolic Pressure	60	<60		PaCO2	44	>50	
Respiratory Rate	>30	36		WBC	22000	<4000 or >30,000	
Fever	>101.5	104		BUN	16	>20	
Pulse	114	>140		O2Sat	90	<90	

Click here to enter/update lab data

Based on vital sign severity indices, hospitalization is recommended as "Category 4 - Severe"

Please check any of the following conditions that apply:

Ademo

- ☐ Vasopressors needed >4 hours
- ☐ Urine output<20 ml/hr or total <80ml/4hr without explanation
- ☐ Mechanical ventilation required
- ☐ Opacity increase >50% in 48 hrs
- ☐ Bilateral/ multilobe involvement

Hospitalization recommended as "Category 4 -Severe" if any of the above apply.

- ☑ Empyema
- ☐ Meningitis
- ☐ Septic arthritis
- ☐ Endocarditis

Hospitalization as at least Category 3 is suggested if any of above suppurative complications exist:

- ☐ Malnutrition
- ☐ Diabetes Mellitus
- ☑ ETOH Abuse
- ☐ Post Splenectomy
- ☑ COPD or ROAD (Asthma)
- ☐ Vomiting, Dehydration

- ☐ Chronic Renal Failure
- ☐ Hospitalized within Year
- ☐ Altered Mental Status
- ☐ Suspicion of Aspiration
- Age over 65
- Patient's age 66

Above are significant comorbidity factors

Review indications

The next screen displays information transferred from the history and physical, key information transfer, or progress note with areas for addition of other relevant information needed for the community-acquired pneumonia protocol according to American Thoracic Society guidelines. Information that has not yet been added can be entered here.

FIGURE 13-12 Hospitalization Threshold Screen

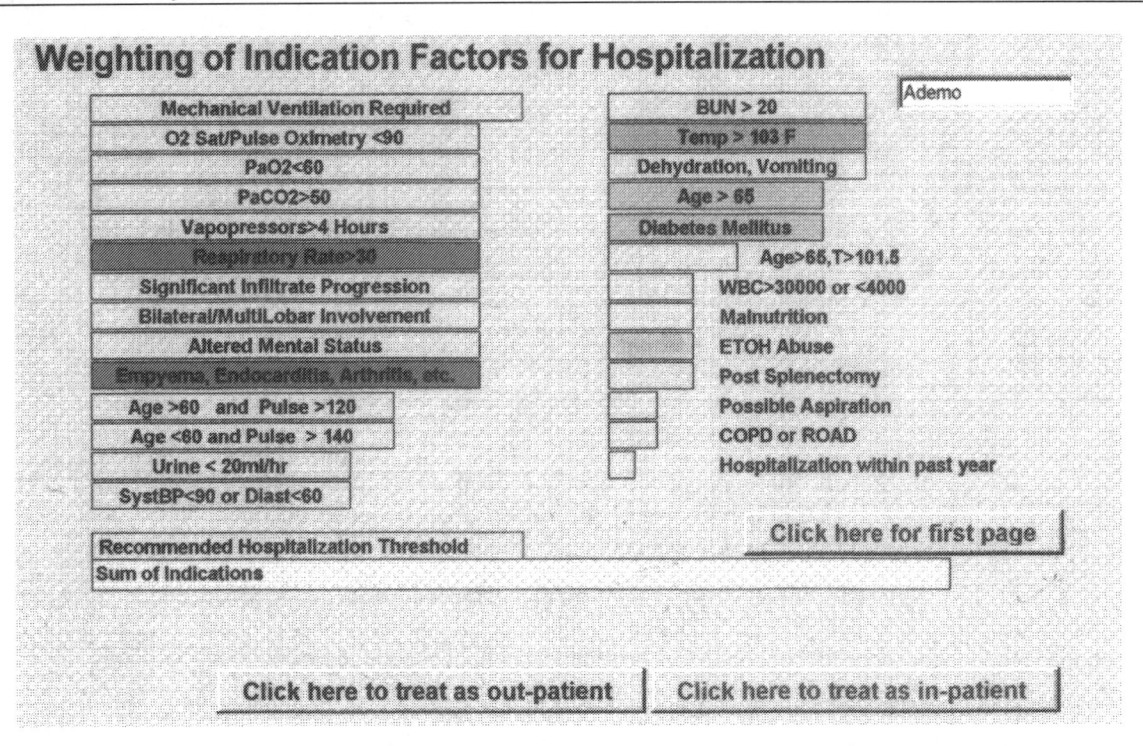

Weighting of Indication Factors for Hospitalization

Ademo

- Mechanical Ventilation Required
- O2 Sat/Pulse Oximetry <90
- PaO2<60
- PaCO2>50
- Vapopressors>4 Hours
- Respiratory Rate>30
- Significant Infiltrate Progression
- Bilateral/MultiLobar Involvement
- Altered Mental Status
- Empyema, Endocarditis, Arthritis, etc.
- Age >60 and Pulse >120
- Age <60 and Pulse > 140
- Urine < 20ml/hr
- SystBP<90 or Diast<60

- BUN > 20
- Temp > 103 F
- Dehydration, Vomiting
- Age > 65
- Diabetes Mellitus
- Age>65,T>101.5
- WBC>30000 or <4000
- Malnutrition
- ETOH Abuse
- Post Splenectomy
- Possible Aspiration
- COPD or ROAD
- Hospitalization within past year

Recommended Hospitalization Threshold
Sum of Indications

Click here for first page

Click here to treat as out-patient   Click here to treat as in-patient

This screen shows recommendations for hospitalization as calculated from the weighted criteria listed on the previous screen. Any positive indicators will appear in bright orange, showing their inclusion in the total weighting sum. A pink line under the Recommended Hospitalization Threshold will appear wider and deeper depending on the total sum. Any sum past the right side margin of the Recommended Hospitalization Threshold box indicates that the patient should be considered for hospitalization according to the community-acquired pneumonia guidelines.

FIGURE 13-13 Outpatient Treatment Selection Screen

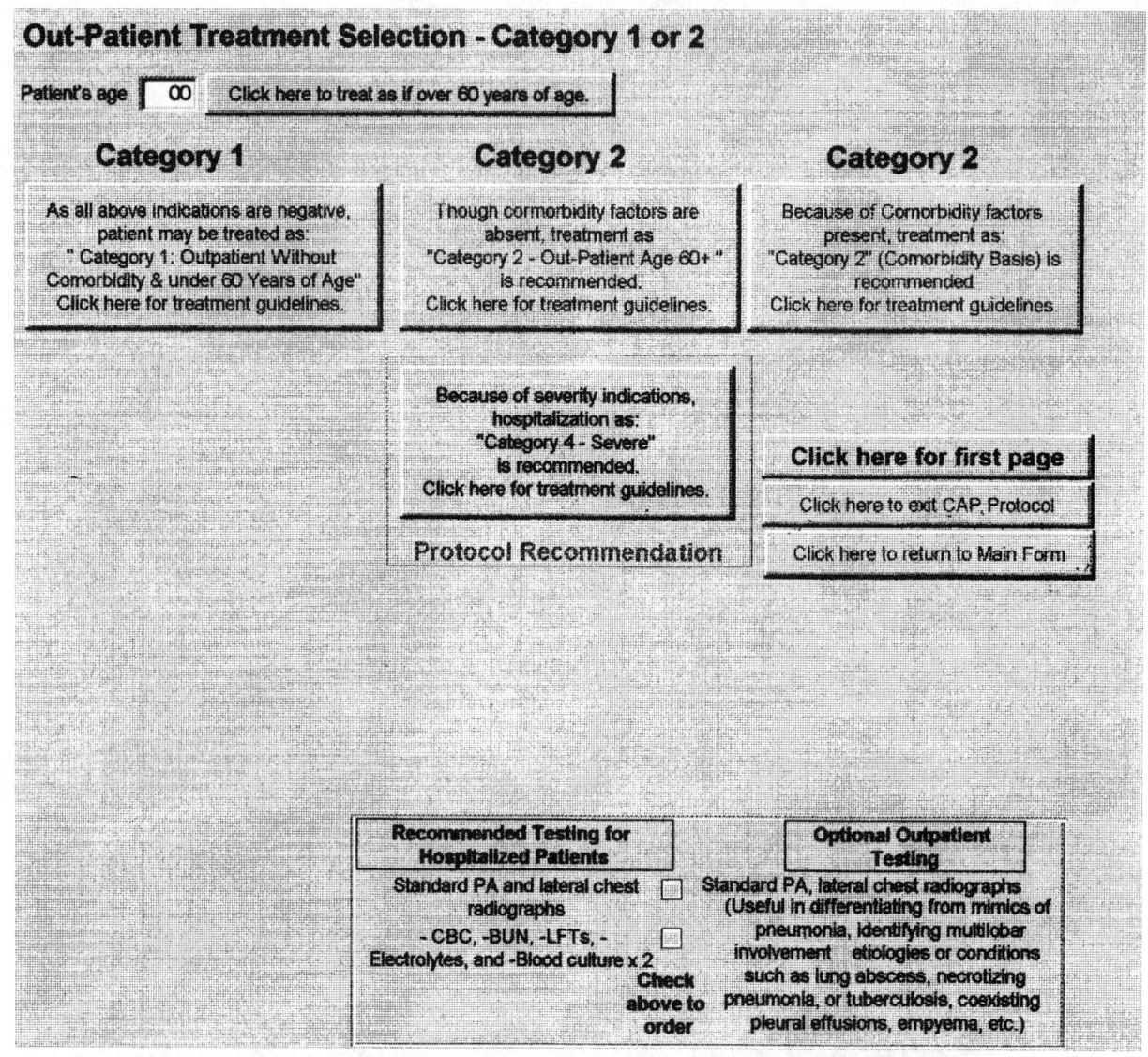

Choices of outpatient treatment options according to severity category are given on this screen. The category recommended by use of the community-acquired pneumonia guidelines is automatically highlighted with a red outline. Alerting the physician may encourage documentation of reasons for choices outside of the recommendations.

- Use the modules included in the hospital's clinical computer system that will be instituted in the future.
- Add a module to the CAP computer program.
- Document variances manually on paper for later input into the computer system.

Collecting, Reporting, and Analyzing Outcome Data

The CAP computer program automatically gathers outcome data for all patients. It will allow AMI physicians to analyze outcome data in a variety of ways. For example, the PatRec system will eventually be designed to provide information about an individual physician's practice patterns and patient outcomes as compared with regional and

FIGURE 13-14 Inpatient Physician Order Sheet for Patients with Community-Acquired Pneumonia

Patient Name:	Able, Arr Wee
Date of Birth:	1/3/44
Allergies:	No known drug allergies (NKDA)
Admit to:	Dr. Doe
	Regular medical floor/diagnosis: community-acquired pneumonia, category 3
Vitals:	Vital signs q shift
Diet:	Regular diet as tolerated ( ) Other ( )
Activity:	Bed rest with bathroom privileges
Respiratory Orders:	Oximetry or ABGs on room air on admission (circle one)
	O_2 2L NP if O_2 sat < 91%
	and titrate to keep >91%, recheck oximetry qod and wean as tolerated per respiratory protocol
X Rays:	Chest X ray on admission and repeat on hospital days 3 and 5
Lab:	CBC on admission and repeat on days 3 and 5
	SMA6/60 on admission
	Blood culture × 2 (if indicated)
	Sputum gram stain (if cough productive)
	AFB culture and isolation (if TB suspected)
Meds:	Continue patient's prehospitalization medications
Antibiotics:	Erythromycin (500 mg qid × 10d)
	Cefuroxime 750 mg IV q 8 hours

Jane M. Doe, M.D.   3/30/96

national norms. A series of measures will be used to determine the outcome of patients managed according to the CAP guidelines. These measures include:

- Time from first medical intervention until patient returns to normal temperature
- Time from start of IV antibiotic until transition to oral antibiotic
- Time from first visit to discontinuation of active management (including follow-up physician visits)
- Hospital length of stay
- Time from first visit to patient's return to subjective health (the time at which the patient believes that maximum expected function has returned)
- Time from first visit until patient returns to normal activity
- Mortality rate
- Complication rates
- Patient satisfaction
- Physician satisfaction
- Avoidance of hospitalization
- Estimated dollars spent in managing the pneumonia episode of care

Data for these measures will be captured in the PatRec computerized information system to enable ongoing performance assessments to evaluate issues such as:

FIGURE 13-15 Outcomes Data Collection Screen

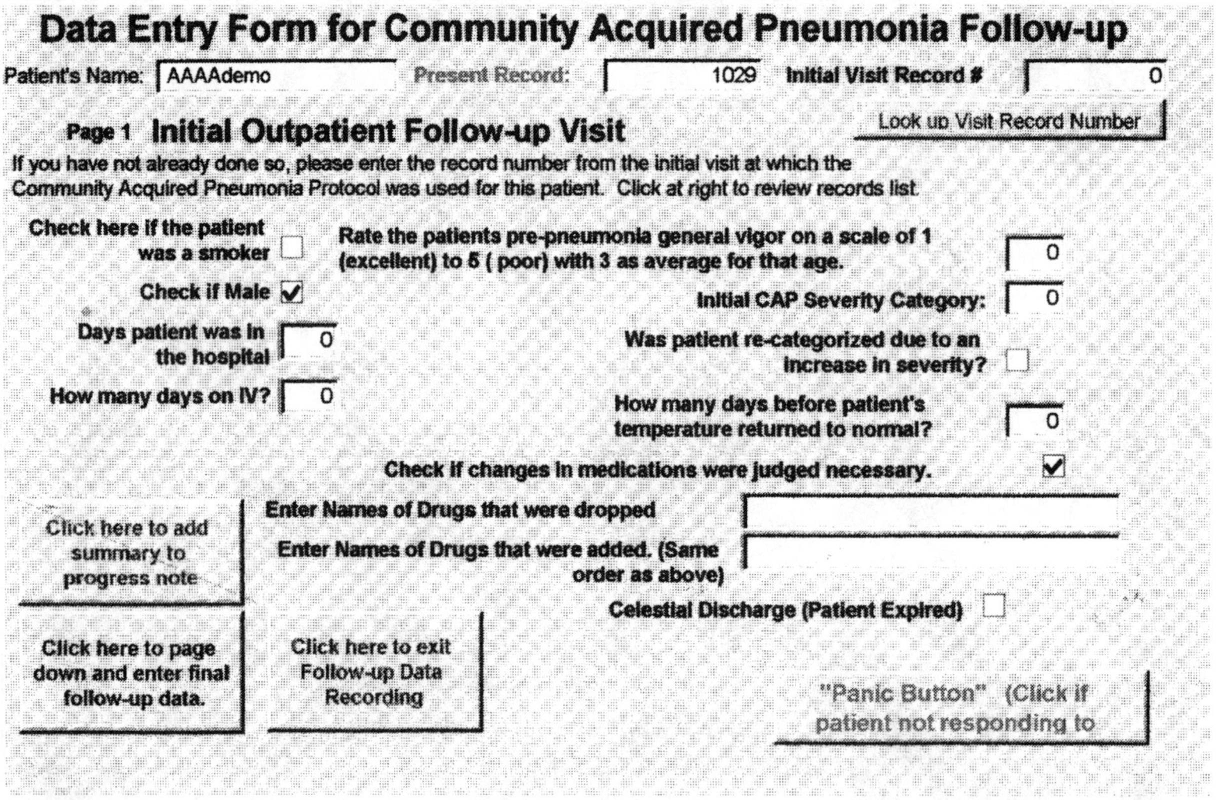

Data Entry Form for Community Acquired Pneumonia Follow-up

Patient's Name: AAAAdemo   Present Record: 1029   Initial Visit Record #: 0

Page 1 Initial Outpatient Follow-up Visit   Look up Visit Record Number

If you have not already done so, please enter the record number from the initial visit at which the Community Acquired Pneumonia Protocol was used for this patient. Click at right to review records list.

Check here if the patient was a smoker ☐

Check if Male ☑

Days patient was in the hospital: 0

How many days on IV? 0

Rate the patients pre-pneumonia general vigor on a scale of 1 (excellent) to 5 (poor) with 3 as average for that age. 0

Initial CAP Severity Category: 0

Was patient re-categorized due to an increase in severity? ☐

How many days before patient's temperature returned to normal? 0

Check if changes in medications were judged necessary. ☑

Click here to add summary to progress note

Enter Names of Drugs that were dropped

Enter Names of Drugs that were added. (Same order as above)

Celestial Discharge (Patient Expired) ☐

Click here to page down and enter final follow-up data.

Click here to exit Follow-up Data Recording

"Panic Button" (Click if patient not responding to

Following hospitalization, data is collected in follow-up entry screens by physicians or other designated staff members. This information can potentially also be added automatically to the hospital discharge summary or office note in narrative form.

- The degree to which the guidelines were followed
- Patient management changes that occurred over time as a result of guideline use, for example:
  - Hospital length of stay
  - Use of antibiotics (parenteral versus oral)
  - Ancillary test utilization
  - Time required for patients to return to full function
  - Amount of variation in CAP treatment among community physicians
- Whether adherence to the guidelines improved patients' clinical outcomes
- How IPA-initiated modifications in the guidelines affect physicians' practice patterns
- How physician-initiated modifications in the guidelines affect patient outcomes
- How physicians use clinical practice information when it is made available to them at the point of patient care delivery

To ensure that information is captured on all patients with CAP regardless of where they are receiving care, communication lines have to be established with the hospital and physician providers. The study project coordinators will be alerted to inpatient CAP admissions by notice from cooperating physicians or by the hospital admissions department. Information about CAP patients treated outside the hospital

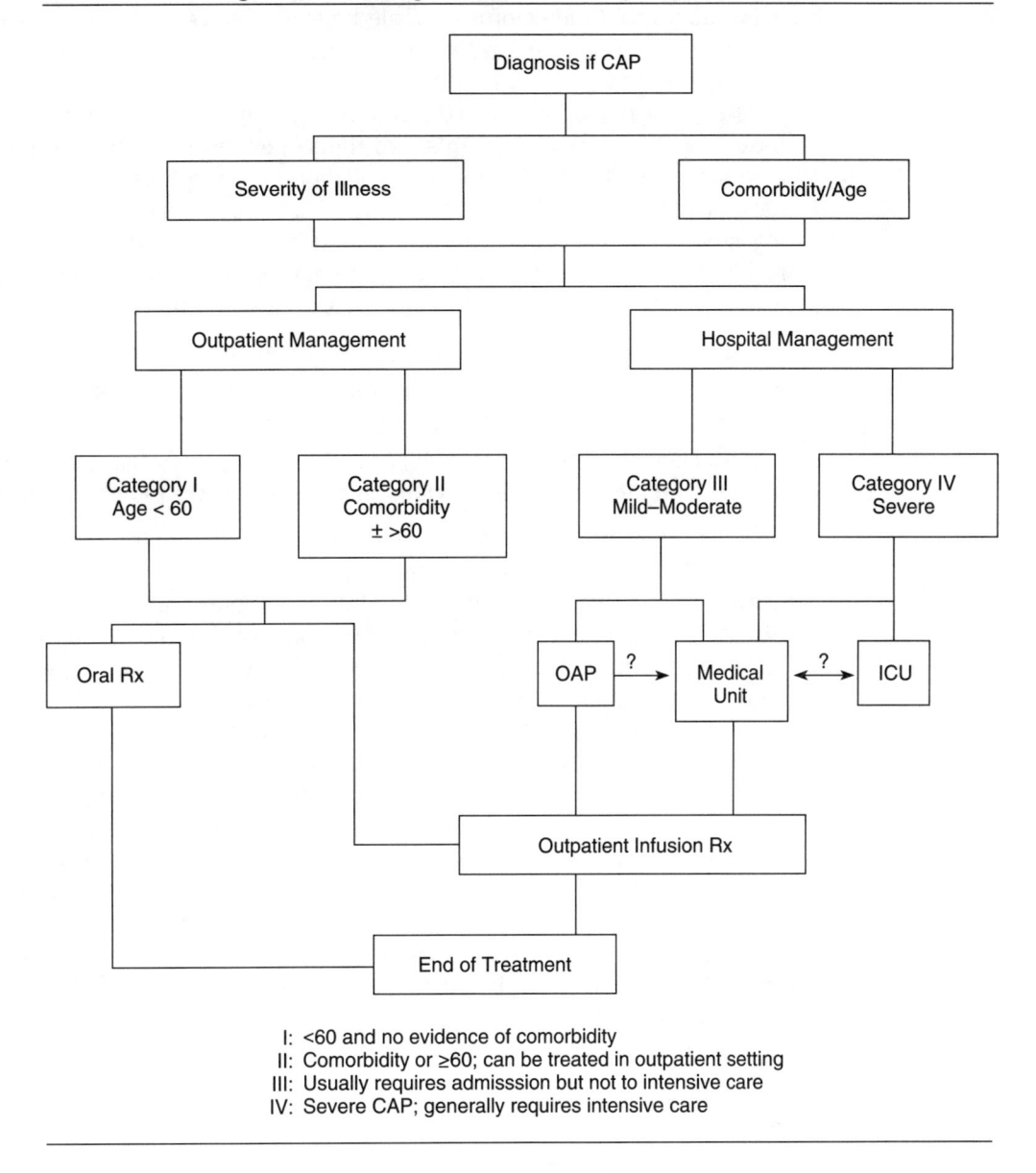

FIGURE 13-16 Algorithm for Management of Community-Acquired Pneumonia

```
                    Diagnosis if CAP
                    /              \
          Severity of Illness    Comorbidity/Age
                    \              /
              ┌──────────┴──────────┐
     Outpatient Management    Hospital Management
          /        \              /           \
   Category I   Category II   Category III   Category IV
   Age < 60     Comorbidity   Mild–Moderate  Severe
                ± >60
        |                        |        ?        |     ?
     Oral Rx                   OAP  ←→  Medical  ←→  ICU
                                         Unit
                         |
                 Outpatient Infusion Rx
                         |
                  End of Treatment
```

I: <60 and no evidence of comorbidity
II: Comorbidity or ≥60; can be treated in outpatient setting
III: Usually requires admisssion but not to intensive care
IV: Severe CAP; generally requires intensive care

is supplied by participating physicians in the community or the emergency care center of the hospital.

The CAP project is in the early phases of data collection. As the process continues improvements are planned, particularly the creation of a PatRec module to transmit CAP records to the project coordinator confidentially. Capture of study data will improve significantly with the distribution of the enhanced PatRec program to local physicians.

SUMMARY

Since the first set of nationally developed clinical practice guidelines were disseminated, there have been many studies on how to garner physician compliance. Computerization has been a favored implementation strategy; however, many older computer systems required complex data input and physician knowledge of DOS-based software programs. Studies often revealed a lack of physician acceptance and use. With recent advancements information systems have become more user friendly, allowing greater ease of input and access.

Recently, physicians have become more enthusiastic about integrating computer-based decision support systems into their practices.[23-25] For example, the quality of care for patients with CAP in three collaborating hospitals in Missouri was shown to have increased through the monitoring of key process indicators, coupled with ongoing analysis and feedback.[26] The implementation of guidelines in that community resulted in a significant reduction in patient mortality and length of stay. Several interesting recommendations were made by the study authors:

- It is important that each set of practice guidelines be tailored to specific user needs.
- Quick reference guides containing recommendations and key findings must be conveniently available to health care providers.
- Physicians will respond favorably to feedback on the quality of their management when the information is provided in a clear, private, and objective manner.

Like many providers who are working toward developing computer-stored patient records, AMI and GFH find themselves somewhere along an evolutionary continuum, using a hybrid system encompassing both computer and paper records. At times the disease management initiative and the design of the integrated information system have created more questions than answers. However, by starting with small projects, health care providers hope to eventually develop larger systems that will meet the needs of all clinicians in all provider sites. Many physicians in active clinical practice in this community are eager to turn their mountains of paper information into computerized patient outcome data that can be used to constantly improve patient care.

The caregivers in the GFH community have the opportunity to create a disease management model that impacts patient care throughout the continuum. This effort takes commitment and focused energy by all parties involved in the delivery of health care, including physicians, the hospital, and the public health agencies. Information systems will play a critical role in linking all aspects of the disease management model and providing outcomes data that caregivers can use to constantly improve their processes. Although the Glens Falls health care community is at the beginning of this long journey, it strongly believes it is on the right road!

References

1. Kanouse, D. E., and others. *Changing Medical Practice Through Technology Assessment: An Evaluation of the NIH Consensus Department Program.* Ann Arbor, MI: Association for Health Services Research and Health Administration Press, 1989.

2. Woolf, S. H. Practice guidelines: a new reality in medicine. III. Impact on patient care. *Archives of Internal Medicine* 153:2646–55, 1993.

3. Greco, P. J., and Eisenberg, J. M. Changing physicians' practices. *New England Journal of Medicine* 329:1271–73, 1993.

4. VanAmringe, M., and Shannon, T. Awareness, assimilation, and adoption: the challenge of effective dissemination and the first AHCPR-sponsored guidelines. *Quality Review Bulletin* 13:397–404, 1992.

5. Grant, J., Hayes, R., Pates, R., and others. HCFA's health care quality improvement program: the medical informatics challenge. *Journal of the American Medical Informatics Association* 3(1):15–26, Jan.–Feb. 1996.

6. Kaegi, L. Meeting update: Using guidelines to change clinical behavior: dissemination through area health education centers and geriatric education centers. *Quality Review Bulletin* 5:165–69, 1993.

7. Lomas, J., Anderson, G., Domnick-Pierre, K., and others. Do practice guidelines guide practice? *New England Journal of Medicine* 321(19):1306–11, 1989.
8. Pearson, S., Goulart-Fisher, D., Lee, T., and others. Critical pathways as a strategy for improving care: problems and potential. *Annals of Internal Medicine* 123:941–48, 1995.
9. Sullivan, F., and Mitchell, E. Has general practitioner computing made a difference to patient care? A systematic review of published reports. *British Medical Journal* 311:848–52, Sept. 30, 1995.
10. Epstein, R., and Sherwood, L. From outcomes research to disease management: a guide for the perplexed. *Annals of Internal Medicine* 124:832–37, 1996.
11. Harris, J. Disease management: new wine in new bottles? *Annals of Internal Medicine* 124:838–42, 1996.
12. Greenfield, S., Niederman, M., Wernsing, D., and others. Impact of health outcomes on clinical practice: focus on infectious disease. *Infections in Medicine* 13(suppl. B), Mar. 1996.
13. Hussein, T. The nurse case manager in acute care settings: job description and function. *JONA* 23(10):53–61, Oct. 1993.
14. Johnson, K., and Proffitt, N. A decentralized model for case management. *Nursing Economics* 13(3):142–51, 165, 1995.
15. American Thoracic Society Ad Hoc Committee of the Scientific Assembly on Microbiology, Tuberculosis, and Pulmonary Infections. Guidelines for the initial management of adults with community-acquired pneumonias: diagnosis, assessment of severity, and initial antimicrobial therapy. *American Review of Respiratory Disease* 148:1418–26, 1993.
16. Fang, G., Fine, M., Orloff, J., and others. New and emerging etiologies for community-acquired pneumonia with implications for therapy. *Medicine* 69(5):307–16, 1990.
17. Fine, M., Smith, M., Carson, C., and others. Prognosis and outcomes of patients with community-acquired pneumonia. *JAMA* 275(2):134–41, 1996.
18. Dillon-Bader, V., and others. Results of Ceftriaxone-to-Ceftizoxime switch program for treatment of uncomplicated community acquired pneumonia. *Formulary* 31(3):221–29, 1996.
19. Roberts, R., Rosof, B., Thompson, R. Practice guidelines: coping with information overload. *Patient Care*, Feb. 29, 1996.
20. Banks, N. J. Constructing algorithm flowcharts for performance measure evaluation. In: *Using Clinical Practice Guidelines to Evaluate Quality of Care.* Vol. 2, *Methods.* Rockville, MD: U.S. Department of Public Health and Human Services, Public Health Service, Agency for Health Care Policy and Research, Mar. 1995.
21. Niederman and others.
22. U.S. Congress, Office of Technology Assessment. *Protecting Privacy in Computerized Medical Information* (OTA-TCT-576). Washington, DC: U.S. Government Printing Office, Sept. 1993.
23. Evans, R. S., and others. Improving empiric antibiotic selection using computer decision support, *Archives of Internal Medicine* 154:878–84, 1994.
24. Hayward, R. S. A., and others. Implementing preventive care guidelines: information tools for the clinician. *Mayo Clinic Visit,* July 1992.
25. Norman, L. A., and Hardin, P. A. Computer-assisted outcomes management in the ambulatory care setting. In: P. L. Spath, editor. *Medical Effectiveness and Outcomes Management: Issues, Methods and Case Studies.* Chicago: American Hospital Publishing, 1996.
26. Fortune, G., Elder, S., Jaco, D., and others. Opportunities for improving the care of patients with community acquired pneumonia. *Clinical Performance and Quality Health Care* 4(1):41–43, 1996.

CHAPTER 14

Linking Expert Systems to Outcomes Analysis

H. Edmund Pigott, Greg Alter, and Deborah L. Heggie

Expert systems are computerized information systems that attempt to interpret patient information using expertise captured in a computerized database known as a *knowledge base*. Knowledge engineers design these rule-based expert systems by interviewing medical experts and constructing decision rules and scoring algorithms based on the experts' practical experiences and insights, institutional policies, and the medical research literature. A typical rule used within a computerized system for ventilators might read, "If a patient's spontaneous breathing rate changes by more than 10 percent and the change is larger than 5 breaths per minute and the breathing rate is between 0.5 and 70 breaths per minute and the ventilator mode was changed within the last minute, then bring the change to the attending physician's attention."[1]

Implementing expert systems within behavioral health care services is an alluring and frightening prospect. In general, behavioral health has lagged behind other specialties in recognizing the importance of explicitly linking critical patient variables to the differential treatment decision-making process. This failure has stymied progress in the delivery of effective behavioral health services, as well as muted society's recognition of the value such services provide.[2] Furthermore, it undermines behavioral health's quest for parity in health care insurance benefits.

Despite the wealth of empirically sound treatment outcomes research, few such findings filter down to influence actual practice on a widely used and consistent basis. Even when consensus-based guidelines explicitly recommend a particular treatment regimen, caregivers often fail to consider these suggestions.[3,4] Historically, practitioners have overemphasized the "art" of clinical practice and minimized their ability to stabilize service delivery in behavioral health care because of the "unique" circumstances of each patient.[5]

This fundamental professional bias preserves practitioners' decision-making autonomy and protects many from rigorously examining the soundness of their clinical decisions. During or before treatment, authoritative rationales can be generated for almost any clinical decision. This results in wide variance in clinical practice across providers within an organization and even for the individual providers themselves.

In general, managed care organizations have been unable to decrease variance in the clinical and resource allocation decision-making process. Case managers in managed care organizations depend on providers for the information necessary to make treatment authorization decisions. It has been the authors' experience that this information exchange is subject to possible distortions at multiple points due to a variety of factors, including:

- Providers' clarity in organizing and presenting information
- The interpersonal dynamic between providers and case managers and type of day they have had
- Case managers' reactions to providers and their secondhand impressions of patients
- Providers' reluctance to appeal denials for fear of being identified as "managed care unfriendly" and of the potential economic consequences to themselves and their organizations
- Organizational pressures faced by case managers and providers when making inappropriate or high-cost level-of-care decisions

These factors cause widely divergent types and costs of care, and treatment outcomes, for patients with similar conditions. Furthermore, such variance impedes continuous clinical improvement efforts because it is difficult (if not impossible) to reliably identify and repeat those processes that resulted in superior care.[6]

Inconsistencies and flaws in clinical judgment were first documented by psychologist Paul Meehl in his 1954 book *Clinical versus Statistical Prediction: A Theoretical Analysis and Review of the Evidence*. Meehl discovered what 4 decades of subsequent research has overwhelmingly proved: clinical judgment is inferior to empirically based approaches to diagnosis and treatment planning. This research has generally shown that behavioral health professionals' personal biases, overreliance on intuition, and quick decision making based on inadequate information often clouds clinical judgment when it is being applied to specific patients.[7]

These realities are implicitly acknowledged by the tradition of peer supervision within all behavioral health professions. The very nature of assessing and treating people struggling with life's problems can cloud the judgment of even the most experienced clinicians. Too often, providers and case managers form quick hypotheses while assessing clinical situations and *then* look for supportive evidence. Like most people, behavioral health professionals tend to find what they are looking for. In this process, evidence contrary to their initial hypothesis is all too often either ignored or discounted, and alternative explanations for all available data are not fully considered.[8]

THE ROLE OF EXPERT SYSTEMS IN DECISION MAKING

Computers do not suffer from biased decision making. However, this fact is not meant to imply that findings from any expert system should be rigidly applied. The goal of an expert system is to provide more complete and accurate information quickly to the clinician. By improving clinical decision making, improved patient outcomes are expected. Expert systems by definition have limitations. There will always be clinical situations that require the professional to select (or deselect) other treatment components based on additional data or a different interpretation of the available data. In psychiatry, for example, it is generally agreed that the decision-making process should be one that balances individualized clinical acumen and information derived from empirical studies of groups of patients.[9]

The use of expert systems still plays two vital roles. First, the system forces professionals to be explicit and thoughtful about why they are making "nonroutine" decisions. This thought process alone enhances the quality of care. Second, if such decisions result in superior patient outcomes, this knowledge can be incorporated into treatment protocol updates, thereby making it more likely to be repeated for future patients with similar profiles.

THE ROLE OF EXPERT SYSTEMS IN CONTINUOUS QUALITY IMPROVEMENT

The primary purpose of clinical expert systems is to reduce variation in independent variables (the host of clinical and resource allocation decisions that together constitute treatment) so that dependent variables (treatment outcomes) become more directly interpretable. By reducing variance in clinical decision making organizations are better able to reliably identify and repeat those clinical processes that result in superior outcomes while discarding less effective practices.[10]

At this core, reducing variance in the implementation of independent variables is the foundation of true continuous quality improvement. W. Edwards Deming, the father of the continuous quality movement, was relentless in such a focus. Deming's genius was in assisting Japanese companies to stabilize, and reduce variance in, manufacturing processes (independent variables) to ensure production of consistent products (dependent variables, or "outcomes"). Deming recognized that the essence of manufacturing was its ability to replicate the production of products.[11] The foundation of replication is stabilized operations creating a near perfect cause-and-effect relationship between known production processes, on the one hand, and product quality and production cost, on the other. Deming observed that reducing variability in operations improves quality and productivity. This situation occurs because as the number of variables decreases, the opportunity to clearly identify and widely implement superior processes increases proportionally. When operations are stabilized, companies can statistically analyze process and outcome data to identify specific operational components for refinement. Such an interative formula yields substantial improvements in productivity and quality over time.

Deming's concepts are not foreign to health caregivers; in fact, they form the basis of the five steps of scientifically sound treatment outcomes research:[12]

1. Clearly define the independent variables, or the components of treatment, that investigators are able to measure and manipulate.
2. Define the critical characteristics of the patient for whom treatment is intended.
3. Measure the consistency of the treatment's implementation.
4. Collect relevant dependent variables, or outcomes, that investigators believe will be differentially affected by providing, or not providing, treatment.
5. In treatment outcome studies, the final step is analyzing the data and writing up the report.

Unlike a true continuous quality improvement process, most treatment outcome studies end at this point.

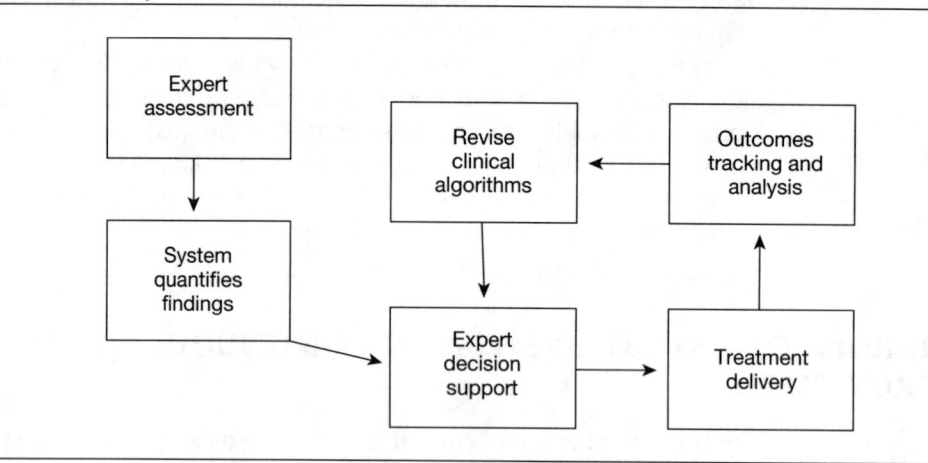

FIGURE 14-1 Clinical Quality Improvement Model That Links Expert Systems to Outcomes Analysis

```
Expert
assessment
     |
     v
System                Revise              Outcomes
quantifies  ----->    clinical   <-----   tracking and
findings              algorithms          analysis
                        |                    ^
                        v                    |
                      Expert              Treatment
                      decision   ----->   delivery
                      support
```

LINKING EXPERT DECISION SUPPORT SYSTEMS TO OUTCOMES ANALYSIS

A clinical quality improvement model linking the use of expert decision support systems to outcomes analysis is illustrated in figure 14-1. Critical assessment information is analyzed to identify the most appropriate treatment plan for a specific patient based on available data. The model then links the prospective focus of expert systems with the retrospective rigor of outcomes analysis to foster the ongoing refinement of the knowledge-based rules and decision algorithms.

Traditionally, the building of a health care expert system required "experts" to translate their knowledge to programmers, who then replicated the experts' decision-making process in a software format using various scoring algorithms. Any changes to the resulting software required additional programming time and expense. A number of such "hard-coded" expert systems have been built for behavioral health care to assist providers in diagnosing patients[13] and making level-of-care decisions.[14]

Use of "authoring tools" is a different approach to building software applications. Authoring tools enable nonprogrammers to build software applications without possessing any software programming expertise. The relationship between the authoring tool and the resulting applications is analogous to that of any software authoring tool that can be used to create specific "products" (or applications) within defined parameters. For example, a word processor is an authoring tool for building an infinite number of document applications (résumés, letters, treatment plans, manuscripts, and so on); and while a word processor is a robust document authoring tool, it does not work well as a spreadsheet or database manager.

Authorware is one such authoring tool that can be used by nonprogrammers to build interactive instructional software programs for providers.[15] Unfortunately, Authorware and similar authoring tools do not allow nonprogrammer developers to integrate scoring algorithms and decision rules into their software programs. This obstacle makes such tools incapable of building expert system applications without the assistance of programming experts.

PATHware is an expert system authoring tool that can be used to build point-of-care decision support applications for health care providers. As an authoring tool, PATHware can be used to build a limitless number of expert system, disease management, and outcomes tracking applications without requiring the creators to have any software programming expertise. Such applications can include complex scoring algorithms and decision rules that replicate an "expert" decision-making process based on available data. This allows the content experts to rapidly build, implement, and continually refine their applications without having to go through an iterative knowledge exchange process with programmers.

The resulting PATHware-authored applications are accessed by clinicians at the point of care either in a client-server environment or via the Internet and secure intranets. PATHware-authored applications can also be embedded into larger software systems such as computerized medical records and managed care and practice management systems.

HOW ONE BEHAVIORAL HEALTH CARE ORGANIZATION IS LINKING EXPERT DECISION SUPPORT AND OUTCOMES ANALYSIS

Pacific Applied Psychology Associates, Inc. (PAPA), is an integrated behavioral health delivery system serving eight counties in northern California. PAPA has more than 350,000 covered lives in its capitated HMO contracts as well as approximately 300,000 covered lives in preferred provider contracts. To provide care for these clients, PAPA has more than 200 behavioral health professionals in its provider network.

Since 1992 PAPA has been using a computerized medical application whose claims, reporting, credentials, and intake functions it has customized. PAPA's information system is now undergoing transition to an integrated system that will include clinical decision support tools offering advice to the clinician regarding diagnosis, testing, and treatment. These software tools will be available to the 200 PAPA providers through a combined local area network and intranet environment.

PAPA chose to first implement an expert system that will assist its network providers in making more consistent level-of-care decisions for psychiatric patients in crisis. To accomplish this task, PATHware's application of the Crisis Triage Rating Scale (figure 14-2) is being integrated into PAPA's computerized medical records and practice

FIGURE 14-2 Crisis Triage Rating Scale

Question 1: How dangerous is this patient?

1. Expresses or hallucinates homicidal or suicidal ideas or has recently made a serious attempt
2. Same as 1, but ideas or behavior are ego-dystonic and no current signs of violent behavior
3. Expresses suicidal or homicidal ideas with ambivalence or has made only ineffective gestures
4. Some suicidal or homicidal ideation or behaviors, or history of same, but wishes to control such behaviors
5. No suicidal or homicidal ideation or behavior nor history of same

Question 2: How much social support does this patient have?

1. No family, friends, or others, nor can social service agencies provide the level of immediate support needed.
2. Some support might be mobilized, but its effectiveness will be limited
3. Support system potentially available, but significant difficulties exist in mobilizing it
4. Interested family, friends, or others, but some question exists of ability or willingness to help
5. Interested family, friends, or others able and willing to provide support needed

Question 3: To what degree is the patient able and willing to cooperate?

1. Unable to cooperate or actively refuses cooperation
2. Shows little interest in, or comprehension of, efforts being made on his or her behalf
3. Passively accepts intervention maneuvers being made on his or her behalf
4. Wants to get help but is ambivalent or motivation is not strong
5. Actively seeks outpatient treatment; willing and able to cooperate

Source: Reprinted, with permission, from Bengelsdorf, H., Levy, L. E., Emerson, R. L., and others. A crisis triage rating scale: brief dispositional assessment of patients at risk for hospitalization. *Journal of Nervous and Mental Disease* 172(7): 424–30, July 1984.

management system. The Crisis Triage Rating Scale was selected for the assessment because it is a public domain instrument with established reliability and validity for assessing high-risk psychiatric patients.[16] The authors of this rating system found that those who scored below a median point on the scale required hospitalization, while those who scored above this point were suitable for crisis intervention as outpatients.

Level-of-Care Decision Support

PAPA's network providers will complete the Crisis Triage Rating Scale as part of the patient intake process. For network providers, access to this rating system on line will:

- Reduce the amount of time needed for completing treatment authorization requests
- Improve the consistency of level-of-care determinations
- Enhance provider confidence in the treatment authorization process

Once the Crisis Triage Rating Scale is completed for an individual patient, PATHware quantifies the results using the rating scale's scoring algorithm and provides a patient score. This score is considered by the provider in selecting the appropriate level of care for the patient. Providers are not required to accept the level-of-care recommendation made by the Crisis Triage Rating Scale. If they disagree with the recommendation, a free text field is provided for recording the provider's rationale for choosing a different level of care.

In all situations (provider agrees with the decision or provider disagrees), the PATHware program initiates an E-mail message to a PAPA case manager to inform him or her of the case, its disposition by the provider, and the appropriate case management criteria to be applied (for example, inpatient versus intensive outpatient versus standard outpatient criteria). The case manager E-mails back to the provider a confirmation of the services authorized.

Treatment Decision Support

Initially, PAPA will use PATHware only to enhance consistency in level-of-care decision making in its provider network. It plans to extend its PATHware use during 1997–98 to implement a number of expert system–driven clinical pathways. Developing such clinical pathways will encourage PAPA's protocol development team, made up of select network providers, to establish explicit links between presenting patient variables and more specific differential clinical decision making. Identifying and quantifying patient variables that influence such decision making will be critical in PAPA's development of expert system–driven clinical pathways.

For example, the protocol development team will use research findings and consensus provider opinion to answer the following questions about the care of depressed patients:

- Which patients are appropriate for cognitive-behavioral therapy, versus interpersonal therapy, versus distress tolerance training, versus a trial on medication alone, or medication in combination with one of the above?
- Which patients are appropriate for individual treatment, versus marital or family, versus group therapy, or some combination thereof?
- Which patients can have their initial medication evaluation performed by their primary care physicians (PCPs) or psychiatric nurse practitioners (PNPs), and which require a psychiatric evaluation? At present, 75 percent of all antidepressant medications are prescribed by PCPs with no rational triaging mechanism in place.

- Which depressed patients require long-term antidepressant therapy (managed by the patient's PCP, versus PNP, versus psychiatrist?) versus just a 4- to 6-month medication trial?
- Among depressed suicidal patients, which can be safely managed with a "no-harm" agreement, telephone monitoring, or multiple weekly contacts to manage their risk level, and which require an inpatient admission?
- Among substance-abusing depressed patients, which should first have a 4- to 6-week period of sobriety prior to initiation of depression treatment, and which will likely benefit from antidepressant therapy right away?

Even when more sophisticated, information-driven pathways are available, providers will not be expected to rigidly adhere to them. PAPA recognizes that there will always be clinical situations that require the provider to select (or deselect) recommended treatment components. The purpose of the pathway is to make these clinical "deviations" a conscious decision. If pathway deviations are ultimately identified as more efficient choices or as choices that lead to superior outcomes, they will be incorporated into future pathways revisions.

Outcomes Analysis

PAPA will store in its relational database the PATHware-recommended level of care, the level of care actually delivered, and the specific treatment components. These data will be used for aggregate outcomes analysis. At regularly scheduled intervals select outcome measures will be analyzed. By combining clinical outcomes data with service delivery data, PAPA's providers will be able to continually evaluate the validity of the expert system. In PAPA's situation, this includes assessing:

- The frequency of patients' being "bumped up" to a higher level of care during the first week of treatment. When this situation occurs, the accuracy of the expert system's level-of-care determination will be questioned.
- The rate of provider concurrence or nonconcurrence with the expert system's recommended level of care
- Patient readmission or relapse rates compared with industry norms
- The quality of clinical outcomes for patients

By conducting statistical analysis of information in this database, PAPA hopes to be able to predict the treatment course, cost, and resulting outcomes for patients with different risk severity profiles. Once this database captures enough historical data, a second PATHware-authored expert system will be implemented that triggers a request for consultation when patients are not progressing as predicted based on their profile.

An analysis of the database also can identify those patients whose risk profiles— and resulting clinical pathway—produce less-than-optimal outcomes. With such knowledge, PAPA can seek outside consultation for targeted pathway revisions. The relational database will also be used to identify critical elements in provider practice patterns that yield better patient outcomes. These elements can be incorporated into the pathways used for managing future patients. Because the pathways will be built using PATHware's expert system authoring tool, modifications will be easy to make.

SUMMARY

Expert systems have several advantages over traditional paper-based clinical pathways. Unlike traditional pathways, an expert system contains rules and decision algorithms that incorporate knowledge and judgment about the health problem at hand and alternative tests and treatments for it. These are built into the expert-based systems in the form of "if-then" decision rules as well as scoring algorithms, such as "If the patient's potassium is less than 3.0 mEq/dl and the patient is on digoxin, then the clinician should consider ordering potassium supplementation."[17] A recent review of systematic studies of the impact of point-of-care expert systems on clinician behavior reports generally positive effects.[18] Expert systems have also been shown to be useful in reminding clinicians of overlooked diagnosis and treatment alternatives and for interpreting and filtering information.[19] Traditional clinical pathways have not proved to be as powerful in their prospective decision support capabilities.

Expert systems also allow for capture of important process and outcome data. For example, by documenting in the computer their rationale for divergent practices, PAPA providers are also providing the information necessary for analyzing process and outcomes. Ultimately, the purpose of clinical pathways is to enable their rapid obsolescence through constant, knowledge-based updating. These updates are best accomplished by linking the prospective focus of expert systems with the retrospective rigor of outcomes analysis to accelerate advances in all aspects of health care service delivery, including behavioral health. No expert system will ever completely replace the provider's experience, memory, and judgment in clinical decision making. As caregivers gather more information about which treatment interventions truly "work" for a given health problem, marked deviations from established clinical paths will become less justifiable. However, there will continue to be room for variation in the judgmental application of treatment protocols to individual patients in particular settings and locations. Expert-based computer systems must be viewed as aids to clinician experience and judgment—not as substitutes for them.

References

1. East, T. D., Young, W. H., and Gardner, R. M. Digital electronic communication between ICU ventilators and computers and printers. *Respiratory Care* 37(9):1113–23, 1992.
2. Pigott, H. E. Computer decision-support as a clinicians' tool. In S. S. Sharfstein and R. K. Schereter, editors. *Managing Care, Not Dollars—Using the Continuum of Care.* Washington, DC: American Psychiatric Association Press, in press.
3. Ramseier, F. Our knowledge is patchwork: survey on the adherence to international guidelines concerning acute and long-term therapy in recurrent depressions and diseases in the schizophrenic field. *Schweiz Rundsch Med Prax* 24(85):792–97, June 11, 1996.
4. Zisselman, M. H., Rovner, B. W., and Shmuely, Y. Benzodiazepine use in the elderly prior to psychiatric hospitalization. *Psychosomatics* 37(1):38–42, Jan.–Feb. 1996.
5. Pigott, H. E. Linking outcomes analysis to critical clinical pathways. *Behavioral Healthcare Tomorrow* 4(1):59–61, Jan.–Feb. 1995.
6. Pigott, H. E., and Broskowski, A. Outcomes analysis: guiding beacon or bogus science? *Behavioral Health Management* 15(3):22–24, 1995.
7. Sleek, S. Ensuring accuracy in clinical decisions. *APA Monitor* 27(4):32–33, Apr. 1996.
8. Sleek, p. 33.
9. Goldner, E. M., and Bilsker, D. Evidence-based psychiatry. *Canadian Journal of Psychiatry* 40(2):97–101, Mar. 1995.
10. Bultema, J. K., Mailliard, L., Getzfrid, M. K., and others. Geriatric patients with depression: improving outcomes using a multidisciplinary clinical path model. *Journal of Nursing Administration* 26(1):31–8, Jan. 1996.
11. America's quality coaches. *CPI Purchasing Magazine,* 22–26, Mar. 1986.
12. Lind, 1753, quoted in Pocock, S. *Clinical Trials: A Practical Approach.* New York City: Wiley, 1983.

13. Coler, M., and Vincent, K. Coded nursing diagnoses on axes: a prioritized, computer-ready diagnostic system for psychiatric/mental health nurses. *Archives of Psychiatric Nursing* 1:125–31, 1988.
14. Gray, G., and Glazer, W. Psychiatric decision making in the 90s: the coming era of decision support. *Behavioral Healthcare Tomorrow* 3(1):47–54, 1994.
15. Crosbie, J., and Kelly, G. A computer-based personalized system of instruction course in applied behavior analysis. *Behavior Research Methods and Computers* 25:366–70, 1993.
16. Bengelsdorf, H., Levy, L. E., Emerson, R. L., and others. A crisis triage rating scale: brief dispositional assessment of patients at risk for hospitalization. *Journal of Nervous and Mental Disease* 172(7):424–30, July 1984.
17. Gibson, R. F., and Middleton, B. Health care information management systems to support CQI. In: S. D. Horn and D. S. P. Hopkins, editors. *Clinical Practice Improvement: A New Technology for Developing Cost-Effective Quality Health Care.* New York City: Faulkner and Gray, 1994, p. 109.
18. Johnston, M. E., and others. Effects of computer-based clinical decision support systems on clinician performance and patient outcome: a critical appraisal of research. *Annals of Internal Medicine* 120(2):135–42, Jan. 15, 1994.
19. Berner, E. S., and others. Performance of four computer-based diagnostic systems. *New England Journal of Medicine* 330(25):1792–96, June 23, 1994.

INDEX

Accepted practices, 226
Active and accountable family participation, 165, 169–70
Addictions Severity Index, 14–15
Administrative information systems, 183
Advanced practical nurse (APN)
 community based, 99
 in heart failure clinic, 87
 multidisciplinary disease management role, 91–92
Aggregate performance analysis, 29
Aggregate variance analysis, 78, 185–86
Allied health, 215
All Patient Refined-Diagnosis-Related Groups system, 211
Anterior laminectomy, 222
Assessment
 in home health care, 133, 135
 in multidisciplinary care planning, 108–9
Authoring tools, 256–57
Authorware, 256
Automated information systems. *See* Information systems

"Bad apples" approach, 39
BASIS-32 (Behavior and Symptom Identification Scale-32), 10, 14, 17
 results made available in real time, 12, 27, 29, 33
 sample form, 18–19
 sample report, 20–22
Beck Depression Inventory, 13–14
Bed rounds, 113–14, 121, 123
Behavioral health care
 expert systems in, 253–54, 257–59
 for geriatric patients, 117–18
 patient and family satisfaction with, 11
 performance measurement in, 9–34
Benchmarks
 externally-derived practice guidelines as, 47
 in geriatric evaluation and management program, 117, 118
 for home care paths, 141
 for outcomes data, 49
"Best practice" standards, 53, 117
Brief Symptom Inventory (BSI), 14

Cardiac catheterization, 201–12
Cardiac rehabilitation, 87–88
Cardiac rehabilitation nurse, 92
Cardiac surgery
 clinical pathways in, 164–65
 proactive pathway model for, 166–69
 reducing practice variation in open heart surgeries, 53–69
Cardiovascular radical outcome method (CV-ROM), 165–73
 clinical nurse coordinator–case manager in, 164, 165, 171–72
 family empowerment in, 166–67, 169, 176
 information system for, 172–73
 operational problems of, 177
 performance measurement for, 173–76
 in very complex cardiac surgery patients, 175–76
Care Connection, 79, 96
Care guides, 199
Care management. *See also* Case management
 care coordination, 78, 79
 interdisciplinary development model of, 72
 multidisciplinary initiative for, 71–101
 service-line model of, 78
 unit-based model of, 78
Care management coordinator, 78, 91
CAREVUE™ clinical information system, 54, 61, 68–69
Case management. *See also* Case managers
 advantages of, 146
 clinical paths compared with, 160
 defined, 147
 development of model, 146–57
 in disease management initiatives, 227–29
 early program difficulties, 157
 effectiveness measures for, 160–61
 in home care, 145–62
 ideal information system for, 182–86
 information system selection, 188–94
 integrated system at Bristol Medical Center, 214–15, 224
 in multidisciplinary disease management, 78–79
 patient selection for, 153–54, 229, 231
 staffing requirements for, 154–57
Case managers
 in cardiac surgery, 164, 165, 171–72
 as change agents, 229
 in geriatric evaluation and management program, 120
 in home care, 147–53, 161
 information requirements of, 181–82, 254
 in integrated case management system, 214–15
 job descriptions for, 148–51, 172, 230
 in multidisciplinary care planning, 106
Catholic Healthcare Initiatives, 77–78
Cause-and-effect diagrams
 for congestive heart failure, 82, 83
 for coronary artery bypass grafts, 57, 59
Center for Epidemiologic Studies Depression self-rating scale, 14
Champion physicians
 in clinical practice guideline implementation, 39, 41
 in disease management initiative, 84
 in geriatric evaluation and management program, 120, 124
Chart audit process, 25
Chart Audit tool, 17, 23–24
Charting by exception, 141
Chest pain, 222, 223
Chronic diseases, 80
Chronic obstructive pulmonary disease, clinical pathway for, 224, 233
Claims management systems, 182–83
Client records. *See* Patient records
Clinical algorithms
 in clinical practice guideline presentation, 37, 41–42
 for congestive heart failure, 86, 89
Clinical information systems. *See also* Information systems
 case management system integration with, 183
Clinical judgment, 253–54, 260
Clinical nurse coordinator–case manager (CNC-CM), 164, 165, 171–72
Clinical outcomes. *See also* Patient outcomes
 as component of quality, 11

263

Clinical outcomes (*continued*)
  in geriatric evaluation and management program, 124
  measurement instruments for, 13
  measurement of, 12, 96–97
  patient satisfaction correlating with, 11
Clinical paths. *See also* Interdisciplinary pathways; Path variance
  administrative liaisons for path teams, 223
  automation of analysis of, 217–18
  for cardiac surgery, 164–65
  care guides at Hinsdale Hospital, 199–201
  case management compared with, 160
  for chest pain, 222, 223
  for chronic obstructive pulmonary disease, 224, 233
  clinical quality improvement taken beyond, 1–6
  for community-acquired pneumonia, 233, 237–40
  for congestive heart failure, 74–75, 86
  copaths, 137, 138
  for coronary artery bypass graft, 66–67
  cost of development, 144
  development teams, 2, 72
  expert system–driven paths, 258–59
  generic medical pathways, 73–74, 76–77
  for home care, 97–98, 129–44, 220
  implementation difficulties with, 225–26
  implementation in disease management initiative, 232–34
  improvement goals not addressed by, 145
  information system module for, 184–86
  in integrated case management model, 215–17
  interactive pathways, 164–65, 176
  merging of, 185
  and multidisciplinary care planning, 103–4, 107, 121
  nurse-oriented models for, 71, 141
  paper-based, 177, 182, 225, 259–60
  PathPlan 2000 information system, 214, 217
  patient-record interface, 201–5
  for patients, 93, 94
  practice pattern variation affecting, 53, 65, 68
  proactive pathway model, 166–69
  process variation affecting, 9
  and record documentation systems, 103–4
  stakeholders in, 215
  surgical pathways, 73–74
  templates for, 184
  as total quality management tool, 1, 2
  typical initiative for, 2
Clinical practice guidelines (CPGs), 35–51
  acceptance of, 39, 47, 236, 249–50
  for acute pharyngitis-tonsillitis, 42
  for community-acquired pneumonia, 233, 235–36
  for congestive heart failure, 39
  development guidelines for, 46–49
  disease management based on, 229–32
  dissemination of, 43
  hindrances to development of, 38–40
  implementation barriers, 226–27
  information system for, 48–49
  investment-to-benefit ratio of, 47–48
  liability concerns, 43–44
  operational definition of, 37
  physician subgroups for creating, 73
  presentation format for, 41–42
  reasons for using, 36
  reporting performance measurement data, 45–46
  topic selection for, 40–41
Clinical quality improvement. *See also* Continuous quality improvement; Total quality management
  change as resulting from, 5
  characteristics of successful initiatives, 3–4
  focusing on known or suspected problems, 2
  performance measurement as tool for, 9–34
  stages of, 4–5
  taking beyond paths, 1–6
Clinician- and patient-completed measurement instruments, 14–15
Clinician-reported measurement instruments, 14
Clinician-reported outcomes, 12
Clinicom™ documentation system, 201, 205
Clinton Memorial Hospital Home Health Agency (Wilmington, OH)
  case management in, 145–62
  clinical pathway initiative of, 130–44
Community-acquired pneumonia (CAP)
  algorithm for management of, 249
  clinical path for, 233, 237–40
  clinical practice guidelines for, 233, 235–36
  information system in management of, 241–50
  physician order sheet for, 247
  statistical analysis of patients with, 236
Community health specialists, 92, 95–96
Community settings
  case management services in, 147
  congestive heart failure care in, 99
Computers. *See* Information systems
Confidentiality, of patient-satisfaction survey responses, 25
Congestive heart failure (CHF)
  case management and clinical paths compared, 160
  clinical pathway for, 74–75
  clinical practice guideline for, 39
  disease management initiative for, 79–100
  as highest volume diagnosis for inpatient care, 80
  home care for, 130, 134, 136
  outcome improvement through automation, 220
  patient instruction sheet for, 95
  patient pathway for, 93, 94
  typical patient profile, 81
Continuing education, 94–96, 226
Continuous quality improvement (CQI). *See also* FOCUS-PDCA model of continuous improvement
  clinical practice guidelines for, 36
  expert systems in, 255
  in practice pattern analysis, 53–55
  as stakeholder in clinical path process, 215
  team training in, 69
Copaths, 137, 138
Coronary artery bypass graft (CABG), sedation practice variation in, 54–65
Costs
  charge comparison for percutaneous transluminal coronary angioplasty, 211
  of clinical path development, 144
  cost-effectiveness of home care paths, 140–41
  a cost-efficient path variance database, 199–212
  of data retrieval and analysis, 68
  for open heart surgery patients, 65, 68
  variance analysis of, 185, 186
Crisis Triage Rating Scale, 257–58
Critical pathway method (CPM). *See also* Clinical paths
  strengths and weaknesses of, 163

Dashboard report, 45
Data. *See also* Databases; Data collection; Information
  data entry, 187, 210, 217, 250
  transforming into information, 27, 29–31
Databases
  a cost-efficient path variance database, 199–212
  existing databases, 212
  nonintegrated databases, 48–49
  relational databases, 187, 259
  report generation from, 183–84
Data collection
  automation of, 68–69, 246–49
  centralization of, 223–24
  for clinical practice guidelines, 49
  minimizing burden of, 212
  for path variance analysis, 77, 78, 208–10, 216–17
  in performance measurement, 17, 25
  for practice pattern variation reduction, 54, 56, 68–69
Data entry, 187, 210, 217, 250
Decision making
  clinical judgment in, 253–54

continuing education replacing personal experience in, 226
critical question for patient discharge, 165, 169
expert systems in, 254–55
fact-based, 4, 36
Decision Support Systems' PathPlan 2000, 214, 217
Deming, W. Edwards, 36, 255
Depression Technology of Patient Experience, 15
Discharge, critical question of decision on, 165, 169
Discharge planning, 108, 110, 184
Disease management
  case management in, 227–29
  continuing education for, 94–96
  defined, 79
  documentation tools for, 90
  goal of, 81
  guideline-based, 229–32
  human resources in, 90–93
  information systems for, 225–51
  multidisciplinary initiative for, 71–101
  regional model for, 227
  treatment guideline creation, 86
Documentation. *See also* Patient records
  Clinicom™ documentation system, 201, 205
  for disease management initiatives, 90
  exception-based documentation, 75, 185
  for home care, 131–37
  integration of, 75
  of outcome progress, 184
  of variances, 113–14

Empowerment of family and patient
  advanced practical nurses providing, 92
  in cardiac surgery, 166–67, 169
  rationale for, 84
Exception-based documentation, 75, 185
Expert systems, 253–61
  advantages of, 259–60
  authoring tools for creating, 256–57
  in behavioral health care, 253–54, 257–59
  clinical pathways driven by, 258–59
  in continuous quality improvement, 255
  in decision making, 254–55
  defined, 253
  PATHware authoring tool, 256–59
  traditional method of creation, 256

Facility profiling, 30
Fact-based decision making, 4, 36
Falls risk evaluation, 55, 59, 61, 63, 119
Family empowerment. *See* Empowerment of family and patient
Financial management systems, 182–83
Focus group interviews, 15, 16
FOCUS-PDCA model of continuous improvement
  in coronary artery bypass patient sedation, 54–65
  Plan-Do-Check-Act model, 10–11, 37, 54–65
Fractured hip, 104, 222
Frail elderly persons, 116
Functional outcome measurement data, 44–45

General family nursing interventions, 169
Generic medical pathways, 73–74, 76–77
Geriatric evaluation and management (GEM), 114–25
  defined, 104
  development process, 115–20
  integrating with multidisciplinary care planning, 103–27
  program evaluation, 123
  program tools, 121
Global Assessment of Functioning (GAF) scale, 14
Goals. *See* Improvement goals

Handheld computers, 187
HBOC TrendStar™ system, 208, 211
Health Level Seven (HL-7), 186
Health status data, 44–45
Heart failure clinic, 87
Hewlett Packard (HP) CAREVUE™ clinical information system, 54, 61, 68–69
Hip fracture, 104, 222
Hip replacement, total, 222
HL-7 (Health Level Seven), 186
Holistic approach, 172
Home care
  case management in, 145–62
  clinical pathways for, 97–98, 129–44, 220
  interdisciplinary paths for, 141–43
  performance improvement in, 137–41
  in regional disease management model, 227
  variance in outcomes in, 137, 139
  visit nurses, 150, 152, 157, 161
Home care service days, 160–61
Horizontal matrix format, 72
Hospital-initiated case management, 145
Hospitalization threshold, 245
Human-to-computer interface, 187

Improvement goals
  administrative and clinical leaders defining, 2
  defining, 11–12
  as environmentally aligned, 3
  those not addressed by care paths, 145
Information. *See also* Data; Information systems
  rapid growth of, 226
  transforming data into, 27, 29–31
Information systems, 179–261. *See also* Expert systems
  automating pathway variance analysis, 213–24, 244–46
  for cardiovascular radical outcome method, 172–73
  CAREVUE™ clinical information system, 54, 61, 68–69
  clinical path module, 184–86
  with clinical practice guidelines, 48–49
  Clinicom™ documentation system, 201, 205
  cost-efficient path variance database, 199–212
  desirable system functions, 188, 190
  for disease management, 225–51
  goals of, 188, 189
  hardware, 187
  HBOC TrendStar™ system, 208, 211
  HL-7, 186
  ideal case management system, 182–86
  integrated design in, 240–49
  key vendor issues, 192–93
  laptop computers, 187, 217
  links of, 240
  PathPlan 2000 clinical path system, 214, 217
  PatRec program, 235, 241–49
  performance measurement requirements for, 32
  priority-setting form for software, 190, 191
  product demonstrations, 193–94
  request for information (RFI) for vendors, 190
  selecting a system, 181–97
  Starting Line™ database, 29
  technical issues in selection of, 186–87
  Transition Systems, Inc., 78
  Windows™ technology, 186–87
Insulin-dependent diabetes mellitus (IDDM), 130, 138
Interactive pathways, 164–65, 176
Interdisciplinary collaboration. *See also* Interdisciplinary pathways; Multidisciplinary care plans
  in clinical path analysis, 216
  in successful quality improvement initiatives, 4
Interdisciplinary development model of care management, 72
Interdisciplinary pathways, 71–101
  as case management strategy, 214
  congestive heart failure team, 81
  design teams for, 73
  development of, 72–75
  discipline-specific requirements for, 73
  for home care, 141–43
  variances in, 75–78
Interface, computer
  human-to-computer, 187
  between patient record and clinical path systems, 201–5
  as system-selection issue, 186
Intervention summary, 90

Judgment, clinical, 253–54, 260
Juran, Joseph, 2–3, 36

Key indicators, 77, 79, 250
Knowledge base, 253, 260

Laptop computers, 187, 217
Length of stay
  automatic variance reporting of, 185, 186
  for cardiac surgery patients, 163, 164–65, 173–75
  for congestive heart failure patients, 81, 83, 86, 96, 98, 220
  for coronary artery bypass patients, 55, 57, 64, 65, 68
  critical question of patient discharge decision, 165, 169
  for geriatric patients, 117, 124
  in home care programs, 140, 154–55, 160–61
  reports on, 210, 211
  for top 10 ranked Medicare DRGs, 228
  variance in, 111
Level-of-care decisions, expert systems support for, 257–58, 259
Liability
  family empowerment reducing, 176
  minimizing concerns of clinical practice guidelines, 43–44
Living With Heart Failure Questionnaire, 96

Managed care
  continuous quality improvement tools for, 36–37
  learning curve for, 40
  preparing for, 226–27
Mayo Mini-Mental Status, 55, 59, 60, 62
MBC Corporate Patient Satisfaction Survey, 17
Measurement instruments, selection of, 13–17
Measurement of performance. *See* Performance measurement
Meehl, Paul, 254
Messaging standards, 186
Micromanagement, to systems management from, 9–11
Microsoft Access™, 241
Mission and ministry department, 92–93
Multidisciplinary care plans (MCPs)
  case managers, 106
  development process for, 104
  integrating geriatric evaluation and planning with, 103–27
  nature of, 107–14
  organizational structure and support processes for, 104–7
  program manager, 106
  project teams, 106
  variance management, 109–14

Multidisciplinary collaboration. *See* Interdisciplinary collaboration
Myocardial infarction, 220, 222

Narrative charting, 141
Noncompliance reports, 30, 31
Nurse case managers. *See* Case managers
Nurse-oriented models, 71, 141
Nurses
  advanced practical nurses, 87, 91–92, 99
  cardiac rehabilitation nurses, 92
  primary care nurses, 92, 146
  PRN nurses, 161
  proactive pathways benefiting, 171
  as stakeholders in clinical path process, 215
  visit nurses, 150, 152, 157, 161

Objectives. *See* Improvement goals
Occupational therapy, 141, 142, 143
Office visits, 40
On-line analytical processing (OLAP), 184
Open heart surgeries, reducing practice variation in, 53–69
OQ-45.1, 14
Otitis media, 40, 48, 49–50
Outcomes analysis. *See also* Clinical outcomes; Patient outcomes; Performance measurement
  automated report of, 221
  benchmarks for, 49
  expert systems in, 253–61
  five steps of, 255
  information systems in, 246–49
Outlier physicians, 39
Outpatient care
  clinical practice guidelines for improving, 35–51
  upward trend in, 225

PathPlan 2000 clinical path information system, 214, 217
Path variance
  aggregate variance analysis, 78, 185–86
  automating analysis of, 213–24, 244–46
  computerized report of, 219
  cost-efficient database for, 199–212
  data collection for analysis of, 77, 78, 208–10, 216–17
  data reporting and analysis for, 210–12, 217–18
  in interdisciplinary pathways, 75–78
  reporting forms for, 200, 204, 216
  selection of data for analysis of, 206–8
PATHware authoring tool, 256–59
Pathway development teams, 2, 72
Pathway templates, 184
Patient care coordination, 78, 79
Patient education, 93–94, 111, 112

Patient-focused care model of service delivery, 78
Patient information sheet, 25, 27
Patient outcomes. *See also* Clinical outcomes; Patient satisfaction
  automating data collection for, 244
  automation enhancing improvements in, 218–22
  cardiovascular radical outcome method improving, 175
  documentation of, 184
  with home care, 129
  measuring variation in, 44–45
  outcomes analysis report, 221
  performance measurement as first step for managing, 10
  quality-of-life measures, 96–97
Patient profiles, 183
Patient progress chart, 170
Patient records
  audit worksheet to gather information from, 16
  clinical path integration with, 103–4
  clinical path interface, 201–5
  clinical practice guidelines improving, 44
  computerization of, 42, 236, 244
  data collection from, 54
  information flow using computerized, 244
  PatRec program, 235, 241–49
Patient-reported measurement instruments, 13–14
Patient-reported outcomes, 12
Patients. *See also* Patient outcomes; Patient records; Patient satisfaction
  assessment tools for, 108
  clinical paths for, 93, 94
  education for, 93–94, 111, 112
  empowerment of, 84, 92, 166–67, 169
  self-care skills, 145, 160
  as stakeholders in clinical path process, 215
Patient satisfaction
  with case management in home care, 160
  clinical outcomes correlating with, 11
  measurement instruments, 15–16, 21–22
  measurements of, 12–13
PatRec program, 235, 241–49
Peer review, 38–39
Peer-to-peer presentations, 73
Percutaneous transluminal coronary angioplasty (PTCA), 201–12
Performance improvement. *See also* Improvement goals
  automation enhancing, 218–22
  clinical pathways in, 79
  in geriatric evaluation and management program, 123–24
  for home care, 137–41
  strategies for, 10–11, 84
Performance measurement
  for cardiovascular radical outcome method, 173–76

for case management in home care, 160–61
in clinical practice guideline programs, 45–46
defining measurement process, 17, 25–27
as first step for managing patient outcomes, 10
for home care, 140, 160–61
human system requirements, 32
identifying measurements, 12–13
information system requirements, 32
major steps in, 25, 27, 28
measurement instrument selection, 13–17
in multidisciplinary disease management initiative, 96–97
as quality improvement tool, 4, 9–34
standardization formula for, 49
Pharyngitis-tonsillitis, 40–41, 42, 44, 49–50
Physical therapy, 108, 111, 141, 143
Physician orders
in computerized patient record system, 241–42, 247
generated from clinical paths, 185
preprinted, 75, 205, 207
Physicians. *See also* Champion physicians
clinical practice guideline acceptance by, 39, 47, 236, 249–50
clinical practice guideline creation by, 73
collaboration with administration, 214
continuing education in disease management, 94
in guideline-based disease management, 231–32
outlier physicians, 39
peer review, 38–39
peer-to-peer presentations of pathways, 73
as sponsors of disease management initiative, 91
as stakeholders in clinical path process, 215
Plan-Do-Check-Act model, 10–11
in clinical practice guideline development, 37
for coronary artery bypass sedation practices, 54–65
Pneumonia. *See also* Community-acquired pneumonia
multidisciplinary care plans for, 104
path variance in, 220

Posterior laminectomy, 222
Practice pattern variation
continuous quality improvement approach to, 53–55
patient diversity causing, 39
reducing in open heart surgeries, 53–69
Preprinted physician orders, 75, 205, 207
Pressure ulcer potential (PUP), 116, 123
Primary care, multidisciplinary disease management in, 98–99
Primary care nurses, 92, 146
PRN nurses, 161
Proactive pathway model, 166–69
Process variance. *See also* Path variance; Practice pattern variation
automated system for charting, 185
clinical practice guidelines for reducing, 43
factors producing legitimate, 9
measurement of, 44–45
negative and positive, 111, 137
in patient care, 163
three categories of, 111–13
Protocols, for congestive heart failure, 86
Provider input, 25, 26
Psychiatric Symptom Assessment Scale, 14
Psychological services, 92–93

Quality. *See also* Clinical quality improvement
factors in, 11
Quality-of-life measures, 96–97

Ramsey Sedation Scale, 55, 59, 61
Readmissions
of cardiac surgery patients, 164, 175
for congestive heart failure, 220
of coronary artery bypass patients, 68
Records. *See* Patient records
Relational databases, 187, 259
Residents, continuing education in disease management, 95
Role modeling, 171

Sedation management, for coronary artery bypass patients, 54–69
Self-care skills, 145, 160
Service-line model of care management, 78

SF-36, 14, 44–46
Shewhart cycle. *See* Plan-Do-Check-Act model
Short-stay pathway, for congestive heart failure, 86, 88
Sinusitis, 40, 49–50
Software. *See* Information systems
Specialty clinics and services, 87
Speech therapy, 141, 143
Starting Line™ database, 29
Structured interviews, 16
Surgery. *See also* Cardiac surgery
surgical pathways, 73–74
System interface capabilities, 186
Systems, information. *See* Information systems
Systems management, from micromanagement to, 9–11

Technical performance, measurement of, 12, 15
Telemanagement, 88–89, 90
Total hip replacement, 222
Total quality management (TQM)
clinical paths as tool for, 1, 2
components of, 2–3
critical pathway method, 163
Transition Systems, Inc. (TSI), 78
Treatment decision, expert systems support for, 258–59
TrendStar™ system, 208, 211
23-hour chest pain, 222, 223

Unit-based model of care management, 78
Utilization, as component of quality, 11
Utilization measurements, 12
instruments for, 13
in multidisciplinary disease management, 97, 98

Variance. *See* Process variance
Visit nurses, 150, 152, 157, 161

Wall-mounted documentation screens, 187
Windows™ technology, 186–87

Zander, Karen, 1